A BIBLIOGRAPHY OF NURSING LITERATURE
1859-1960

To

MARY CARPENTER

Director in the Education Division
Royal College of Nursing and National Council
of Nurses of the United Kingdom

A BIBLIOGRAPHY
OF NURSING LITERATURE
1859-1960

WITH AN HISTORICAL INTRODUCTION

Edited and Compiled by
ALICE M. C. THOMPSON, F.L.A.

LONDON
THE LIBRARY ASSOCIATION
FOR THE ROYAL COLLEGE OF NURSING
AND NATIONAL COUNCIL OF NURSES OF THE UNITED KINGDOM
IN ASSOCIATION WITH
KING EDWARD'S HOSPITAL FUND FOR LONDON
1968

Published by
The Library Association
7 Ridgmount Street, London, W.C.1
for
The Royal College of Nursing

© 1968 Royal College of Nursing
SBN: 85365 470 0

Text set in 8 point Times New Roman,
'Monotype' Series 327

Printed and bound in England by
STAPLES PRINTERS LIMITED
at their Rochester, Kent, establishment

ACKNOWLEDGMENTS

THANKS must first be made to the King Edward's Hospital Fund for London which, by a most generous grant, made possible the existence of this bibliography.

Secondly thanks must go to the Rockefeller Foundation and to the Council of the Royal College of Nursing and National Council of Nurses of the United Kingdom, to the first for making it possible, by the award of a Travelling Fellowship, for the Editor to visit medical and nursing libraries in the Eastern United States to collect material for this bibliography and to the second for making possible a subsequent tour which extended to the Pacific Coast and to Canada.

The Editor is indebted to two former members of the staff of the Library of Nursing—to Mrs. Carol Sawers for help in transcription and to Mrs. Sheila Harvey for proof-reading. This list of acknowledgments would be incomplete without reference to the invaluable secretarial assistance of Miss Margaret Ollis.

To Mr. Alfred Brandon, Editor of the *Bulletin of the Medical Library Association* I am grateful for permission to include the introductory chapter on "The Literature of Nursing" which was first printed in *Bulletin of the Medical Library Association*, April 1964.

Finally I must thank all those, both librarians and nurses in the United States and Canada who not only made me so welcome, but who also put the resources of their libraries at my disposal.

ALICE M. C. THOMPSON
Editor

Royal College of Nursing and
National Council of Nurses of the United Kingdom

CONTENTS LIST

SPECIALTIES OF KNOWLEDGE AND PRACTICE

HOSPITALS

PREFACE

IT is but comparatively recently that the literature of nursing has developed and this bibliography is an attempt to bring together all the material written for nurses and about the nursing profession.

The work of the nurse now merges with that of so many others that the books she must use extend far beyond the literature of the profession itself and the multitude of books which nurses must use but which are not written expressly for them are, for obvious reasons, excluded.

Florence Nightingale's *Notes on nursing, what it is and what it is not*, published in 1859 as the first book for nurses, forms a suitable starting point and all major publications of the following hundred years are included. The bibliography is arranged in a simple form, working always from the general subject to its specific aspect. All sections are subdivided alphabetically by the aspect of the subject.

The literature is covered by five main sections
  History
  Biography
  The profession of nursing
  Specialities of knowledge and practice
  Hospitals

Entries are included only if reference is made to nursing.

A small number of references throughout the bibliography because of the information contained in the books, pre-date 1859. Editions are given where known. There are few double entries. Where no place of publication appears it may be assumed to be the U.K.

An author index has been excluded deliberately since no more than a dozen authors appear on more than one page of the bibliography. This is essentially a guide to what has been written about nursing.

As far as is known this is the first bibliography of nursing. It is hoped that nurses and librarians alike will find it worthy of a place on library shelves.

ALICE M. C. THOMPSON

Royal College of Nursing and
National Council of Nurses of the United Kingdom
May 1968

INTRODUCTION

THIS Bibliography of Nursing Literature, the first in its field, surveys the work of a momentous century. Modern nursing began with the publication of Florence Nightingale's *Notes on nursing* in 1859. Miss Thompson takes this as the starting point for her work and continues the story down to 1960, by which time nursing had become established nationally and internationally as one of the great professions, having reached this position almost entirely through the efforts of its own members. It is not perhaps generally realized, but the writings analyzed here demonstrate clearly that nurses have consistently through those hundred years aimed at and achieved the improvement of their own professional education and intellectual equipment.

The Bibliography is based primarily on the literature under Miss Thompson's charge in the Library of the Royal College of Nursing, which is in fact Britain's national nursing library and one which she has developed into an active centre of service and research. Miss Thompson has had opportunities to examine also the nursing libraries of Canada and the United States and has availed herself of their resources to supplement those available at home.

I have no doubt that this Bibliography will become a standard work of reference wherever there is need for knowledge of nursing literature. The effort which Miss Thompson has voluntarily devoted to this work has been encouraged thoughout by the Council of the Royal College of Nursing. As Chairman of the Library Advisory Group of the College I have been privileged to watch the Bibliography growing and am proud to be asked to introduce it.

W. R. LeFanu

FOREWORD

ON behalf of the Royal College of Nursing and National Council of Nurses of the United Kingdom, I welcome this *Bibliography of nursing literature*. We take especial pleasure in its having been published under the College imprint, and are proud that most of the works in it are to be found in the Library of Nursing.

The College owes a debt of gratitude to the King Edward's Hospital Fund for London, without whose generosity the Bibliography could not have been undertaken.

THEODORA TURNER
President
Royal College of Nursing and
National Council of Nurses
of the United Kingdom

THE DEVELOPMENT
OF THE LITERATURE OF NURSING

"THE importance of being able to read can never be overvalued in anyone who is in charge of the sick. Indeed it should be a *sine qua non* that they should be able to read and write. How many of our present nurses this single requirement would cut off." So wrote Dr. Aeneas Munro in 1873,* thirteen years after the opening of the Nightingale School at St. Thomas's Hospital in London, the first nurse training school ing England. The fifteen women who were admitted when the school opened in July 1860, and who were to lay the foundation of a new profession, were specially selected for their potentialities as leaders. These were educated women, but for many years the nursing of patients continued, for the most part, to be done by women recruited from the working, and therefore illiterate, class. It must be remembered that in Great Britain the reform of nursing antedates compulsory primary education by ten years.

The growth of a profession can be measured by its literature. One of the hallmarks of a profession is that it has educational standards; and it is a natural corollary that the demand for education engenders a demand for books.

Early text books were few, and usually written by doctors. Nursing education was rudimentary and the course of teaching limited to one year. In 1873 only four usable text books were known and when in 1900 Dr. Anna Hamilton published her thesis "Considerations sur les infirmieres des hospitaux" she included a list of 198 nursing text books in ten languages, including five in Latin. These books have lost all but historic interest. In 1928 the International Council of Nurses collected some fresh information on the subject. The list of books in 18 languages which the Council published in its Journal, included only three out of Dr. Hamilton's original 198. Two remarks preface the International Council of Nurses compilation—"most of the books which appeared in the last century and many of those which came out between 1900 and 1910 are not now obtainable" and "in many countries, schools of nursing employ books published abroad, especially where there is a language in common. For instance, most of the British Dominions depend for books upon Great Britain and the United States".

At the present day books covering all aspects of nursing are published in all the principal languages. The growth of the literature can be gauged when we know that the Library of the Royal College of Nursing and National Council of Nurses of the United Kingdom, which was founded in 1921 with a stock of 178 books listed in the Committee Minutes as "one text book for nurses, four for midwives and 173 on medical and surgical subjects" now has a stock of approximately 19,000 volumes and 2,000 pamphlets as well as 250 current periodicals.

There are reasons for the short history of nursing literature as compared with the literature of medicine, and a brief survey of the development of nursing may explain this.

Nursing was primarily a vocation, the province of the religious orders. Nursing, like other manual arts was learnt by practice. Emphasis was less on the physical than on the spiritual welfare of the patient. The military-monastic system of nursing under the Knights of St. John of Jerusalem and other orders of Knights Hospitallers was probably better equipped to meet the nursing needs of the day than most modern amateurs would be. Large numbers of wounded men on a battlefield, need swift attention and it is in the interest of all that those caring for them should know something of first aid. Military camp and feudal castle which trained the hospitallers, both men and women, did not create a "bookish" type of education and little is known of the techniques used.

Between the 12th and 16th centuries a series of organizations was formed, all predominantly religious in motive but differing in method from the religious orders in that members went out from the Mother House into the homes of the sick and needy. The secularization of nursing had begun. As the feudal system declined a new prosperous middle class of merchants and traders emerged to take over some responsibility for the welfare of their own townspeople and to build and support their own charitable institutions. Thus we have the founding of almshouses and what have been called "Houses of Pity".

The study of medicine developed with the Renaissance and the great age of social and intellectual awakening. Women, alas, had little share in the opportunities offered to the men, and those engaged in nursing appear to have benefitted little from this revival of learning. Paradoxically one of the darker periods of nursing comes at a time when medical science was reviving.

A rudimentary nurse-training began when St. Vincent de Paul founded the French Sisters of Charity in the 17th century. Being both a social reformer of vision and an educator, he saw that reliable, trained workers were needed for the care of the sick and he developed a plan of recruitment and training which has something in common with our present system of nurse-training; characterized by a probationary period, followed by a period of instruction and study before practical work in the community was begun. Unfortunately this excellent system did not flourish beyond the death of its progenitor.

Two centuries later the Fliedners, Frederic and Caroline, founded a similar school for deaconesses at Kaiserswerth in Germany. To this school came Florence Nightingale.

Nursing then was primarily a vocation, practised under a strong religious influence and, as so often happens with a vocation, blind devotion stultifies progress. With the dissolution of the monasteries such

* Aeneas Munro *The science and art of nursing the sick*, 1873.

nursing of the sick as there was, lay in the hands of the unlettered, the vicious, and the drunken. No soil could have been less productive of literature.

With the advent of Florence Nightingale, the first nursing leader appears on the scene.

Florence Nightingale took some of the best features of the Kaiserswerth training, adapted them for use in the school she founded at St. Thomas's Hospital, and lifted nursing right out of the sphere of the Church, to start it on its career as a branch of medical service run by a secular staff.

The Nightingale School set out to train leaders for the nursing profession. Women like Lucy Osburn who founded the nursing profession in Australia, or Alice Fisher who, as Matron at the Blockley Hospital in Philadelphia continued the reform of American nursing begun by Clara Barton. But for many years after the founding of the Nightingale School nurses generally were recruited from the illiterate working class. Essentially a practical skill, practised by those lacking the ability to write, nursing possessed few books, and those few were usually written at an elementary level by doctors.

There is little evidence that doctors, even as recently as the 19th century were concerned about the system of nursing or made any attempt to improve the preparation of nurses. Manuals on the home care of the sick and the nursing of children were written by doctors, but these were intended for domestic use, and would have been useless to the servant class of nurse since few, if any, could read or write.

The statutory recognition of nursing which required a standard of education for entry to the profession and which laid down a syllabus of training, and the improvement of nurses' working conditions which led therefore to the recruitment of better educated women caused a significant increase in professional books. But statutory recognition did not come in England until 1919.

Of all the text books written for nurses we need consider only one. The first book written has not been surpassed in expression of sound common sense. *Notes on nursing, what it is and what it is not* was published by Florence Nightingale in 1859. All is there, the observation of the sick, noise in the sickroom, sleep, diet, psychology (properly confined to a single telling chapter) and a chapter of advice to the patient's relatives delightfully entitled "Chattering hopes and advices". The 20th century nurse, starting on her career with all her qualifications, would not find as much common sense in any other nursing book written during the past 100 years. Compare the economic prose style of the book with the florid phraseology of many modern text books which by their circumlocution make even the simplest procedure appear complicated.

Florence Nightingale is a phenomenon. It is not always realized that her work for nursing was but a small part of what she accomplished during her life. Administrator, statistician, philosopher, nurse, a leader and a martinet, born into an unassailable position of social and political influence, she is possibly the most remarkable woman known to history. The Nightingale literature is vast; not least her own correspondence. Her two outstanding biographers Sir Edwin Cook (1913) and Mrs. Cecil Woodham-Smith (1950) have each written a definitive life of Florence Nightingale. Cook is of particular value for he not only lists chronologically all books about Florence Nightingale and all her own writings, but gives particulars of pictorial presentations of his subject, paintings, drawings and sculptures with their location. Cecil Woodham-Smith's book is based on Nightingale and Verney family papers which were not available to Sir Edwin Cook, and contains much on Florence Nightingale not found elsewhere.

The profession went under the microscope of investigating committees at an early stage. From 1890–1892 the Parliamentary Committee appointed to consider the administration and staffing of the Metropolitan Hospitals made its report: a detailed exposition of nursing conditions in the London hospitals at that time, with verbal evidence of matrons and nursing superintendents given in full.

A second report containing much on the education of nurses appeared in 1905 as the deliberations of a Parliamentary Committee on the State Registration of Nurses. Opposition from the doctors was bitter. "I firmly believe", said Mr. Sidney Holland of the London Hospital, "that if registration were to pass it would lead nurses to consider themselves as belonging to what is called 'a profession'. The tendency would be to think themselves much more the colleagues of the doctors instead of simply carriers out of the orders of doctors, in fact they would be a pseudo-scientific kind of person." Mr. Holland continued, "It is a very great danger when a nurse thinks herself an amateur doctor . . . the other side (the nurses) is always talking about nursing being a 'profession' and 'graduates' in nursing just as they do in America." In such a climate it is understandable that the literature of nursing did not develop.

These two reports are major sources of information on nursing in England nearly three-quarters of a century ago. Subsequent reports made by the *Lancet* Commission in 1934 and the Ministries of Health and Education in 1939 and 1947 enquire into the recruitment and training of nurses and set out sound proposals, which have never been implemented. Comparable reports in the United States of America are those on "Nursing and nursing education in the United States"—a report of a survey made in 1923 by the Committee for the Study of Nursing Education, and the final report of the "Committee on the Grading of Nursing Schools" published in 1934. Between them these reports give a fairly complete picture of nursing in these two countries over the past 75 years.

Histories of nursing proliferate, but two are outstanding. *A general history of nursing* by Lucy Seymer, first published in 1932, is an extremely erudite and thorough work and it is not quite matched in excellence by the American book *A history of nursing*, published in four volumes by Adelaide Nutting and Lavinia Dock in 1912.

While nursing text books did not develop in any numbers until a statutory training was set up, nursing periodicals have, from the earliest days of the profession been of vigorous growth. That eminent American nurse, Adelaide Nutting, has said "let no one ignore the journals of a country. The first faltering steps towards organization, legislation and education are always found in a little sheet or journal."

The first magazine of a national scope was the English *Nursing notes*, appearing in 1887. Sub-titled "A practical journal for nurses: being the journal of the Workhouse Infirmary Nursing Association and the Midwives Institute and Trained Nurses Club" the journal gave particular prominence to District Nursing. Clinical articles by doctors were also published and very full reports of events in the world of nursing. Over the years increasing space was given to midwifery matters and in 1921 the title was changed to *Nursing notes and midwives chronicle*. Eventually "Nursing Notes" was removed from the head of the title and *The midwives chronicle and nursing notes* continues to flourish as the official journal of the Royal College of Midwives, a professional organization for midwives founded in 1881.

A few months after the appearance of *Nursing notes* the *Nursing mirror and midwives journal* made its bow in London in 1888. This journal is and always has been owned by a commercial firm. It has one of the largest circulations of any nursing journal, carries good clinical articles and is very much *au courant* with nursing affairs.

The year 1888 was a notable one for the production of new nursing journals. As well as the *Nursing mirror*, the *Nursing record* appeared in England and *The trained nurse and hospital review* in the United States of America.

It would be difficult to find a better source for material on the evolution of nursing as a profession in Great Britain than the *Nursing record*. Sub-titled "A journal for nurses, a chronicle of hospital and institutional news, and a review of women's work", it appeared at a time when nurses were beginning to feel the need to organize themselves into associations, to seek for recognition and to establish their status. The first issue contains a full report of the first meeting of the British Nurses Association acclaimed by the journal in an editorial as "a serious effort, which we think will eventually be crowned with success . . . to place upon a satisfactory footing the large body of 15,000 nurses in the United Kingdom." At the first meeting it was unanimously agreed that a British Nurses Association be formed and that among its objects should be the following: the obtaining of "a Charter that will enable the Association to examine and register nurses and to confer degrees, the devising of annuity and sick funds for nurses . . ." and so on. Here are the beginnings of a profession, history in the making, typical of the kind of material which appeared in the *Nursing record*. Few clinical articles were published, the emphasis being always on nursing as a profession rather than on techniques. In 1893 the journal was bought by Ethel Bedford Fenwick, a forceful, indeed militant, personality, who fought long and hard for the state registration of nurses and who founded the International Council of Nurses. The journal which became *The British journal of nursing* in 1903 was edited by Mrs. Bedford Fenwick until her death in 1947 and was the medium through which she transmitted her forceful views and ideas on nursing.

The journal was the official journal of the British College of Nurses, founded by Mrs. Bedford Fenwick. In later years the standard of the journal declined and it ceased publication in 1956. For thirty years the journal was published with an excellent index, but issues of the last thirty years lack an index.

The trained nurse was for ten years the sole nursing and hospital journal in the United States of America, and, until the founding of the *American Journal of Nursing* in 1900, the official journal of the national nursing association of America.

Included in every monthly issue was a supplement called "The Hospital". Each supplement, with occasional exceptions, dealt with a single hospital and is a mine of hospital history. Contents of the main part of the journal at first tended to be rather chatty and articles on "Tea in health and sickness", "How to wash the baby" and "Let us refrain from gossip", are to be found in an early issue.

The magazine always served the interests of the nurse working in industry and included a section for the nurse working in this specialty. With the change of name in 1951 *The trained nurse* became *Nursing World* until its unfortunate demise in 1960.

European nursing journals appeared as early as those of England and America. Holland published *Tijdschrift voor Ziekenverpleging* in 1890. Most countries of the world have had for many years a national association for nurses, countries presently emerging have too, and all have produced a nursing journal. One of the earliest was the *Australian nurses journal*, first published in 1903 and still flourishing. Canada followed in 1905 with *The Canadian nurse*. Since 1959 there has also appeared a French edition *L'Infirmière Canadienne*. Sweden and Denmark published journals early in the century which are still appearing. South America, South Africa, China, India, Japan, Zambia and the Philippines and all European countries have nursing periodicals—a catalogue of nursing journals "from China to Peru". Most are of a good calibre, but good or not each and every one is the source of information on the history and progress of nursing in each country.

The American journal of nursing, founded in 1900, is the first magazine to be owned and published by a national association of nurses. The journal concerns itself with all fields of the nursing profession and has a strong interest in nursing education. The index, published annually and in five-yearly cumulative volumes, is notable for its clarity.

The English *Nursing times* was first published in 1905, the second of the two existing English nursing journals. It began as a venture by Messrs. Macmillan who are still the publishers. The first editorial stated ". . . this journal will report news without bias, and its columns will be open to all experts on non-political matters. The journal will be written chiefly by nurses for nurses." In its earlier days the journal was distinguished by its comprehensive and conscientious reporting of nursing politics. Latterly more clinical material has been included. The early volumes again are valuable for the nursing historian. In 1926 the *Nursing times* became the official journal of the Royal College of Nursing but paradoxically, its views were not necessarily those of the College. The *Nursing times* is no longer the official journal of The Royal College of Nursing and National Council of Nurses of the United Kingdom which now publishes a news sheet for its members called *Nursing standard*.

Two notable journals for a special interest group are *The American association of industrial nurses journal* first published in 1944, and the English *Journal for industrial nurses* now *Occupational health*. First published in 1949 by the Nuffield Department of Occupational Health in the University of Manchester, the journal has been published, since 1955, by the *Nursing times* in association with the Occupational Health Section of the Royal College of Nursing and National Council of Nurses of the United Kingdom. Both journals are good, but the second takes pride of place with its first class articles on occupational health.

The first magazine for public health nurses has had a chequered career. *The visiting nurse quarterly* was published in America in 1909. It was published under this title until 1913 and from then until 1918 as *The public health nursing quarterly*. From 1918–1931 it was published monthly as *The public health nurse*, and as *Public health nursing* from 1931–1953. Up to this time it has been the official journal of the National Organization for Public Health Nursing, but in 1953 the periodical became the official journal of the National League for Nursing and the title was changed to *Nursing outlook*, which title is still retained. As the official journal of the League it is now concerned very much with nursing education and training.

There is no English journal specially for the public health nurse. Both the *Nursing times* and the *Nursing mirror* carry articles on public health and publish public health issues from time to time. The monthly *District nursing* founded as recently as 1956 is for the nurse engaged in home visiting.

Nursing research is a comparatively new field of nursing. Its development was earlier and swifter in the United States of America than elsewhere and some 15 years ago The National League for Nursing and the American Nurses Association jointly sponsored a new periodical *Nursing research*, the only journal dealing with this facet of nursing. This appears quarterly and publishes original papers on nursing research and research method. The periodical also publishes from time to time lists of university theses on nursing research with their location and their availability on inter-library loan. A second, and possibly more important branch of the periodical's coverage is that an abstracting service, made possible by a grant from the United States Public Health Service, is undertaken for the journal by the Institute of Research and Service in Nursing Education at Teachers College, Columbia University. The abstracts cover nursing education, nursing research and selected nursing services. A notable issue, for example, abstracted public health reports published in the English language. British as well as American journals are abstracted. The periodical has an annual index, which is issued cumulatively every four years. This journal underlines the amount of research into nursing that is now being undertaken.

The International Council of Nurses publishes the only international journal. The Council was founded in 1899 by Mrs. Bedford Fenwick and the first, very modest, *Bulletin* appeared in 1924 and ran for six issues. In 1925 at the International Council of Nurses Congress in Finland the decision was taken to publish a larger magazine and from 1926–1929 *The I.C.N.* was published quarterly from the Headquarters of the Council in Geneva. From 1930–1939, a change of name gave us the *International nursing review*, published, with the exception of 1935, six times a year with articles in English, French and German. Publication was suspended during the second world war when the Council moved its Headquarters to New York. From New York the *International nursing bulletin* was published quarterly from 1945. The Council is now established in Geneva and publishes the *International nursing review* (a reversion to an earlier title) four times a year. The Council also publishes periodically in one volume what are called "National reports". Although not strictly a periodical this publication is important since information on educational requirements for entry to nursing, standards of nurse-training and contents of syllabuses as extant in all member countries are contained therein.

Surveying all this material we naturally ask "where are the guides to this literature, where the indices, where the bibliographies?". This is a sea that is virtually uncharted.

The *Index medicus* and the *Cumulative index to hospital literature* contain some references to nursing. A *Cumulative index to nursing literature* issued originally in 1956–1960 by the Librarians of three nurse-training schools in California, is now published in bi-monthly issues and as an annual cumulative volume by the Seventh Day Adventist Hospital Association. This however includes periodical literature only, and that only from 1956.

The Yale University School of Nursing Project on nursing research is shortly to flower into a four-volume index. This index contains chiefly periodical literature and research reports. Two volumes have been published to date. In 1960 the American Journal of Nursing Company published an *International nursing index*.

The development of nursing education and nursing libraries, the increasingly complex task of the nurse which follows the increasingly complex content of medicine and the growth of nursing research make some control of this literature essential.

This Bibliography is intended as a guide to the first hundred years of nursing literature.

ALICE M. C. THOMPSON

Royal College of Nursing and
National Council of Nurses of the United Kingdom

HISTORY OF NURSING

GENERAL WORKS

ABBOTT, MAUDE E. SEYMOUR
Lectures on the history of nursing, Part I (Lectures I-IX with addenda). Montreal, McGill University Publications, 1924.
(With descriptive list of lantern slides.)

CALDER, JEAN MCKINLAY
The story of nursing. Methuen, 1954.
2nd edn., 1958.
3rd edn., 1960.

DOCK, LAVINIA L., *and* STEWART, ISABEL MAITLAND
A short history of nursing from the earliest times to the present day. New York, Putnam, 1920.
2nd edn., 1925.
3rd edn., 1931
4th edn., 1938.
[Later editions published as "A history of nursing," by Isabel M. Stewart and Anne L. Austin.]

ARCHIBALD, —
The evolution of fever nursing in Glasgow, a lecture given to the Glasgow Branch of the College of Nursing.... Glasgow, the Glasgow Branch of the College of Nursing, 19?.

AUSTIN, ANNE L.
The historical method in nursing. *Nursing Research*, Feb. 1958, p. 4-10.

AUSTIN, ANNE L.
History of nursing source book. New York, Putnam, 1957.

BETT, W. R.
A short history of nursing. Faber, 1960.

DOCK, LAVINIA L.
State registration. *British Journal of Nursing*, Feb. 2, 1905, p. 148-51.

DODGE, BERTHA SANFORD
The story of nursing. Boston, Little, Brown, 1954.

FRANK, SISTER CHARLES MARIE
Foundations of nursing. Philadelphia, Saunders, 1953.
2nd edn., 1959.

FRANK, SISTER CHARLES MARIE
The historical development of nursing: emphasizing the cultural background of the race and the influence of philosophy and religion on the healing arts. Philadelphia, Saunders, 1953.

GOLDER, CHRISTIAN
History of the deaconess movement in the Christian church. Cincinatti, Jennings and Pye, 1903.

GOODNOW, MINNIE
Outlines of nursing history. Philadelphia, Saunders, 1916.
2nd edn., 1919.
3rd edn., 1923.
4th edn., 1928.
5th edn., 1933.
6th edn., 1938.
7th edn., 1942, entitled "Nursing history in brief".
8th edn., 1949.
9th edn., 1953.
10th edn., 1958, entitled "History of nursing", ed. Josephine A. Dolan.

GUTHRIE, DOUGLAS
Nursing through the ages. *Nursing Mirror*, [195?].

HAMPTON, ISABEL A., *and others*
Nursing of the sick, 1893: papers and discussions from the International Congress of Charities, Correction and Philanthropy, Chicago, 1893. New York, McGraw-Hill, 1949.

History of nursing and sociology, compiled by a Sister of Charity of Emmitsburg, Maryland. Bridgport, Connecticut, 1929.

HUGHES, M. F.
A pageant of nursing. Leicester, Brockhampton Book Co., 1942.

JAMIESON, ELIZABETH MARION, *and* SEWALL, MARY
Trends in nursing history: their relationship to world events. Philadelphia, Saunders, 1940.
2nd edn., 1944.
3rd edn., 1949.
4th edn., 1954.
5th edn., 1959.

JENSEN, DEBORAH MACLURG
A history of nursing. St. Louis, Mosby, 1943.
2nd edn., 1950, entitled "History and trends of professional nursing".
3rd edn., 1955.
4th edn., 1959.

Leaves from the annals of the Sisters of Mercy. 3 vols. New York, Catholic Publication Society, 1881-83.
Vol. I. Ireland.
Vol. II. England, the Crimea, Scotland, Australia and New Zealand.
Vol. III. America.

LIU, JAMES K. C., *and* STEPHENSON, GLADYS E.
An outline of the history of nursing. Shanghai, for the Nurses' Association of China, by Kwang Hsueh Publishing House, 1936.
[Written and paged in Chinese.]

MORISON, L. J., *and* FEGAN, ANNA C.
History of nursing, an outline. Philadelphia, Davis, 1942.

MORTEN, HONNOR
From a nurses' note-book. Scientific Press, 1899.

MURPHY, DENIS G.
They did not pass by: the story of the early pioneers of nursing. Longmans Green, 1956.

NUTTING, M. ADELAIDE, *and* DOCK, LAVINIA L.
A history of nursing: the evolution of nursing systems from earliest times to the foundations of the first English and American training schools for nurses. 4 vols. New York, Putnam.
Vols. 1 & 2, 1907.
Vols. 3 & 4, 1912.

PAVEY, AGNES E.
The story of the growth of nursing as an art, a vocation and a profession. Faber, 1938.
2nd edn., 1944.
3rd edn., 1951.
4th edn., 1953.
5th edn., 1959.

PILLERS, MARJORIE E.
The lamp, a pageant of nursing. Liverpool, Benington, 1943.

ROBINSON, VICTOR.
White caps: the story of nursing. Philadelphia, Lippincott, 1946.

SELLEW, GLADYS, *and* NUESSE, C. J.
A history of nursing. St. Louis, Mosby, 1946.
2nd edn., 1951.

SEYMER, LUCY RIDGELY
A general history of nursing. Faber, 1932.
2nd edn., 1949.
3rd edn., 1954.
4th edn., 1957.

SHRYOCK, RICHARD HARRISON
The history of nursing: an interpretation of the social and medical factors involved. Philadelphia, Saunders, 1959.

STEPHENSON, GLADYS E.
A short outline of nursing history. Shanghai, for the Nurses' Association of China, Kwang Hsueh Publishing House, 1936.

STONEY, A. H.
In the days of Queen Victoria—memories of a hospital nurse. Bristol, Wright, 1931.

TOOLEY, SARAH A.
The history of nursing in the British Empire. Bousfield, 1906.

WALSH, JAMES J.
The history of nursing. New York, Kenedy, 1929.

WISCONSIN STATE NURSES' ASSOCIATION
Nursing through the ages: a pictorial history. [Madison], The Association, 1938.

WORCESTER, ALFRED
Nurses and nursing. Cambridge, Mass., Harvard University Press, 1927.
[Contains articles on nursing in the old world and the new: on Florence Nightingale, A. L. Pringle, The First American Training School.]

HISTORY OF NURSING IN OTHER COUNTRIES

AUSTRALIA

[ANDERSEN, CAROLINE E.]
The story of bush nursing in Victoria.
[Melbourne, The Victorian Bush Nursing Association, 1951?]

BOWE, E. J.
The story of nursing in Australia since Foundation Day: 8th Annual Oration, Sept. 8, 1960, at the New South Wales College of Nursing. The College, 1960.

SOUTH AUSTRALIAN TRAINED NURSES' CENTENARY COMMITTEE
Nursing in South Australia: the first hundred years 1837-1937. Adelaide, The Committee, 1939.

CANADA

CHITTICK, RAE
Forty years of growing. Canadian Nurse, Jan. 1957, p. 29-34.

GIBBON, JOHN MURRAY, and MATHEWSON, MARY S.
Three centuries of Canadian nursing. Toronto, Macmillan, 1947.

CHINA

STEPHENSON, GLADYS E.
The story of Christian nursing in China. (195—).

FINLAND

JARVI, K.
Hospital nursing in Finland. Bulletin of the California State Nurses Assoc., Jan. 1959, p. 6-7.

GERMANY

KENEALY, ANNESLEY
In a cholera hospital at Hamburg. Nursing Record, Sept. 22, 1892, p. 785-6.

VICTORIA HOUSE NURSE TRAINING SCHOOL, FRIEDRICHSHAIN KRANKENHAUS, BERLIN
Nursing in Germany: pioneer work by the Empress Frederick. Nursing Record, Jan. 25, 1902, p. 69-70.

INDIA & PAKISTAN

BLEAKLEY, ETHEL
Meet the Indian nurse. Zenith Press, n.d.

WILKINSON, A.
A brief history of nursing in India and Pakistan. Delhi, Trained Nurses Assn. of India, 1958.

ITALY

GIUNTI, I. DI T.
Notes on the history of nursing care with special reference to Italy. International Nursing Review, May 1957, p. 12-15.

NEW ZEALAND

LAMBIE, M. I.
A wealth of information: facts relating to our nursing history which every nurse should know. New Zealand Nursing Journal, July 1960, p. 8-17.

MACLEAN, HESTER
Nursing in New Zealand: history and reminiscences. Wellington, N.Z., Tolan, 1932.

NEW ZEALAND
The Hospital Nurses' Registration Act. Nursing Record, Nov. 23, 1901, p. 416-7.

NEW ZEALAND. DEPARTMENT OF HEALTH
Historical development of nursing in New Zealand, 1840-1946. Wellington, Dept. of Health [1947].

PHILIPPINES

TUPAS, ANASTACIA
History of nursing in the Philippines and Manila. [Manila] Univ. Press, 1952.

SOUTH AFRICA

Editorial commemorating State Registration of Nurses in Cape Colony. Nursing Record, Sept. 17, 1891, p. 145-7.

SWEDEN

DILLNER, ELISABET
The stave of mercy: a pageant play of tableaux . . . trans. by Ronald de Wolfe. [Swedish Nurses' Association, 1949.]

LOBBAN, M.
Nursing museum in a Swedish hospital. Nursing Mirror, Oct. 5, 1956, p. viii-ix.

TURKEY

SEHSUVAROGLU, B. N.
A survey of nursing in Anatolian Turks and nursing history. Tip Fakultesi Mecmurasi, 1960, p. 247-50.

UNITED KINGDOM

ABEL-SMITH, BRIAN
A history of the nursing profession. Heinemann, 1960.

AMBERG, EMIL
State registration of nurses. British Journal of Nursing, June 18, 1904, p. 494-6.

BARNETT, R. P.
Speech made when moving the second reading of the Nurses Registration Bill in the House of Commons, March 28th. British Journal of Nursing, April 5, 1919, p. 217-29.

BONHAM-CARTER, HENRY
Is a general register for nurses desirable? Nursing Record, Sept. 6, 1888, p. 301-4.

BREAY, MARGARET
Nursing in the Victorian era. Nursing Record, June 19, 1897, p. 493-502.

BRITISH JOURNAL OF NURSING
Deputation of anti-registrationists at the Privy Council Office. *British Journal of Nursing*, June 23, 1906, p. 499-501.

BRITISH MEDICAL ASSOCIATION
Memorandum on the Bills for State Registration of Nurses, prepared respectively by the Association for the State Registration of Trained Nurses and the Royal British Nurses' Association. *British Journal of Nursing*, June 11, 1904, p. 472-3.

BRITISH NURSES ASSOCIATION
Circular sent to the Chairmen of the Committees of Management of Hospitals throughout the United Kingdom having nurse training schools attached, suggesting the foundation of a Registration Council. *Nursing Record*, Nov. 21, 1889, p. 284-5.

CENTRAL COMMITTEE FOR THE STATE REGISTRATION OF NURSES
Correspondence between the Committee and the College of Nursing on the nurses registration bill. *British Journal of Nursing*, Dec. 2, 1916, p. 447-54.

CENTRAL COMMITTEE FOR THE STATE REGISTRATION OF NURSES
Deputation to the Home Secretary. *British Journal of Nursing*, Aug. 8, 1914, p. 115-22.

CENTRAL COMMITTEE FOR THE STATE REGISTRATION OF NURSES
State legislation and the College of Nursing. *British Journal of Nursing*, Sept. 16, 1916, p. 238-40.
[A report of negotiations between the Committee and the College of Nursing which took place in the hope of agreeing upon a joint Bill.]

COLLEGE OF NURSING
College of Nursing opposes the nurses' petition to the Prime Minister. *British Journal of Nursing*, June 9, 1917, p. 398-9.

COLLEGE OF NURSING
Conference on State Registration. *British Journal of Nursing*, April 1, 1916, p. 292-300.

CONFERENCE ON STATE REGISTRATION OF NURSES
Conference between representatives of various nursing bodies and the Parliamentary Bills Committee of the B.M.A. held on 14th Jan. 1896: Report of Proceedings. *Nursing Record*, Jan. 18, 1896, p. 55-7.

COPE, Z.
Evolution of the sister tutor. *Nursing Times*, Dec. 9, 1955, p. 1388-91.

CRAWFORD, J. A.
The reasons for the state registration of trained nurses. *Nursing Record*, Aug. 25, 1900, p. 149-50.

FENWICK, ETHEL GORDON
The Nurses' Registration Act. *British Journal of Nursing*, Jan. 10, 1920, p. 20-2.

FENWICK, ETHEL GORDON
The nursing profession and the Board of Trade. *British Journal of Nursing*, Jan. 22, 1916, p. 73-5, Jan. 29, 1916, p. 94-9.

FENWICK, ETHEL GORDON
The organisation and registration of nurses. *Nursing Record*, April 12, 1902, p. 284-7.

FOX, E. M.
What the twentieth-century nurse may learn from the nineteenth. *British Journal of Nursing*, Nov. 26, 1910, p. 432-4, Dec. 3, 1910, p. 447-9.

BENNETT, B. A.
The evolution of the nursing profession in Britain.
(1) 19th and early 20th centuries.
(2) From First to Second World War.
(3) Post-war period.
(4) Present trends.
Nursing Mirror, May 13, 1960, p. 588-90; May 20, 1960, p. 681-3; May 27, 1960, p. 778-9; June 3, 1960, p. 867-8.

HALDANE, ELIZABETH
The British nurse in peace and war. Murray, 1923.

HART, MARGARET H.
Pre-reformation nurses in England. Murray, [193?].

HOLLAND, SYDNEY
Manifesto against state registration. *British Journal of Nursing*, March 26, 1904, p. 246-8.

HOSPITALS ASSOCIATION. JOINT SECTIONAL COMMITTEE OF REGISTRATION
Report, and extracts of comments in the *Lancet* and *Manchester Guardian*. *Nursing Record*, May 3, 1888, p. 51-3.

LANCET
The registration of trained nurses. *Nursing Record*, July 11, 1889, p. 22-4.

LAURENCE, E. C.
A nurse's life in war and peace. Smith, Elder, 1912.

MACDONALD, ISABEL
Queens in nursing history: a memento of Coronation year. Royal British Nurses' Association, 1953.

Nursing progress in the nineteenth century. *Nursing Record*, Dec. 29, 1900, p. 512-8.

POOLE, HENRIETTA.
The reasons for the state registration of trained nurses. *Nursing Record*, Aug. 18, 1900, p. 131-3.

SOCIETY FOR THE STATE REGISTRATION OF TRAINED NURSES
A reply to the manifesto compiled by Sydney Holland. *British Journal of Nursing*, March 26, 1904, p. 248-50.

SOCIETY FOR THE STATE REGISTRATION OF TRAINED NURSES
Proceedings of a public meeting held at Morley Hall on May 30th organised by the Society. *Nursing Record*, June 7, 1902, p. 453-8.

SOCIETY FOR THE STATE REGISTRATION OF TRAINED NURSES
Memorandum prepared by Miss Isla Stewart and presented to the Public Health Committee of the House of Commons. *British Journal of Nursing*, April 16, 1904, p. 310-2.

SOCIETY FOR THE STATE REGISTRATION OF TRAINED NURSES
A meeting to discuss the R.B.N.A.'s redrafted Bill for State Registration. *British Journal of Nursing*, Jan. 27, 1906, p. 73-6.

SOCIETY FOR THE STATE REGISTRATION OF TRAINED NURSES
Meeting to discuss the College of Nursing Conference on State Registration. *British Journal of Nursing*, April 8, 1916, p. 316-7.

SOCIETY FOR THE STATE REGISTRATION OF TRAINED NURSES
Deputation to the Prime Minister in support of state registration. *British Journal of Nursing*, May 22, 1909, p. 406-11.

TOOGOOD, F. SHERMAN
The reasons for the state registration of trained nurses. *Nursing Record*, Aug. 11, 1900, p. 109-12.

UNITED STATES

ALLEN, DOTALINE E.
History of nursing in Indiana. Indianapolis, Wolfe, 1950.

BOYD, LOUIE CROFT
State registration for nurses. Philadelphia, Saunders, 1911. 2nd edn., 1915.

BRECKINRIDGE, MARY
Wide neighbourhoods: a story of the Frontier Nursing Service. New York, Harper, 1952.

CHRIST, EDWIN A.
Missouri's nurses: the development of the profession, its associations and its institutions. Jefferson City, The Missouri State Nurses Assn., 1957.

DAUGHTERS OF CHARITY OF ST. VINCENT DE PAUL,
LOS ANGELES
One hundred years of service—the Daughters of Charity of St. Vincent de Paul 1856-1956. Los Angeles, 1956.

GARDNER, CAROLINE
Clever country: Kentucky mountain trails. New York, Revell, 1931.

KENNEALLY, C. MILDRED
Nurses and nursing in the Confederacy. Reprinted from *Southern Hospital*, April 1942.

MERRILL, BERTHA ESTELLE
The trek from yesterday: a history of organized nursing in Minneapolis, 1883-1936. Minneapolis Nurses Association, 1944.

NEW YORK STATE
A Bill for the registration of nurses of New York State. *British Journal of Nursing*, March 28, 1903, p. 252.

NORTH CAROLINA STATE
An act to provide for the registration of trained nurses. *British Journal of Nursing*, April 18, 1903, p. 314.

POOLE, ERNEST
Nurses on horseback. New York, Macmillan, 1932.

ROBB, ISABEL HAMPTON
Presidential address to the National Associated Alumnae of the United States on the importance of state registration. *Nursing Record*, Nov. 24, 1900, p. 415-8.

ROBERTS, MARY MAY
American nursing: history and interpretation. New York, Macmillan, 1954.

RODABAUGH, JAMES H., *and* RODABAUGH, MARY JANE
Nursing in Ohio: a history. Columbus, Ohio, The Ohio State Nurses Assn., 1951.

THOMS, ADAH B., *compiler*
Pathfinders: a history of the progress of colored graduate nurses with biographies of many prominent nurses. New York, Kay Printing House, 1929.

TRENHOLME, LOUISE IRBY
History of nursing in Missouri. Columbia, The Missouri State Nurses' Assn., 1926.

WEST, ROBERTA MAYHEW
History of nursing in Pennsylvania. Philadelphia, Pennsylvania State Nurses' Assn., 1926.

WOOLSEY, ABBY HOWLAND
A century of nursing, with hints toward the organization of a training school and Florence Nightingale's historic letter on The Bellevue School, Sept. 18, 1872, and Hospitals and Training Schools: report to the Standing Committee on Hospitals of the State Charities Aid Association, New York . . . 1876 . . . to which is added Founding of the Bellevue Training School for Nurses, chapter VI, "Recollections of a happy life", by Elizabeth Christophers Hobson, New York, Putnam, 1916. New York, Putnam, 1950.

WOOLSEY, JANE STUART
Hospital days. New York, Van Nostrand, 1870.

WORCESTER, ALFRED
Nurses for our neighbours. Boston, Houghton, Mifflin, 1914.

WYCHE, MARY LEWES
History of nursing in North Carolina. Chapel Hill, University of Carolina Press, 1938.

HISTORY SPECIAL ASPECTS

AIR FORCE NURSING

MARTIN, A. M.
We earn our wings. *American Journal of Nursing*, July 1957, p. 894-6.

PRINCESS MARY'S ROYAL AIR FORCE NURSING SERVICE
In
REXFORD-WELCH, S. C., *editor*
The Royal Air Force Medical Services.
Vol. 1. Administration. H.M.S.O., 1954.
[Contains a chapter giving the pre-war and war history of the Princess Mary's Royal Air Force Nursing Service.]

SLATTERLEY, L. C.
Air Force nurses progress towards the space age. *Military Medicine*, July 1960, p. 482-8.

ARMY NURSING

ARKLE, ANNIE
The Indian Army Nursing Service. *British Journal of Nursing*, Sept. 6, 1902, p. 196-7.

AUSTRALIAN ARMY NURSING SERVICE
Lest we forget. Melbourne, The Australian Army Nursing Service, 1944.

BEITH, JOHN HAY
One hundred years of army nursing: the story of the British Army Nursing Services from the time of Florence Nightingale to the present day. Cassell, 1953.

BRODRICK, ALBINIA L.
Correspondence between Miss Brodrick and the War Office on the shortage of trained nurses for the troops. *British Journal of Nursing*, June 5, 1915, p. 482-3.

BROWNE, SIDNEY
The Army Reserve and Territorial nurse; the naval nurse; Lady Minto's Indian nurses.
See
NURSING TIMES
The nurse and the nation: a survey of her position in the State today. *Nursing Times*, Nov. 5, 1910, p. 904-31.

BROWNE, SIDNEY
The military nurse at home and abroad.
See
NURSING TIMES
The nurse and the nation: a survey of her position in the State today. *Nursing Times*, Nov. 5, 1910, p. 904-31.

CUTBUSH, EDWARD
Observations on the means of preserving the health of the soldiers and sailors—and on the duties of the medical department of the army and navy with remarks on hospitals and their internal enlargement. Philadelphia, Dobson, 1808.
[Contains instructions to matrons and nurses.]

DOBSON, JESSIE
The army nursing service in the eighteenth century. *In:* Annals of the Royal College of Surgeons of England, vol. 14, June 1954.

EVATT, G. J. H.
A corps of volunteer female nurses for service in the army hospitals in the field, with suggestions as to the incorporation of the nursing profession. *Nursing Record*, Aug. 4, 1900, p. 95-6, and Aug. 11, 1900, p. 112-3.

FLIKKE, JULIA O.
Nurses in action, the story of the Army Nurse Corps. Philadelphia, Lippincott, 1943.

LATTIMORE, J. G.
The transition from medical training to patient care. *Medical Technician's Bulletin*, Sept.-Oct., 1959, p. 191-4.

LOCH, CATHERINE G.
The Indian Army Nursing Service. *Nursing Record*, Sept. 12, 1896, p. 204-5; Sept. 19, 1896, p. 225-7; Sept. 26, 1896, p. 244-5.

MATRONS' COUNCIL
Account of a deputation to the War Office to lay before the Under Secretary of State for War suggestions of a practical nature in reference to army nursing reform. *Nursing Record*, April 6, 1901, p. 270; April 27, 1901, p. 331-5.

NATIONAL COUNCIL OF TRAINED NURSES OF GREAT BRITAIN
AND IRELAND
Resolution and statement sent to the Secretary of State
for War expressing dissatisfaction with the organisation
of the nursing of sick and wounded soldiers in military
auxiliary hospitals at home and abroad. *British Journal of
Nursing Supplement*, Jan. 30, 1915, p. i-vii.

The nurse and the V.A.D. members. Interesting views for
military matrons. *Nursing Times*, May 26, 1917, p. 624-7.

ODIER, LUCIE
Some advice to nurses and other members of the medical
services of the Armed Forces. Geneva, International
Committee of the Red Cross, 1951.

QUEEN ALEXANDRA'S IMPERIAL MILITARY NURSING SERVICE
In
CREW, F. A. E., *editor*
The army medical services.
Administration Volume II. H.M.S.O., 1955.
[Contains a chapter giving the history of the army nursing
services.]

QUEEN ALEXANDRA'S IMPERIAL MILITARY NURSING SERVICE
A qualification for military Matrons. Examination of
Sisters for the rank of Matron, Queen Alexandra's
Imperial Military Nursing Service. *British Journal of
Nursing*, Mar. 10, 1906, p. 196-7.

ROBERTS, MARY MAY
Yesterday, today: [The Army Nurse Corps]. Washington,
D.C., U.S. Army Nurse Corps, 1955.

ROGAN, JOHN
Military medical services in the reign of Elizabeth I.
Nursing Mirror, May 1, 1959, p. 349-50.

ROSS, JOHN W.
Lessons drawn from practical professional experience with
trained women nurses in military service. *British Journal
of Nursing*, Feb. 28, 1903, p. 168-9, and Mar. 7, 1903,
p. 187-8.

STIMSON, JULIA Catherine
The forerunners of the American army nurse. Reprinted
from the *Military Surgeon*, Feb. 1926.

STIMSON, JULIA CATHERINE
History and manual of the Army Nurse Corps. *Army
Medical Bulletin*, 1937, No. 41.

U.S. DEPARTMENT OF THE ARMY. OFFICE OF THE SURGEON
GENERAL. TECHNICAL LIAISON OFFICE
Highlights in the history of the Army Nurse Corps.
Washington, Govt. Printing Office, n.d.

WAR OFFICE
Appointment to the nursing service of the army. *Nursing
Record*, July 2, 1891, p. 18-19.

WARD, IRENE
F.A.N.Y. Invicta. Hutchinson, 1955.
[The history of the First Aid Nursing Yeomanry in two
world wars.]

WATT, PHOEBE F.
The work of the Indian Army Nursing Service. *British
Journal of Nursing*, Sept. 13, 1902, p. 214-5.

DEACONESSES AND SISTERHOODS

CLARE, SAINT
St. Clare and her order: story of seven centuries, edited by
the author of "The Enclosed Nun". Mills & Boon, 1912.

DOYLE, ANN
Nursing by religious orders in the United States (1809-
1928). Reprinted from the *American Journal of Nursing*,
vol. XXIX:
Part I, July 1929.
Part II, Aug. 1929.
Part III, Sept. 1929.
Part IV, Oct. 1929.
Part V, Nov. 1929.
Part VI, Dec. 1929.

HOLLOWAY, S. W.
The All Saints' Sisterhood at University College Hospital,
1862-99. *Medical History*, April 1959, p. 146-56.

HOWSON, JOHN SAUL
Deaconesses or the official help of women in parochial
work and in charitable institutions; an essay reprinted
with large additions from the *Quarterly Review*, Sept. 1860.
Longmans Green and Roberts, 1862.

JAMESON, ANNA BROWNELL
Sisters of charity, Catholic and Protestant, abroad and at
home. Longmans, 1855.

JAMESON, ANNA BROWNELL
Sisters of charity, Catholic and Protestant, and the com-
munion of labour. Boston, Ticknor & Fields, 1858.

POTTER, HENRY GODMAN
Sisterhoods and deaconesses at home and abroad. New
York, Dutton, 1873.

REINHART, ANNA
A memorial: the Kaiserswerth Deaconesses at Alexandria.
Alexandria, Kaiserswerth Deaconesses' Hospital, [1932].

ROBINSON, JANE MARIE
Deaconesses in Europe and their lessons for America.
New York, Hunt & Eaton, 1889.

THOBURN, JAMES MILLS
The deaconesses and their vocation. New York, Hunt and
Eaton, 1893.

WHEELER, HENRY
Deaconesses: ancient and modern. New York, Hunt &
Eaton, 1889.

DOMICILIARY NURSING

ANDERSON, GENEVIEVE
An oversight in nursing history. *Journal of History of
Medicine*, Summer 1948, p. 417-26.
[London Epidemiological Society's efforts to encourage
health visiting.]

ANDREWS, —
History and development of the Ranyard nurses, nursing
branch of the London Biblewomen and Nurses Mission,
25 Russell Square, London, W.C. A reprint from a paper
read by Miss Andrews before the Jubilee Congress of
District Nursing in Liverpool, May 1909.

BRAINARD, ANNIE B.
The evolution of public health nursing. Philadelphia,
Saunders, 1922.

BUCKINGHAMSHIRE COUNTY COUNCIL. NORTH BUCKS
TECHNICAL EDUCATION COMMITTEE
Health at home: report of the training of the rural health
missioners, and of their village lecturing and visiting.
Winslow, Bucks. County Council, 1892.
[Reprint entitled "Reproduction of a printed report . . .
containing letters from Miss Florence Nightingale on
health visiting. . . , 1911.]

BUNFORD, ALICE M.
Ninety years a mission, 1857-1947. The Ranyard Mission,
1947.

CENTRAL COUNCIL FOR DISTRICT NURSING IN LONDON
History of the Central Council for District Nursing,
London, 1914-44. The Council, [194-].

COPE, ZACHARY
Florence Nightingale and district nursing. *District
Nursing*, Nov. 1958, p. 179-80.

EASTWOOD, C. G.
The Public Health Service: its history and work. *Nursing
Mirror*, June 10, 1955, p. 721-2; June 17, 1955, p. 799-800;
June 24, 1955, p. xiii-xiv; July 1, 1955, p. v-vi; July 8, 1955,
p. vi-vii; July 15, 1955, p. x; July 22, 1955, p. ii-iii and xii.

FULMER, HARRIET
History of visiting nurse work in America. *Nursing
Record*, June 21, 1902, p. 496-8, and June 28, 1902, p. 515.

GREENWOOD, F. J. L.
The evolution of the health visitor. *Nursing Times*, Feb. 10, 1917, p. 160-3, and Feb. 17, 1917, p. 186-8.

HUGHES, AMY
History of district nursing in England and other countries. Report of Jubilee Congress on District Nursing. Queen Victoria's Jubilee Institute, 1909.

HUGHES, AMY
The origin, growth and present status of district nursing in England. *Nursing Record*, May 10, 1902, p. 370-2, and May 17, 1902, p. 391-3.

HUGHES, AMY
The origin and present work of Queen Victoria's Jubilee Institute for Nurses.
In
HAMPTON, ISABEL A., *and others*
Nursing of the sick, 1893.

JUBILEE CONGRESS OF DISTRICT NURSING
Report and proceedings of the Jubilee Congress of District Nursing held at Liverpool, 12-14 May, 1909. Liverpool, Marples, 1909.

LESSON, G.
District nursing in Manchester ninety years ago. *Nursing Times*, Jan. 25, 1957, p. 104-5.

LONDON BIBLEWOMEN AND NURSES MISSION
The district nurses of the London Biblewomen and Nurses Mission. *British Journal of Nursing*, June 9, 1906, p. 455-8.

Metropolitan and National Association for providing trained nurses for the sick poor; Report of the sub-committee of reference and enquiry. London, 1875.

PLATT, ELSPETH
The story of the Ranyard Mission, 1857-1937. Hodder & Stoughton, 1937.

POOLE, ERNEST
Nurses on horseback. New York, Macmillan, 1932.
[The work of the Kentucky Frontier Nursing Service.]

QUEEN VICTORIA'S JUBILEE INSTITUTE FOR NURSES
Regulations as to the training and engagement of district nurses for the sick poor. *Nursing Record*, July 24, 1890, p. 44-5.

QUEEN VICTORIA'S JUBILEE INSTITUTE FOR NURSES
Statement as to the past and present position of Queen Victoria's Jubilee Institute for Nurses. *Nursing Record*, July 17, 1890, p. 34-5.

QUEEN'S INSTITUTE OF DISTRICT NURSING
Survey of district nursing in England and Wales: information obtained and compiled by the Queen's Institute of District Nursing. The Institute, 193?.

RATHBONE, WILLIAM
Sketch of the history and progress of district nursing from its commencement in the year 1859 to the present date. . . . Macmillan, 1890.

STOCKS, MARY
A hundred years of district nursing. Allen & Unwin, 1960.

WALD, LILLIAN D.
The house on Henry Street. New York, Henry Holt, 1915.
[Describes the work done by visiting nurses in child and youth welfare in East Side New York in the 1890s.]

WALD, LILLIAN D.
Windows on Henry Street. Boston, Little, Brown, 1934.
[A continuation of "The House on Henry Street".]

NAVAL NURSING

JACKSON, W. L.
We've reached the golden year. *American Journal of Nursing*, May 1958, p. 671-3.
[Navy Nurse Corps 50th anniversary.]

NURSING MIRROR
Nursing in the Navy. *Nursing Mirror*, July 27, 1956, p. iv-vi.

NURSING RECORD
Regulations for the Staff of Nursing Sisters in the Royal Naval Hospitals. *Nursing Record*, July 2, 1891, p. 7-9.

NURSING RECORD
Regulations for the Staff of Nursing Sisters in the Royal Naval Hospitals. *Nursing Record*, June 21, 1902, p. 493-4.

QUEEN ALEXANDRA'S ROYAL NAVAL NURSING SERVICE
Regulations for Queen Alexandra's Royal Naval Nursing Service. *British Journal of Nursing*, Nov. 29, 1902, p. 437-9.

QUEEN ALEXANDRA'S ROYAL NAVAL NURSING SERVICE
New regulations. *British Journal of Nursing*, Sept. 9, 1911, p. 207-8.

QUEEN ALEXANDRA'S ROYAL NAVAL NURSING SERVICE RESERVE
Regulations for Queen Alexandra's Royal Naval Nursing Reserve. *British Journal of Nursing*, Jan. 14, 1911, p. 28-9.

SINGER, C.
An eighteenth-century naval ship to accommodate women nurses. *Medical History*, Oct. 1960, p. 283-7.

SPEER, THEODORE V.
Nursing on the hospital ship "Solace". *Nursing Record*, Dec. 30, 1899, p. 532-5.

UNITED STATES, DEPARTMENT OF THE NAVY. BUREAU OF MEDICINE AND SURGERY. NURSING DIVISION
Annotated history of the Nurse Corps, U.S. Navy. Washington, Govt. Printing Office, 1957.

NURSE-MIDWIFERY

HUMFREY, MARIAN
The monthly nurse: her origin, rise and progress. *Nursing Record*, May 21, 1891, p. 267-72.

MATERNITY CENTER ASSOCIATION, NEW YORK
Twenty years of nurse-midwifery, 1933-1953. New York, Maternity Center Association, [1955].

SHOEMAKER, SISTER M. THEOPHANE
History of nurse-midwifery in the United States. Washington, Catholic University of America Press, 1947.

OCCUPATIONAL HEALTH NURSING

CHARLEY, IRENE H.
The birth of industrial nursing: its history and development in Great Britain. . . . Bailliere, Tindall & Cox, 1954.

HOLMES, K. M.
History of industrial nursing up to date. 1931.

LUCAL, M. W.
Industrial nursing—A history. A brief history of American industrial nursing. *American Association of Industrial Nurses Journal*, Feb. 1958, p. 14-16.

POOR LAW NURSING

BARTON, ELEANOR C.
The evolution of poor law nursing. *British Journal of Nursing*, Aug. 23, 1913, p. 149-51, and Aug. 30, 1913, p. 170-1.

BARTON, ELEANOR C.
The history and progress of poor law nursing. Law and Local Government Pubs. Ltd., [1926].

BODLEY, —
State aid for poor law nurses. *British Journal of Nursing*, Jan. 13, 1912, p. 25-6.

COBBE, FRANCES POWER
Workhouse sketches. *Macmillan's Magazine*, vol. III (Nov. 1860-April 1861), p. 448-61.
[Contains an account of the nursing provided in workhouses.]

Friendly letter to under-nurses of the sick—especially in unions, by a lady. London, 1861.

HALDANE, ELIZABETH S.
Nursing in Scottish poor houses. *British Journal of Nursing*, July 5, 1902, p. 14-15.

JULIAN, E. E.
The need of nursing reform in workhouse infirmaries. *Nursing Record*, Jan. 28, 1899, p. 70-2.

Lady nurses for the sick poor in our London workhouses. Report of proceedings at the Strand Union's Board of Guardians, Sept. 4, 1866. London, 1866.

LANCET SANITARY COMMISSION FOR INVESTIGATING THE STATE OF THE INFIRMARIES OF WORKHOUSES
The findings of the Lancet Commission for investigating the care of the sick in the workhouse infirmaries, presented, among other matters, observations of the conditions in nursing and suggested appropriate remedies. *Lancet*, July 1, 1865, p. 14-22.

LANDALE, E. J. R.
Nursing in a workhouse infirmary: some of the nurses' difficulties. *Nursing Record*, Jan. 6, 1894, p. 6-8.

LOCAL GOVERNMENT BOARD
The abolition of pauper nursing in Irish workhouse infirmaries. *Nursing Record*, Oct. 16, 1897, p. 309.

MOLLETT, M.
On an unpopular branch of our profession (workhouse infirmary nursing). *Nursing Record*, Feb. 20, 1890, p. 90-3, and Feb. 27, 1890, p. 100-2.

TWINING, LOUISA
The history of workhouse reform.
In
HAMPTON, ISABEL A., *and others*
Nursing of the sick, 1893.

TWINING, LOUISA
Notes of six years' work as guardian of the poor, 1884-1890.
[Includes the regulations developed by the Poorlaw Board and the Local Government Board relating to nursing in workhouse infirmaries.]

TWINING, LOUISA
Workhouses and pauperism and women's work in the administration of the poor law. 1853.

WILKIE, C. B. S.
The best means of providing and training nurses for the indoor poor. *Nursing Record*, Feb. 25, 1899, p. 150-1, and Mar. 4, 1899, p. 170-2.

[WILSON, T.]
Nursing in workhouses and workhouse infirmaries. University Press, n.d.

WOOD, C. J.
The present position of poor law nursing. *Nursing Times*, June 10, 1905, p. 91-2.

WORKHOUSE INFIRMARY NURSING ASSOCIATION
Memorial to the Local Government Board, with appendices on suggested rules for nurses, and nursing in workhouse sick wards. *Nursing Record*, July 20, 1893, p. 20-3.

PSYCHIATRIC NURSING

DEUTSCH, ALBERT
The mentally ill in America: a history of their care and treatment from colonial times. New York, Columbia University Press, 1946.

GODDARD, L.
The history of mental nursing. *British Journal of Nursing*, Nov. 1952, p. 106-7; Dec. 1952, p. 121; June 1953, p. 77; July 1953, p. 88-9; Nov. 1953, p. 130-1.

HUNTER, R. A.
In the mental hospital. The rise and fall of mental nursing. *Lancet*, Jan. 14, 1956, p. 98-9.

JONES, KATHLEEN
Lunacy, law and conscience, 1744-1845: the social history of the care of the insane. Routledge & Kegan Paul, 1955.

SANTOS, ELVIN H., *and* STAINBROOK, EDWARD
A history of psychiatric nursing in the nineteenth century. *Journal of the History of Medicine and Allied Sciences*, Vol. 4, No. 1, Winter 1949.

RED CROSS & THE ORDER OF ST. JOHN OF JERUSALEM

AMERICAN NATIONAL RED CROSS SOCIETY
American Red Cross nursing service. Washington, the Society, n.d.

BARK, EVELYN
Time to kill. Hale, 1960.
[Recollections of a woman who has spent a lifetime in the service of the Red Cross.]

BARTON, CLARA
The Red Cross in peace and war. Meriden, Conn., Journal Publishing Co., 1912.

BARTON, CLARA
The story of the Red Cross. New York, Appleton-Century-Crofts, 1904.

BEST, S. H.
The story of the British Red Cross. Cassell, 1938.

BICKNELL, ERNEST P.
Pioneering with the Red Cross. New York, Macmillan, 1935.

BILLINGTON, MARY FRANCES
The Red Cross in war: woman's part in the relief of suffering. Hodder & Stoughton, 1914.

BOARDMAN, MABEL T.
Under the Red Cross flag at home and abroad. Philadelphia, Lippincott, 1915.
2nd edn., 1917.

BRITISH RED CROSS SOCIETY AND THE ORDER OF ST. JOHN OF JERUSALEM
Red Cross and St. John: the official record of the humanitarian services of the war organization of the British Red Cross Society and Order of St. John of Jerusalem, 1939-1947; compiled by P. G. Cambray and G. G. B. Briggs. British Red Cross Society, 1949.

DOCK, LAVINIA L., *and others*
History of American Red Cross nursing. New York, Macmillan, 1922.

DULLES, RHEA FOSTER
The American Red Cross: a history. New York, Harper, 1950.

DUNANT, J. HENRY
A memory of Solferino. Cassell, for the British Red Cross Society, 1947.

ELLIMAN, V. B.
American Red Cross Nursing Services; 50th anniversary. *Nursing Outlook*, March 1959, p. 148-51.

FLETCHER, N. CORBET, *compiler*
The St. John Ambulance Association: its history and its part in the ambulance movement. St. John Ambulance Assn., [1929].

GLADWIN, MARY E.
The Red Cross and Jane Arminda Delano. Philadelphia, Saunders, 1931.

GREENBIE, MARJORIE BARSTOW
Lincoln's daughters of mercy. New York, Putnam, [1944].
[The story of the U.S. Sanitary Commission—the forerunner of the American Red Cross.]

GUMPERT, MARTIN
Dunant: the story of the Red Cross. Eyre & Spottiswoode, 1939.

KERNODLE, PORTIA B.
The Red Cross nurse in action, 1882-1948. New York, Harper, [1949].

KING, E. J.
The grand priory of the Order of the Hospital of St. John of Jerusalem in England: a short history. [Fleetway Press], 1924.

LEAGUE OF RED CROSS SOCIETIES
Red Cross Nursing: report presented to the XIV International Red Cross Conference, The Hague, Oct. 1928. Paris, The League, 1928.

PEARSON, E.
British Red Cross Nursing Service—at home and abroad. *Nursing Times*, April 29, 1955, p. 456.

PICKETT, SARAH ELIZABETH
The American National Red Cross: its origin, purposes and service. New York, Century, 1923.

UNIFORMS

ADAMS, RALPH, *and others*
New fashions in surgical attire. *American Journal of Nursing*, Aug. 1959, p. 1102-7.

CENTRAL HEALTH SERVICES COUNCIL. STANDING NURSING ADVISORY COMMITTEE
Report of a sub-committee on the design of nurses' uniforms. H.M.S.O., 1959.

KELLY, C. W.
What nurses want in a uniform. *American Journal of Nursing*, Oct. 1957, p. 1282-4.

KNOWLES, L. N.
The collar that became a cap. *American Journal of Nursing*, Sept. 1958, p. 1246-8.

LOCKERBY, F. K.
Nursing fashion note; new uniform design for hospital merger. *Hospital Management*, July 1957, p. 44-5.

MICHAELS, ROBERTA
What's new in uniforms. *R.N.*, Mar. 1958, p. 52-9, 94-100.

NEWCASTLE REGIONAL HOSPITAL BOARD
Report on design of nursing uniforms. The Board, 1954.

NURSING MIRROR
The nurse's uniform. *Nursing Mirror*, Dec. 20, 1957, p. 868.

NURSING TIMES
The nurse and her outfit in hospital, on district, in private and midwifery work, in government service, and abroad. *Nursing Times*, Nov. 13, 1909, p. 920-33.

NURSING TIMES
The nurse and her uniform. *Nursing Times*, Oct. 7, 1955, p. 1111-2.

NURSING TIMES
Nurses' uniform, new American ideas. *Nursing Times*, Oct. 7, 1955, p. 1128-30.

ROBSON, P. L.
Nurses' uniforms. (1) Standards and patterns. *Nursing Mirror*, Nov. 11, 1960, p. 541-2.

SMITH, MARION E.
Uniforms. *Nursing Record*, Sept. 5, 1896, p. 183-5.

THE TERRITORIAL FORCE NURSING SERVICE
Uniform. *British Journal of Nursing*, May 27, 1911, p. 415.

Why a cap? A short history of nursing caps from some schools organised prior to 1891. Philadelphia, Lippincott, 1940.

WAR NURSING

ALCOTT, LOUISA MAY
Hospital sketches, camp and fireside stories. Boston, Redpath, 1863.
Cambridge, Mass., University Press, 1869.
Boston, Roberts, 1895.
Boston, Little, Brown, 1902.

ALCOTT, LOUISA MAY
Hospital sketches, edited by Bessie Z. Jones. Cambridge, Mass., Belknap Press of Harvard University Press, 1960.

ALOYSIUS, SISTER MARY
Memories of the Crimea. London, Burns, 1897.

ARCHARD, THERESA
G.I. Nightingale: the story of an American army nurse. New York, Norton, 1945.

BARTON, GEORGE
Angels of the battlefield, an history of the labors of the Catholic sisterhoods in the late Civil War. Philadelphia, Catholic Pub. Co., 1897.

BEAUCHAMP, PAT
Fanny went to war. Routledge, 1940.
[The story of the First Aid Nursing Yeomanry during the first world war.]

BOWDEN, JEAN
Grey touched with scarlet: the war experiences of the Army Nursing Sisters. Hale, 1959.

BOWSER, THEKLA
The story of British V.A.D. work in the Great War. Melrose, 1917.

BRITISH MEDICAL JOURNAL
[Crimean hospitals.] *British Medical Journal*, Jan. 23, 1960, p. 268.

CLINT, M. B.
Our bit: memories of war service by a Canadian nursing-sister. Montreal, Royal Victoria Hospital, 1934.

CROY, PRINCESS MARIE DE
War memories. Macmillan, 1932.

CUMMING, KATE
A journal of hospital life in the confederate army of Tennessee from the Battle of Shiloh to the end of the war. Louisville, Kentucky, Morton, 1866.

CUMMING, KATE
Kate: the journal of a confederate nurse, edited by Richard Barksdale Harwell. Louisiana State Univ. Press, 1959.

DEARMER, MABEL
Letters from a field hospital; with a memoir of the author by Stephen Gwynn. Macmillan, 1915.

EDGE, GERALDINE, *and* JOHNSTON, MARY E.
The ships of youth: the experiences of two army nursing sisters on board the hospital carrier "Leinster". Hodder & Stoughton, [1945].

EDMONDS, S. EMMA E.
Nurse and spy in the Union Army. Hartford, Conn., W. S. Williams, 1867.

EVELYN, GEORGE PALMER
A diary of the Crimea, edited by Cyril Falls. Duckworth, 1954.

FEDDEN, MARGUERITE
Sisters' quarters, Salonika. Grant Richards, 1921.

FITZGERALD, —
The Edith Cavell nurse from Massachusetts. A record of one year's personal service with the British expeditionary force in France (Boulogne, The Somme, 1916-17), with an account of the imprisonment, trial and death of Edith Cavell. Boston, Butterfield, 1917.

FITZROY, YVONNE
With the Scottish nurses in Roumania. Murray, 1918.

GIBBS, PETER
Crimean blunder: the story of war with Russia a hundred years ago. Frederick Muller, 1960.

GOODMAN, MARGARET
Experiences of an English sister of mercy. Smith, Elder, 1862.

GOWING, TIMOTHY
Voice from the ranks: a personal narrative of the Crimean campaign by a sergeant of the Royal Fusiliers. . . . Ed. by Kenneth Fenwick. Folio Society, 1954.

HAMMARLUND, MABEL
The United States army nurse in Korea. *Nursing Outlook*, April 1955, p. 208-10.

HARRISON, ADA, *editor*
Grey and scarlet: letters from the war areas by army nursing sisters on active service. Hodder & Stoughton, 1944.

HAWKINS, DORIS M.
Atlantic torpedo: the record of twenty-seven days in an open boat following a U-boat sinking. Gollancz, 1943.

HENRIETTA, SISTER
War nursing in South Africa, 1901. *British Journal of Nursing*, Sept. 27, 1902, p. 254-6.

HOLLAND, MARY A. GARDINER, *compiler*
Our army nurses: interesting sketches, addresses and photographs of nearly one hundred of the noble women who served in hospitals and on battlefields during our Civil War. Boston, Wilkins, 1895.

HUTTON, I. EMSLIE
With a woman's unit in Serbia, Salonika and Sebastopol. Williams & Norgate, 1928.

JEFFREY, BETTY
White coolies. Sydney, Angus & Robertson, 1954.
[The story of the Australian Army nursing sisters who were in Malaya with the 8th Division A.I.F. in 1941-42 and who were taken prisoner by the Japanese.]

JORDEN, ELLA
Operation mercy. Muller, 1957.

KIRKCALDIE, R. A.
In gray and scarlet. Melbourne, Alexander McCubbin, [1922].

A LADY
Ismeer: or Smyrna and its British hospital in 1855. Madden, 1856.
[An account of hospital and nursing conditions in the Crimea, written by a woman who volunteered for service.]

LIVERMORE, MARY A.
My story of the war; a woman's narrative of four years' personal experience as a nurse in the Union army and in relief work at home, in hospitals, camps and at the front, during the war of rebellion. With anecdotes, pathetic incidents and thrilling reminiscences portraying the lights and shadows of hospital life and the sanitary service of the war. Hartford, Conn., Worthington, 1889.

LOCKE, E. I. J.
Post-war letters of a V.A.D. nurse. Stockwell, 1933.

LONGMORE, T.
The sanitary contrasts of the British and French armies during the Crimean War. Charles Griffin, 1883.

LUARD, K. E.
Unknown warriors—extracts from the letters of K. E. Luard . . . nursing sister in France 1914-1918. Chatto & Windus, 1930.

McCAUL, ETHEL
Under the care of the Japanese War Office. Cassell, 1904.

McLAREN, BARBARA
Women of the war. Hodder & Stoughton, 1917.
[An account of the work of English women in many fields of work during the first world war. A considerable section deals with nursing.]

MILLARD, SHIRLEY
I saw them die: diary and recollections of Shirley Millard, edited by Adele Comandini. Harrap, 1936.

MILLER, JEAN DUPONT
Shipmates in white. New York, Dodd, Mead, 1944.

MITCHINER, PHILIP HENRY, *and*
MACMANUS, EMILY ELVIRA PRIMROSE
Nursing in time of war. Churchill, 1939.
2nd edn., 1943.

MOORE, FRANK
Women of the war: their heroism and self-sacrifice. Hartford, Conn., Scranton, 1866.

MRS. H.
Three years in field hospitals of the army of the Potomac. Philadelphia, Lippincott, 1867.

NEWCOMB, ELLSWORTH
Brave nurse: true stories of heroism. New York, Appleton, Century, 1945.

OLNHAUSEN, MARY PHINNEY
Adventures of an army nurse in two wars, edited from the diary and correspondence of Mary Phinney, Baroness Von Olnhausen, by James Phinney Monroe. Boston, Little, Brown, 1903.

OSBORNE, SYDNEY GODOLPHIN
Scutari and its hospitals. Dickinson, 1855.

THE PATRIOT DAUGHTERS OF LANCASTER
Hospital scenes after the battle of Gettysburg, July, 1863. Philadelphia, Ashmead, 1864.

POPE, GEORGINA FANE
Nursing in South Africa during the Boer War. *British Journal of Nursing*, Sept. 20, 1902, p. 232-4.

QUEEN ALEXANDRA'S IMPERIAL MILITARY NURSING SERVICE
Reminiscent sketches 1914-1919. Bale, 1922.

RECICAR, CATHERINE
I nursed aboard a refugee ship. *American Journal of Nursing*, March 1957, p. 300-2.

REDMOND, JUANITA
I served on Bataan. Philadelphia, Lippincott, 1943.

REED, WILLIAM HOWELL
Hospital life in the army of the Potomac. Boston, Spencer, 1866.
[Includes an account of the work of Helen Gilson in the army.]

RICHARDSON, TERESA EDEN
In Japanese hospitals during war-time; fifteen months with the Red Cross Society of Japan (April 1904 to July 1905). Blackwood, 1905.

THE ROVING ENGLISHMAN, *pseud.*
Pictures from the battle fields. Routledge, 1855.

RUNDLE, HENRY
With the Red Cross in the Franco-German war, A.D. 1870-1: some reminiscences. Werner Laurie, [18—].

RUSSELL, W. H.
The war. 2 vols. Routledge, 1855-6.
Vol. I. From the landing at Gallipoli to the death of Lord Raglan. 1855.
Vol. II. From the death of Lord Raglan to the evacuation of the Crimea. 1856.
[The classic account of conditions in the Crimea. By the correspondent of the London *Times*.]

SANDBACH, BETSY, *and* EDGE, GERALDINE
Prison life on a Pacific raider: the adventures of nurse escorts to the first five hundred children evacuated to Australia. Hodder & Stoughton, 1941.

SIMONS, JESSIE ELIZABETH
While history passed: the story of the Australian nurses who were prisoners of the Japanese for three and a half years. Heineman, 1954.

SIMPSON, CORA E.
A joy-ride through China for the N.A.C. Shanghai, Kwang Hsueh, [192?].

SKIMMING, SYLVIA
Sand in my shoes: the tale of a Red Cross welfare officer with the British hospitals overseas in the Second World War. Edinburgh, Oliver & Boyd, 1945.

SMITH, ADELAIDE W.
Reminiscences of an army nurse during the Civil War. New York, Greaves, 1911.

SMITH, LESLEY
Four years out of life. Glasgow, Philip Allan, 1931.

SOYER, ALEXIS
Instructions to military hospital cooks in the preparation of diets for sick soldiers. Eyre & Spottiswoode, 1859.

SOYER, ALEXIS
Soyer's culinary campaign: being historical reminiscences of the late war; with the plain art of cookery for military and civil institutions, the army, navy, public, etc. Routledge, 1857.
[Contains information about Florence Nightingale in its description of the Scutari hospital.]

STEVENSON, ISOBEL
Nursing in the civil war. *In* Ciba Symposia, Summitt, New Jersey, 1941.

STIMSON, JULIA CATHERINE
The army nurse corps. Washington, Govt. Printing Office, 1927. *In* The medical dept. of the U.S. Army in the World War, vol. XIII.

STIMSON, JULIA CATHERINE
Finding themselves; the letters of an American Army chief nurse in a British hospital in France. New York, Macmillan, 1918.

STIMSON, JULIA CATHERINE
Women nurses with the Union Forces during the Civil War. Reprinted from the *Military Surgeon*, Jan.-Feb., 1928.

TERROT, S. A.
Reminiscences of Scutari hospitals, 1854-1855 (from the diary of the late Miss S. A. Terrot). *Nursing Times*, Sept. 11, 1909, p. 741-2; Sept. 18, 1909, p. 761; Sept. 25, 1909, p. 781-2.

THURSTAN, VIOLETTA
Field hospital and flying column: being the journal of an English nursing sister in Belgium and Russia. New York, Putnam, 1915.

WIDMER, C. L.
Grandfather and Florence Nightingale. An account of bread supply to troops in the Crimea. *American Journal of Nursing*, May 1955, p. 569-71.

BIOGRAPHY

COLLECTED BIOGRAPHY

COLE, MARGARET
Women of today. Nelson, 1938.
[Contains chapters on Edith Cavell, Elizabeth Garrett Anderson, Beatrice Webb.]

McGILL UNIVERSITY. SCHOOL FOR GRADUATE NURSES, HISTORY OF NURSING SOCIETY
Pioneers of nursing in Canada. Montreal, Canadian Nurses Association, 1929?

MARSHALL, M. L.
Nurse heroines of the Confederacy. *Bulletin of the Medical Library Association*, July 1957, p. 319-36.

NATIONAL LEAGUE OF NURSING EDUCATION
Early leaders of American nursing. New York, The League, [1923?].
[Helen Borden (Sister Helen)   Anna Caroline Maxwell
Linda Richards   Isabel Adams Hampton
Alice Fisher   Lavinia Lloyd Dock
Lucy Lincoln Drown   Isabel McIsaac
Louise Darche   Sophia F. Palmer
Diana Clifton Kimber   Jane Arminda Delano]

PACIFIC COAST JOURNAL OF NURSING
History sketches of national officers [of nursing organizations]. *Pacific Coast Journal of Nursing*, June 1915.
[Contents:
Annie W. Goodrich   Mary M. Riddle
Genevieve Cooke   Sarah E. Parsons
Clara D. Noyes   Ella Phillips Crandall
Edna L. Foley   Helen Park Creswell
Sophia Palmer   Lydia A. Giberson
M. Adelaide Nutting   Sara E. Sly
Kathrine de Witt   Mathilde Krieger]
C. V. Twiss

PADWICK, CONSTANCE E.
Heroines of healing: a book for readers amongst working girls. London United Council for Nurses' Education, 1915.

PENNOCK, META RUTTER, *editor*
Makers of nursing history: portraits and pen sketches of fifty-nine prominent women. New York, Lakeside Pub. Co., 1928

STEPHENSON, GLADYS E.
Some pioneers in the medical and nursing world. Shanghai, Kwang Hsueh Publishing House, for the Nurses' Association of China, 1924.

WAKEFORD, CONSTANCE
The wounded soldiers' friends—the story of Florence Nightingale, Clara Barton and others. Swarthmore Press, [191?].

Who's Who in the nursing world: the nursing profession year book . . . containing particulars of administrative and examining bodies, colleges, the nursing services, nursing associations, institutions and societies, nurse training schools, clubs, etc., together with details concerning the nursing careers of the leaders of the nursing profession: compiled and edited by H. E. Smithers. Smithers Pub. Co., 1928.

YOST, EDNA
American women of nursing. Philadelphia, Lippincott, 1947.
2nd edn., 1957.
[Contents:
M. A. Nutting   Estelle M. Osborne
Lillian Wald   Florence Blake
Annie M. Goodrich   Anne Prochazka
Mabel M. Stewart   Theodora Floyd
Olivia M. Gowan   Lucile Leone]

INDIVIDUAL BIOGRAPHY

ADAMS, GEORGINA KINNEAR
Matron, Ruchill Fever Hospital, Glasgow. *Nursing Record*, May 11, 1901, p. 372.

AITKENHEAD, M.
Mary Aitkenhead, 1787-1858: founder of the Irish Sisters of Charity, by T. H. Bishop. *Nursing Mirror*, Oct. 24, 1958, p. vii.

ALKIN, ELIZABETH
Elizabeth Alkin, alias Parliament Joan, by J. J. Keevil. Reprinted from *Bull. Hist. Med.*, Vol. XXXI, No. 1, 1957.

ALKIN, ELIZABETH
A Florence Nightingale of the Commonwealth, by Isabel Macdonald. Privately printed. Keighley, Rydal Press, [193?].

ALSOP, H. A.
Matron, Kensington Infirmary. *British Journal of Nursing*, Jan. 3, 1914, p. 7.

ANDERSON, MARGARET
Lady Superintendent, East End Mother's Home. *British Journal of Nursing*, Dec. 21, 1907, p. 502.

APPLEYARD, MARY L.
Matron, Salop Infirmary, Shrewsbury. *British Journal of Nursing*, Feb. 16, 1907, p. 130.

AUSTEN, KATE
Northern nurse, by Elliott Merrick. New York, Scribners, 1947.
[The story of Kate Austen, an Australian nurse working in Labrador.]

BANFIELD, MAUD
Superintendent of the Polyclinic Hospital, Philadelphia. *British Journal of Nursing*, July 5, 1902, p. 13.

BARTON, CLARA
Clara Barton, founder of the American Red Cross, by William Barton. 2 vols. Boston, Houghton, Mifflin, 1922.

BARTON, CLARA
Clara Barton, founder of the American Red Cross, by Helen Dore Boylston. New York, Random House, 1955.

BARTON, CLARA
Founder of the Red Cross movement in America. *British Journal of Nursing*, May 4, 1912, p. 353.

BARTON, CLARA
The life of Clara Barton, by Percy H. Epler. New York, Macmillan, 1915.

BARTON, CLARA
Angel of the battlefield: the life of Clara Barton, by Isabel Ross. New York, Harper, 1956.

BARTON, CLARA
See
WAKEFORD, CONSTANCE
The wounded soldier's friends. . . .

BARTON, CLARA
Clara Barton—daughter of destiny, by Blanche Colton Williams. Philadelphia, Lippincott, 1941.

BARTON, CLARA
Clara Barton, a centenary tribute, by Charles Sumner Young. Boston, Richard C. Badger, 1922.

BARTON, ELEANOR C.
Miss Eleanor C. Barton, Matron of the Chelsea Infirmary. *British Journal of Nursing*, Jan. 28, 1905, p. 69.

BEACHCROFT, CASSANDRA M.
Lady Superintendent of the County Hospital, Lincoln. *Nursing Record*, April 6, 1895, p. 213.

BEATRICE, SISTER
Voice of the past. *Canadian Nurse*, Dec. 1959, p. 1133-8. [Reminiscences of Sister Beatrice of St. John's Hospital, Toronto.]

BICKERDYKE, MARY ANN
Cyclone in calico, the story of Mary Ann Bickerdyke, by Nina Brown Baker. Boston, Little, Brown, 1952.

BICKERDYKE, MARY ANN
Mary A. Bickerdyke, "Mother", by Julia A. Chase. Lawrence, Kansas, Journal Publishing House, 1896.

BICKERDYKE, MARY ANN
Mother Bickerdyke and the soldiers, by Margaret Burton Davis. San Francisco, A. T. Dewey, 1886.

BICKERDYKE, MARY ANN
Mother Bickerdyke as I knew her, by Florence S. Kellogg. Chicago, Unity Publishing Co., 1907.

BICKERTON, —
Matron, Prince of Wales General Hospital, Tottenham. *British Journal of Nursing*, Feb. 7, 1920, p. 81.

BLANCHFIELD, FLORENCE A.
Colonel Florence A. Blanchfield, by Edith A. Aynes. *Nursing Outlook*, Feb. 1959, p. 78-81.

BODLEY, AMY M. E.
Matron, Selly Oak Infirmary. *British Journal of Nursing*, May 30, 1914, p. 487.

BRADLEY, EDITH M.
Matron of the Salford Union Infirmary. *British Journal of Nursing*, Dec. 4, 1909, p. 458.

BREWERTON, HANNAH
Miss Hannah Brewerton, Matron of the English Hospital, Zanzibar. *British Journal of Nursing*, Oct. 13, 1906, p. 288.

BRIDSON, —
Matron, Noble's Hospital, Isle of Man. *British Journal of Nursing*, Sept. 21, 1912, p. 286.

BRINTON, MARY WILLIAMS
My cap and my cape: an autobiography. Philadelphia, Dorrance, 1950.

BUCKINGHAM, MAUDE A.
Matron, Queen's Hospital, Birmingham. *British Journal of Nursing*, April 11, 1914, p. 315.

BURGESS, ELIZABETH CHAMBERLAIN
Elizabeth Chamberlain Burgess, by Isabel M. Stewart. *American Journal of Nursing*, August 1958, p. 1101-5.

BURLEIGH, AMY L.
Matron of the Melbourne Hospital. *Nursing Record*, May 18, 1901, p. 392, and *British Journal of Nursing*, Dec. 13, 1902, p. 477.

BURLEIGH, KATHLEEN LUCRETIA
Miss Kathleen Lucretia Burleigh, Matron, Fountain Fever Hospital, Tooting Graveney. *Nursing Record*, Sept. 9, 1899, p. 210.

BUSHBY, ALICE MARY
Matron, Isolation Hospital, Southampton. *Nursing Record*, Mar. 1, 1902, p. 173.

CADBURY, MARY
The story of a Nightingale nurse, and kindred papers, by M. Christabel Cadbury. Headley, [1939].

CARAMAN, ELIZABETH
Daughter of the Euphrates. New York, Harper, 1939. [Written by an American nurse describing the period 1915-19.]

CAMERON, HELEN
Matron, Royal Hospital for Diseases of the Chest. *British Journal of Nursing*, April 9, 1904, p. 292.

CARSON-RAE, A.
Miss A. Carson-Rae, Secretary of the Irish Nurses' Association. *British Journal of Nursing*, April 30, 1910, p. 349.

CATHERINE OF SIENNA
Saint Catherine of Sienna, by Johannes Jorgensen. New York, Longmans, 1938.

CAVELL, EDITH
Nurse Cavell, the story of her life and martyrdom, Anonymous. Pearson, 1915.

CAVELL, EDITH
See
COLE, MARGARET
Women of today. . . . 1938.

CAVELL, EDITH
The case of Nurse Cavell, from the unpublished documents of the trial . . . interpreted by Ambroise Got. Hodder & Stoughton, [192?].

CAVELL, EDITH
Friend within the gates: the story of Edith Cavell, by Elizabeth Grey. Constable, [1960].

CAVELL, EDITH
Edith Cavell, by A. A. Hoehling. Cassell, 1958. [American edn. called "A whisper of eternity". New York, Yoseloff, 1957.]

CAVELL, EDITH
The martyrdom of Nurse Cavell: the life story of the victim of Germany's most barbarous crime, by William Thomson Hill. Hutchinson, 1915.

CAVELL, EDITH
Nurse Cavell, dog lover, ed. by Rowland Johns. Methuen, 1934.

CAVELL, EDITH
Edith Cavell, by Helen Judson. New York, Macmillan, 1941.

CAVELL, EDITH
Edith Cavell—her life story. A Norfolk tribute, by Herbert Leeds. Jarrolds, 1915.

CLARIDGE, SARAH ALICE
Matron-in-Chief, St. John's Voluntary Aid Detachment. *British Journal of Nursing*, Oct. 3, 1914, p. 260-1.

COLVIN, SARAH TARLETON
A rebel in thought. New York, Island Press, 1944.

COOKE, GENEVIEVE
Miss Genevieve Cooke, editor of the "Nurses' Journal of the Pacific Coast". *British Journal of Nursing*, Jan. 27, 1906, p. 72.

CRAIN, CLARE
We shall rise. New York, Pageant Press, [1955].

CURETON, MARY NEWCOMBE
Matron, Addenbrooke's Hospital, Cambridge. *Nursing Record*, Jan. 7, 1899, p. 10.

CUTLER, BEATRICE
Miss Beatrice Cutler, Assistant Matron, St. Bartholomew's Hospital. *British Journal of Nursing*, May 16, 1908, p. 388.

DARCHE, LOUISE
Superintendent of the New York Training School for Nurses. *Nursing Record*, June 10, 1899, p. 456-8.

DAVIES, J. W.
Matron, Royal Infirmary, Bradford. *British Journal of Nursing*, Oct. 19, 1912, p. 316.

DAVIS, ELIZABETH
Autobiography of Elizabeth Davis, a Balaclava nurse, edited by Jane Williams. 2 vols. Hurst & Blackett, 1857.

DELANO, JANE ARMINDA
Memories of Jane A. Delano, by Mary A. Clarke. New York, Lakeside Pub. Co., 1934.

DE PELCHIN, KEZIA PAYNE
Candle by night: the story of the life and times of Kezia Payne de Pelchin, by Harold J. Matthews. Boston, Bruce Humphries, 1942.
[The story of a pioneer nurse, social worker and teacher in Texas, who nursed during the 1878 epidemic of typhus in Memphis and was head nurse of an early hospital in Houston.]

DIX, DOROTHEA LYNDE
Dorothea Dix, pioneer of mental hospital reform, by Donald Blair. *Nursing Mirror*, Feb. 18, 1955, p. iii-iv.

DIX, DOROTHEA LYNDE
Life of Dorothea Lynde Dix, by Francis Tiffany. Boston, Houghton Mifflin, 1891.

DOCK, LAVINIA LLOYD
Lavinia Lloyd Dock. *Nursing Outlook*, May 1956, p. 298-9.

DOCK, LAVINIA LLOYD
Miss L. L. Dock. *British Journal of Nursing*, April 1, 1922, p. 197.

DOCK, LAVINIA LLOYD
Lavinia Lloyd Dock, nurse, feminist, internationalist, by M. M. Roberts. *American Journal of Nursing*, Feb. 1956, p. 176-9.

DORA, SISTER
See
PATTISON, DOROTHY WYNDLOW

DOUGHERTY, ELLEN
Matron of the Palmerston North Hospital, Wellington, New Zealand. *Nursing Record*, Jan. 25, 1902, p. 68.

D'YONVILLE, MARGUERITE
Mother of universal charity, by M. Aubuchon. *Hospital Progress*, June 1959, p. 86-7.
[Founder of Grey Nuns.]

ELIZABETH OF HUNGARY
Life of Saint Elizabeth of Hungary, Duchess of Thuringia, by the Count of Montalembert, translated by Francis Derring Hoyt. New York, Longmans, Green, 1904.

ST. FABIOLA
St. Fabiola (a fourth-century Roman lady), by W. A. Oddie. *Nursing Mirror*, Jan. 9, 1959, p. 1094.

FARQUARSON, MARTHA DURWARD
Miss Martha D. Farquarson, Matron of the Alfred Hospital, Melbourne, Australia. *Nursing Record*, Oct. 5, 1895, p. 223.

FENWICK, ETHEL GORDON
Ethel Fenwick, by R. M. Hallowes. *Nursing Mirror*, May 13, 1955, p. ii-iii.

FISHER, ALICE
Alice Fisher: chief nurse of the training school for nurses, Philadelphia Hospital; compiled from various sources. Philadelphia, Somer, n.d.

FISHER, ALICE
Alice Fisher, matron and reformer, by Sir Zachary Cope. *Nursing Mirror*, June 27, 1958, p. i and 968.

FORREST, CHRISTINA
Matron, Victoria Nurses' Institute, Bournemouth. *British Journal of Nursing*, May 9, 1908, p. 370.

FOX, A. M.
Matron, City of London Lying-in Hospital. *British Journal of Nursing*, Oct. 5, 1907, p. 282.

FOX, E. MARGARET
Miss E. Margaret Fox, Matron of the Tottenham Hospital. *Nursing Record*, Sept. 21, 1901, p. 227.

FRANGHIADI, MARY
Sister, Military Hospital, Athens. *Nursing Record*, Oct. 8, 1898, p. 288.

FRY, ELIZABETH
Elizabeth Fry, by Irene M. Ashby. Hicks, 1892.

FRY, ELIZABETH
Elizabeth Fry, Quaker heroine, by Janet Whitney. Harrap, 1937.

FULLAGAR, CONSTANCE
Matron, Mercers' Hospital, Dublin. *British Journal of Nursing*, Jan. 17, 1905, p. 53.

GARDNER, MARY
Miss Mary Gardner, Matron of the Birmingham and Midland Sanatorium, Blackwell. *Nursing Record*, Dec. 15, 1900, p. 474.

GARDNER, MARY SEWALL
Mary Sewall Gardner, by Katherine Kent. New York, Macmillan, 1946.

GAVED-WILLS, L.
Lady Superintendent, Hospital Dispensary, Newark-on-Trent. *British Journal of Nursing*, April 4, 1903, p. 265.

GILPIN, FANNY
Scenes from hospital life: being the letters of a probationer nurse. London, 1923.

GITTINS, E. A.
Matron of the Union Infirmary, Beckett Street, Leeds. *British Journal of Nursing*, Feb. 13, 1909, p. 131.

GOODRICH, ANNIE WARBURTON
Annie W. Goodrich: her journey to Yale, by Esther A. Werminghaus. New York, Macmillan, 1950.

GOODRICH, ANNIE WARBURTON
Militant angel, by Harriett Berger Koch. New York, Macmillan, 1951.

GOODRICH, ANNIE WARBURTON
Annie Warburton Goodrich, by Virginia Henderson. *American Journal of Nursing*, Dec. 1955, p. 1488-92.

GOODRICH, ANNIE WARBURTON
President, International Council of Nurses. *British Journal of Nursing*, Nov. 2, 1912, p. 354.

GOOSTRAY, STELLA
Stella Goostray, distinguished administrator, professional leader and good neighbor, by Mary M. Roberts. *American Journal of Nursing*, Mar. 1958, p. 352-5.

GREENLAW, BERTA L.
Matron, Allt-yr-yn Hospital, Newport, Mon. *Nursing Record*, Oct. 20, 1900, p. 315.

GREGORY, A. S.
Alice Sophia Gregory, by Ruth M. Hallowes. *Nursing Mirror*, April 1, 1955, p. v-vi.

HARDY, GLADYS M.
Yes, matron. Beck [195?].

HARRISON, LUCY
Bart's. nurse, R.R.C. *Nursing Record*, Oct. 6, 1900, p. 281.

HEATHER-BIGG, MILDRED
Matron, Charing Cross Hospital. *British Journal of Nursing*, Oct. 17, 1903, p. 307.

HEATHER-BIGG, MILDRED
Matron of Charing Cross Hospital. *British Journal of Nursing*, July 23, 1910, p. 65.

HELY, ANNE EYRE
A Crimean heroine. *Nursing Record*, Jan. 8, 1898, p. 31.

HEZLETT, E.
President, Irish Nurses' Association. *British Journal of Nursing*, May 1, 1920, p. 253.

HOLM, ELIZABETH MOORMAN
My fifty years of professional nursing. Privately printed by the author, 1953.

HOPE, MARY E.
Northward my calling. Toronto, Ryerson Press, 1954.

HUGHES, AMY
General Superintendent of Queen Victoria's Jubilee Institute for Nurses. *British Journal of Nursing*, Aug. 4, 1906, p. 86.

HUGHES, FRANCES
Miss Frances Hughes, Matron, St. Mary Abbott's Infirmary, Kensington. *Nursing Record*, May 4, 1895, p. 295.

HUNT, AGNES
This is my life. Blackie, 1938.
[Privately printed in 1935 by Wilding of Shrewsbury with the title "Reminiscences".]

HUNT, AGNES
Dame Agnes Hunt, by R. M. Hallowes. *Nursing Mirror*, July 29, 1955, p. vi-vii and xiv.

HURLBLATT, EVELYN
Matron, Kendal Memorial Hospital. *Nursing Record*, June 1, 1901, p. 430.

HUXLEY, MARGARET
Lady Superintendent of Sir Patrick Dun's Hospital, Dublin. *Nursing Record*, Jan. 7, 1899, p. 11.

JONES, AGNES ELIZABETH
Memorials of Agnes Elizabeth Jones by her sister, with an introduction by Florence Nightingale. Strahan, 1869?
2nd edn., 1870?
3rd edn., 1871.
4th edn., 1871?
5th edn., 1872.
6th edn., 1872.

JONES, AGNES
Agnes Jones, by R. M. Hallowes. *Nursing Mirror*, Jan. 7, 1955, p. vi-vii.

JOY, EILEEN M.
Matron of the Coombe Lying-in Hospital, President of the Irish Matrons' Association. *British Journal of Nursing*, Jan. 25, 1913, p. 69.

KARLL, AGNES
President, German Nurses' Association. *British Journal of Nursing*, Aug. 27, 1904, p. 167.

KELLY, BRIDGET M.
Matron, Dr. Steevens' Hospital, Dublin. *British Journal of Nursing*, Mar. 31, 1906, p. 252.

KENNY, ELIZABETH
And they shall walk: the life story of Sister Elizabeth Kenny; written in collaboration with Martha Ostenso. Hale, 1951.

KEOGH, IERNE C.
President of the Irish Nurses' Association. *British Journal of Nursing*, April 22, 1911, p. 309.

KINDBOM, HANNA
Superintendent of Nursing, John Sealy Hospital, Galveston, Texas. First Nursing Professor, University of Texas. *Nursing Record*, April 2, 1898, p. 272-3.

KINNEY, DITA H.
Superintendent of the American Army Nurse Corps. *British Journal of Nursing*, July 19, 1902, p. 53.

KNIGHT, GERTRUDE
Matron, General Hospital, Nottingham. *Nursing Record*, Mar. 12, 1898, p. 211.

KOUGH, A. M.
Matron, Bethlem Royal Hospital. *British Journal of Nursing*, Mar. 12, 1904, p. 207.

LABOURE, CATHERINE
Life of Blessed Catherine Laboure, by Ernesto Cassinari. St. Louis, Herder, 1934.

LAMBIE, MARY I.
My story: memoirs of a New Zealand nurse. Christchurch, New Zealand, Peryer, 1956.

LAMONT, MARY
General Superintendent, Queen Victoria's Jubilee Institute, Ireland, and President of the Irish Nurses' Association. *British Journal of Nursing*, April 17, 1909, p. 307.

LANDLES, H. G.
Matron, Ruchill Fever Hospital, Glasgow. *British Journal of Nursing*, Oct. 6, 1906, p. 266.

LATHROP, ROSE HAWTHORNE (MOTHER ALPHONSA)
Mother Alphonsa, by James J. Walsh. New York, Macmillan, 1930.

LAURENCE, E. C.
Matron, Hospital for Women, Chelsea. *Nursing Times*, Mar. 17, 1906, p. 222.

LAWRENCE, ISABEL
Matron, National Hospital for Nervous Diseases, Queen's Square, London. *Nursing Times*, Jan. 20, 1906, p. 56.

LAWSON, MABEL G.
President of the National Council of Nurses. *Nursing Times*, May 8, 1959, p. 559-60.

LAWSON, MARGARET
President of the National Association of Midwives. *British Journal of Nursing*, Oct. 14, 1911, p. 318.

LEES, FLORENCE
Mrs. Dacre Craven (Florence Lees), by R. M. Hallowes. *Nursing Mirror*, Dec. 23, 1955, p. iii-iv.

LOCH, CATHERINE GRACE
Memoir of Miss C. G. Loch, R.R.C. [late Senior Superintendent of the Indian Army Nursing Service], by A. F. Bradshaw. Henry Frowde, 1905.

LOCKITT, MARY A.
Matron, Isolation Hospital, Wimbledon. *Nursing Record*, May 10, 1902, p. 376.

LOUISE DE MARILLAC, SAINT
Life of the venerable Louise de Marillac (Mademoiselle le Gras), foundress of the company of Sisters of Charity of St. Vincent de Paul, by Alice Lady Lovat. Simpkin, Marshall, Hamilton, 1916.

LOUISE DE MARILLAC, SAINT
The life of blessed Louise de Marillac, co-foundress of the Sisters of Charity of Saint Vincent de Paul, by Prince Emmanuel de Broglie: translated from the French by Rev. Joseph Leonard. Burns Oates, 1933.

LOUISE DE MARILLAC, SAINT
Saint Louise de Marillac, by Agnes Richomme, translated by the Daughters of Charity. Paris, editions Fleures, 1959.

LOUISE DE MARILLAC, SAINT
Untrodden paths: the social apostolate of St. Louise de Marillac, by J. P. Sheedy. Sisters of Charity of St. Vincent de Paul, 1958.

LOUISE DE MARILLAC, SAINT
Louise de Marillac, the first Sister of Charity, by M. V. Woodgate. Dublin, Browne & Nolan, 1942.

LUCKES, EVA C. E.
Eva Luckes, by R. M. Hallowes. *Nursing Mirror*, Oct. 26, 1956, p. iii-iv.

LUCKES, EVA C. E.
Eva C. E. Luckes, Matron, the London Hospital, 1880-1919, compiled by Margaret McEwan with assistance from D. M. Landon. Pub. for private circulation by the London Hospital League for Nurses, 1958.

LUCKES, EVA C. E.
Eva C. E. Luckes, by Sydney Holland, Viscount Knutsford. Privately published, 191?.

LYONS, GRETTA
President of the Royal Victorian Trained Nurses' Association. *British Journal of Nursing*, Jan. 11, 1919, p. 19.

McCRAE, ANNABELLA
Boston, Massachusetts General Hospital, Nurses' Alumnae Assoc., *Quarterly Record*, June 1948: Annabella McCrae Memorial Issue.

McGAHEY, S. M.
Matron, Prince Alfred Hospital, Sydney. *Nursing Record*, July 22, 1899, p. 73.

MACINTYRE, K. V.
Matron, Royal Albert Edward Infirmary, Wigan. *British Journal of Nursing*, Oct. 19, 1912, p. 309.

McISSAC, ISABEL
President, American Society for Superintendents of Training Schools for Nurses. *Nursing Record*, June 25, 1898, p. 511.

MACKENZIE, ELIZA
Eliza Mackenzie, the Naval "Miss Nightingale" in the Crimea, by Marjorie Penney. *Nursing Mirror*, Dec. 16, 1960, p. ii-iii and xvi.

MACKENZIE, MARY ARD
Chief Superintendent of the Victorian Order of Trained Nurses for Canada; President of the Canadian National Association of Trained Nurses. *British Journal of Nursing*, Aug. 3, 1912, p. 89.

MACLEAN, HESTER
Miss Hester MacLean, President of the New Zealand Trained Nurses' Association. *British Journal of Nursing*, Sept. 28, 1912, p. 253-4.

MACMANUS, Emily E. P.
Matron of Guys. Andrew Melrose, 1956.

MACQUEEN, KATHARINE STUART
Records of a Scotswoman: Katharine Stuart MacQueen, by Olive Maclehose. Glasgow, Maclehose, Jackson, 1921.

MANCE, JEANNE
The saintly life of Jeanne Mance: first lay nurse of North America, by William Henry Atherton. St. Louis, Catholic Hospital Association, 1945.

MANCE, JEANNE
Jeanne Mance, foundress of the Hôtel-Dieu Hospital, Montreal, pioneer nurse of North America, 1642-1673, by Joseph Kearney Foran. Montreal, Hersea Press, 1931.

MANCE, JEANNE
Jeanne Mance, by H. E. MacDermot. Montreal, *Canadian Medical Association Journal*, 1947.
[Reprinted from the *C.M.A. Jnl.*, vol. 57, 1947, p. 67-73.]

MARIANNE, MOTHER
Mother Marianne of Molokai, by L. V. Jacks. New York, Macmillan, 1935.
[Molokai was a leper settlement in the Hawaiian Islands.]

MARRINER, —
Lady Superintendent, Sunderland Nursing Institute. *British Journal of Nursing*, April 4, 1903, p. 265.

MATTHEWS, MARY LATHROP WRIGHT
A nurse named Mary: a biography by Alexander Matthews. New York, Pageant Press, 1957.
[A record of an American nurse who did much work in the missionary hospitals of China.]

MATTICK, —
Matron, Children's Hospital, Bristol. *British Journal of Nursing*, June 8, 1912, p. 457.

MEDILL, —
Matron, St. Mary's Hospital, Paddington. *British Journal of Nursing*, April 21, 1906, p. 316.

MEYERS, MARY E.
My hall of memory: reminiscences of a missionary nurse. Epworth Press, 1956.

MILL, CHARLOTTE RICHMOND
Matron, St. George's Hospital, Bombay. *British Journal of Nursing*, Oct. 11, 1902, p. 299.

MILNE, J. H.
Lady Superintendent of the General Hospital, Launceston, Tasmania. *Nursing Record*, April 12, 1902, p. 288.

MINKS, MARGARET
Lady Superintendent, Children's Hospital, Nottingham. *Nursing Record*, April 2, 1898, p. 270.

MOLLETT, M.
Matron, Royal South Hants Infirmary, Southampton. *Nursing Record*, June 25, 1898, p. 513.

MONTGOMERIE, H. L.
Through a ward window: letters from Miss Anne Pennant . . . to Mrs. Darell. . . . Chapman & Hall, 1938.

MORTEN, HONNOR
From a nurse's note-book. Scientific Press Ltd., 1899.

MORTEN, [VIOLET] HONNOR
Miss Honnor Morten. *Nursing Times*, July 26, 1913, p. 855.

MULVANY, MARGARET F.
Matron, Infirmary and Dispensary, Bolton. *Nursing Record*, April 12, 1902, p. 293.

MUSE, MAUDE B.
Maude B. Muse—nurse, educator, author and creative thinker, by B. V. Cunningham and I. M. Stewart. *American Journal of Nursing*, Nov. 1956, p. 1434-6.

MUSSON, ELLEN M.
Matron of the Swansea General and Eye Hospital. *British Journal of Nursing*, Nov. 17, 1906, p. 397. Matron, General Hospital, Birmingham. *British Journal of Nursing*, June 6, 1914, p. 501.

NELSON, SOPHIE CAROLINE
Sophie Nelson: public health statesman, by Stella Goostray. *American Journal of Nursing*, Sept. 1960, p. 1268-9.

NEWMAN, LYDIA
Lady Superintendent of Nursing, Royal Victoria Hospital, Belfast. *Nursing Record*, Sept. 14, 1901, p. 207.

NICHOLSON, ETHEL
Lady Superintendent of the Manchester Children's Hospital, Pendlebury. *British Journal of Nursing*, April 1, 1911, p. 245.

NIGHTINGALE, FLORENCE
Florence Nightingale, probationer, writes her "Curriculum Vitae". *Nursing Mirror*, May 10, 1957, p. xiii and xii.

NIGHTINGALE, FLORENCE
Florence Nightingale as seen in her portraits, by Maude E. Seymour Abbott. Boston, reprinted from the *Boston Medical and Surgical Journal*, Sept. 14, 21 and 28, 1916.

NIGHTINGALE, FLORENCE
Florence Nightingale—statistician, by L. R. C. Agnew. *American Journal of Nursing*, May 1958, p. 664-5.

NIGHTINGALE, FLORENCE
Florence Nightingale, an appreciation, by Mary Aldis, based on a recent biography by Sir Edward Cook . . . paper read at the Fortnightly Club of Chicago, April 2, 1914. New York, National Organisation for Public Health Nursing, [19—].

NIGHTINGALE, FLORENCE
Miss Nightingale at Scutari, by C. T. Andrews. *Nursing Times*, Dec. 30, 1960, p. 1624-6.

NIGHTINGALE, FLORENCE
A lost commander: Florence Nightingale, by Mary Raymond Shipman Andrews. New York, Doubleday, 1929.

NIGHTINGALE, FLORENCE
Florence Nightingale's influence on nursing, by Margaret G. Arnstein. *Bulletin of the New York Academy of Medicine*, July 1956, p. 540-6.

NIGHTINGALE, FLORENCE
Fiery angel: the story of Florence Nightingale, by Ramona Sawyer Barth. Florida, Glade House, 1945.

NIGHTINGALE, FLORENCE
Florence Nightingale's influence on military medicine, by Frank D. Berry. *Bulletin of the New York Academy of Medicine*, July 1956, p. 547-53.

NIGHTINGALE, FLORENCE
A short biography of Florence Nightingale, O.M., by Mary Frances Billington. Neves & Biscoe, 1910 [Reprinted from the *Daily Telegraph* of Aug. 15, 1910.]

NIGHTINGALE, FLORENCE
Florence Nightingale's letters, by W. J. Bishop. *American Journal of Nursing*, May 1957, p. 607-9.

NIGHTINGALE, FLORENCE
Florence Nightingale's message for today, by W. J. Bishop. *Nursing Outlook*, May 1960, p. 246-9.

NIGHTINGALE, FLORENCE
The life of Florence Nightingale, by Edward Cook. 2 vols. Macmillan, 1913.

NIGHTINGALE, FLORENCE
Miss Florence Nightingale and the doctors, by Zachary Cope. *Proceedings of the Royal Society of Medicine*, Nov. 1956, p. 907-14.

NIGHTINGALE, FLORENCE
Florence Nightingale and the doctors, by Zachary Cope. Museum Press, 1958.

NIGHTINGALE, FLORENCE
Florence Nightingale and her nurses, by Zachary Cope. *Nursing Times*, May 13, 1960, p. 597-8.

NIGHTINGALE, FLORENCE
Florence Nightingale: the woman and the legend, by Margaret Goldsmith. Hodder & Stoughton, 1937.

NIGHTINGALE, FLORENCE
Florence Nightingale, by Eleanor Frances Hall. Soc. for Promoting Christian Knowledge, 1920.

NIGHTINGALE, FLORENCE
Florence Nightingale, by Grace T. Hallock and C. E. Turner. New York, Metropolitan Life Insurance Co., 1928.

NIGHTINGALE, FLORENCE
William Ogle of Derby and Florence Nightingale, by Douglas Hubble. *Medical History*, July 1959, p. 201-11.

NIGHTINGALE, FLORENCE
Florence Nightingale, by Ruth Fox Hume. New York, Random House, 1960.

NIGHTINGALE, FLORENCE
Florence Nightingale—a force in medicine, by Henry Mills Hurd. *Johns Hopkins Nurses Alumnae Magazine*, June 1910, vol. 9, no. 2, pp. 68-81.
[An address at the graduating exercises of the nurses' training school of the Johns Hopkins Hospital, May 19, 1910.]

NIGHTINGALE, FLORENCE
Florence Nightingale as a statistician, by Edwin W. Kopf. Boston, American Statistical Assn., 1916.
[Quarterly publication of the American Statistical Assoc., new series, no. 116 (vol. XV), Dec. 1916.]

NIGHTINGALE, FLORENCE
Florence Nightingale, by D. Lammond. Duckworth, 1935.

NIGHTINGALE, FLORENCE
Florence Nightingale: a biography, by Annie Matheson. Nelson, [19—].

NIGHTINGALE, FLORENCE
A little journey to the home of Florence Nightingale, by C. V. Mosby. St. Louis, Mosby, 1938.

NIGHTINGALE, FLORENCE
The life of Florence Nightingale: an abridgement, with additional matter, by Rosalind Nash, of the life in two volumes by Sir Edward Cook. Macmillan, 1925.

NIGHTINGALE, FLORENCE
A sketch of the life of Florence Nightingale, by Rosalind Nash. S.P.C.K., 1937.

NIGHTINGALE, FLORENCE
The commemoration of Florence Nightingale, an oration delivered by Sir George Newman before the General Meeting of the International Council of Nurses, London, July 1937. Florence Nightingale International Foundation, [1937?].

NIGHTINGALE, FLORENCE
Florence Nightingale's philosophy of life and education, by Mildred E. Newton. Stanford, Univ. of California, 1949.

NIGHTINGALE, FLORENCE
Florence Nightingale, 1820-1856: a study of her life down to the end of the Crimean War, by I. B. O'Malley. Thornton, Butterworth, 1931.

NIGHTINGALE, FLORENCE
Florence Nightingale, the wounded soldier's friend, by Eliza F. Pollard. Partridge, [186?].

NIGHTINGALE, FLORENCE
Florence Nightingale, a drama, by Edith Gittings Reid. New York, Macmillan, 1922.

NIGHTINGALE, FLORENCE
Florence Nightingale's place in British history, by F. B. A. Rundall. *Bulletin of the New York Academy of Medicine*, July 1956, p. 536-9.

NIGHTINGALE, FLORENCE
The challenge which faced Florence Nightingale, by C. F. St. John. *Medical Bulletin of the U.S. Army, Europe*, Feb. 1957, p. 28-9.

NIGHTINGALE, FLORENCE
Florence Nightingale, by Lucy Ridgely Seymer. Faber, 1950.

NIGHTINGALE, FLORENCE
The Nightingale jewel, by Lucy R. Seymer. *American Journal of Nursing*, May 1955, p. 549-50.

NIGHTINGALE, FLORENCE
Selected writings of Florence Nightingale: compiled by Lucy Ridgely Seymer. New York, Macmillan, 1954.

NIGHTINGALE, FLORENCE
The writings of Florence Nightingale, an oration delivered before the Ninth Congress of the International Council of Nurses, Atlantic City, 1947, by Lucy Ridgely Seymer. Florence Nightingale International Foundation, [194?].

NIGHTINGALE, FLORENCE
The British army and Miss Nightingale, by Charles Shrimpton. Balignani, 1864.

NIGHTINGALE, FLORENCE
Portraits of Miss Nightingale at St. Thomas's, by Barbara Stephen, contained in the *Nightingale Fellowship Journal*, May 1936, p. 8-11.

NIGHTINGALE, FLORENCE
Florence Nightingale, educator, by Isobel Maitland Stewart. *Teachers' College Record*, Dec. 1939, p. 208-23.

NIGHTINGALE, FLORENCE
Florence Nightingale, by Margaret E. Tabor. Sheldon Press, 1925.

NIGHTINGALE, FLORENCE
The life of Florence Nightingale, by Sarah A. Tooley. Bousfield, 1905.
2nd edn., 1905.
3rd edn., 1906?
4th edn., 1906.

NIGHTINGALE, FLORENCE
The heroine of the East, by A. J. Wallace. Bell & Daldy, 1856.

BIOGRAPHY

NIGHTINGALE, FLORENCE
Florence Nightingale: a biography, by I. C. Willis. Allen & Unwin, 1931.

NIGHTINGALE, FLORENCE
The story of Florence Nightingale, by W. Wintle. Sunday School Union, n.d.

NIGHTINGALE, FLORENCE
Florence Nightingale, 1820-1910, by Cecil Woodham-Smith. Constable, 1950.

NIGHTINGALE, FLORENCE
Lady-in-chief: the story of Florence Nightingale, abridged from her biography, Florence Nightingale, by Cecil Woodham-Smith. Methuen, 1953.

NIGHTINGALE, FLORENCE
Florence Nightingale and the status of women.
In
ALLCHIN, A. M.
The silent rebellion. . . . 1958.

NIGHTINGALE, FLORENCE
Cheering angel: life and work of Florence Nightingale. *MD Medical News Magazine*, vol. 4, no. 3, Aug. 1960, p. 98-103.

NIGHTINGALE, FLORENCE
Letters to nurses from Florence Nightingale, June 1897 and February 1898. (Reprinted for the nurses of the Liverpool Queen Victoria District Nursing Association by E. A. Rathbone.) Liverpool, Lee & Nightingale (Printers), 1913.

NIGHTINGALE, FLORENCE
Florence Nightingale, the soldier's friend.
See also
CLAYTON, ELLEN C.
Notable women.

NIGHTINGALE, FLORENCE
See also
JOWETT, BENJAMIN
Jowett: a portrait with background, by Geoffrey Faber. Faber 1957.

NIGHTINGALE, FLORENCE
See also
WAKEFORD, CONSTANCE
The wounded soldier's friends. . . .

NIGHTINGALE, FLORENCE
See also
WORCESTER, ALFRED
Nurses and nursing, 1927. Chap. IV.

NUTTING, MARY ADELAIDE
Mary Adelaide Nutting, educator and builder, by Willistine Goodsell. *Teachers' College Record*, vol. 27, 1926, p. 382-93.

NUTTING, MARY ADELAIDE
Mary Adelaide Nutting, by S. Goostray. *American Journal of Nursing*, Nov. 1958, p. 1524-9.

O'CONNOR, M. E.
Matron, Napier Hospital, New Zealand. *British Journal of Nursing*, Feb. 27, 1904, p. 165.

OGLE, WILLIAM
William Ogle of Derby and Florence Nightingale, by Douglas Hubble. *Medical History*, July 1959, p. 201-11.

ORR, J. M.
Matron, Auckland Hospital, New Zealand. *British Journal of Nursing*, Sept. 28, 1912, p. 253.

PAGET, ROSALIND
A notable centenary: Dame Rosalind Paget. *Midwives' Chronicle and Nursing Notes*, Jan. 1955, p. 8.

PALMER, SOPHIA F.
Editor-in-Chief of the American Journal of Nursing. *Nursing Record*, June 29, 1901, p. 509-10.

PARK, A.
Matron, General Lying-in Hospital, London. *British Journal of Nursing*, Nov. 23, 1907, p. 423.

PARKER, SYLVIA
Matron of the Cumberland Infirmary, Carlisle. *British Journal of Nursing*, Aug. 5, 1911, p. 112.

PARSON, JESSY S.
Lady Superintendent, Military Hospital, Athens. *Nursing Record*, Oct. 8, 1898, p. 286.

PATTISON, DOROTHY WYNDLOW
Sister Dora Pattison, by R. M. Hallowes. *Nursing Mirror*, Jan. 14, 1956, p. iv-v and 1001.

PATTISON, DOROTHY WYNDLOW
Sister Dora, a biography, by Margaret Lonsdale. Kegan Paul, 1880.

PEARSE, HELEN L.
Matron of the Great Northern Hospital, London. *British Journal of Nursing*, Nov. 4, 1905, p. 373-4.

PEGG, FLORA G.
Matron, Royal Infirmary, Dundee. *British Journal of Nursing*, Dec. 10, 1910, p. 476.

PETER, PAULINE W.
General Superintendent of Queen Victoria's Jubilee Institute for Nurses. *British Journal of Nursing*, Dec. 2, 1905, p. 454.

PHINNEY, MARY, BARONESS VON GENHAUSEN
See
WORCESTER, ALFRED
Nurses and nursing, 1927, Chap. VI.

PINCHARD, SIBYL TREGENNA BIDDULPH
Matron, Children's Hospital, Paddington Green. *Nursing Record*, Oct. 5, 1901, p. 283.

PLUM, WINIFRED
Matron, Victoria Hospital, Folkestone. *British Journal of Nursing*, Dec. 13, 1902, p. 485.

POLDEN, S. EMILY
Matron of the Royal United Hospital, Bath. *Nursing Record*, April 7, 1900, p. 274.

POTTER, MARY
Mary Potter: foundress of the Little Company of Mary, by Rugh Hallowes. *Nursing Mirror*, May 31, 1957, p. vi-vii.

PRESSLAND, DORA
Matron of the Durham County Hospital. *Nursing Record*, Jan. 8, 1898, p. 34.

PRINGLE, ANGELIQUE LUCILLE
See
WORCESTER, ALFRED
Nurses and nursing, 1927, Chap. V.

RAY, MARY E.
Sister-Matron, King's College Hospital. *British Journal of Nursing*, April 7, 1906, p. 273.

REIJNVAAN, JOHANNA PAULINA
Lady Superintendent of the Wilhelmina Hospital, Amsterdam. *Nursing Record*, Jan. 4, 1896, p. 5.

RICHARDS, LINDA
America's first trained nurse, Linda Richards, by Rachel Baker. New York, Julian Messner, 1959.

RICHARDS, LINDA A.
Reminiscences of Linda Richards, America's first trained nurse. Boston, Whitcomb & Brown, 1911.

RICHARDS, LINDA
America's first trained nurse: Linda Richards, 1841-1930, by Isabelle W. Sloan. New York, Columbia University Teachers' College, 1941.

RICHMOND, K. E.
Matron, Birmingham and Midland Hospital for Women. *British Journal of Nursing*, June 13, 191

RIDLEY, MIRIAM
Matron, Hospital for Epilepsy and Paralysis, Portland Terrace, Regent's Park. *Nursing Record*, July 11, 1896, p. 29.

17

ROBB, ISABEL HAMPTON
Mrs. Isabel Hampton Robb, first President of the National Association of American Nurses. *Nursing Record*, April 3, 1897, p. 271.

ROBERTS, MARY M.
Mary M. Roberts, 1877-1959. *Nursing Outlook*, Feb. 1959, p. 72-4.

ROBERTS, MARY M.
Mary M. Roberts—career highlights. *American Journal of Nursing*, March 1959, p. 344-5.

ROBERTS, MARY M.
Mary M. Roberts: spokesman for nursing, by Edith Patton Lewis. *American Journal of Nursing*, March 1959, p. 336-43.

ROBERTS, MARY M.
Executive editor of the American Journal of Nursing Company; friend—nurse—teacher. *Nursing Outlook*, June 1951, p. 342-3.

ROBINS, DAISY
Secretary and Registrar, Royal British Nurses' Association. Suppl. to *Nursing Record*, Mar. 3, 1893, between p. 56-7.

ROGERS, GERTRUDE A.
Miss G. A. Rogers, Chairman of the provisional committee of the National Council of Nurses, and Lady Superintendent of Leicester Infirmary. *British Journal of Nursing*, Jan. 21, 1905, p. 47-8.

ROSS, MARGARET
Memoirs of a private nurse. Glasgow, McNaughton & Sinclair, 1938.

RUMBALL, MARIAN
Sister Marian Rumball, Sister of the Children's Ward, Royal Homeopathic Hospital. *Nursing Record*, July 4, 1896, p. 4.

RUNDLE, M. S.
The first Isla Stewart scholar. *British Journal of Nursing*, Sept. 10, 1910, p. 205.

SATCHWELL, E.
Matron, Royal Hospital, Chelsea. *British Journal of Nursing*, Feb. 17, 1906, p. 131.

SCHRADERS, CATHARINA G.
Catharina Geertruida Schraders of Holland, 1655-1746, by D. S. Greig. *Nursing Mirror*, May 13, 1960, p. iii-iv.

SCOTT, KATHERINE
Matron, Sussex County Hospital. *British Journal of Nursing*, May 18, 1907, p. 372.

SEACOLE, MARY
Living names in Jamaica's history, by Clinton V. Black. Kingston, Jamaica Welfare, 1943.
[Contains a biographical sketch of Mary Seacole.]

SELLON, PRISCILLA LYDIA
Dr. Pusey and Miss Sellon.
In
ALLCHIN, A. M.
The silent rebellion. . . . 1958.

SELLON, PRISCILLA LYDIA
Priscilla Lydia Sellon: the restorer after three centuries of the religious life in the English church, by Thomas Jay Williams. S.P.C.K., 1950.

SERGEANT, MILLICENT
Matron of the Hospital, Devizes. *British Journal of Nursing*, April 14, 1906, p. 295.

SETON, ELIZABETH
An American woman, Elizabeth Seton, by Leonard Teeney. New York, America Press, 1938.

SIBLEY, ANNIE
Matron, Hope Union Infirmary, Salford, Manchester. Supplement to *Nursing Record*, June 1 1893, between p. 264-5.

SMITH, COURTNEY
Assistant Matron, St. Bartholomew's Hospital. *British Journal of Nursing*, July 4, 1903, p. 9.

SMITH, JANE ADELAIDE
Matron, Infirmary, Kingston-on-Thames. *Nursing Record*, June 28, 1902, p. 510.

SMITH, JESSIE
Sister, Military Hospital, Athens. *Nursing Record*, Oct. 8, 1898, p. 287.

SNIVELEY, AGNES
Lady Superintendent, General Hospital, Toronto. *Nursing Record*, Jan. 18, 1902, p. 53.

SOULE, ELIZABETH STERLING
Mrs. Soule of Washington, by H. A. Loughran.
I. Her early career in nursing. *Nursing Outlook*, Sept. 1956, p. 492-6.
II. The University of Washington School of Nursing. *Nursing Outlook*, Oct. 1956, p. 567-72.

SOYER, ALEXIS
Alexis Soyer—chef in the Crimea, by T. H. Bishop. *Nursing Mirror*, Aug. 29, 1958, p. 1633-4.

SPANN, F. PARKER
Matron, Township Infirmary, Beckett Street, Leeds. *British Journal of Nursing*, April 1, 1916, p. 302.

SPARSHOTT, M. E.
Matron, Royal Infirmary, Manchester. *British Journal of Nursing*, Aug. 17, 1907, p. 130.

STEVENSON, LOUISA
President of the Society for the State Registration of Trained Nurses. *British Journal of Nursing*, July 5, 1902, p. 8.

STEWART, ISLA
Matron, St. Bartholomew's Hospital. *British Journal of Nursing*, April 16, 1910, p. 306.

STEWART, ISLA
Isla Stewart: her life and her influence on the nursing profession, by Rachel Cox-Davies. National Council of Trained Nurses of Great Britain and Ireland, 1912.

STEWART, ISABEL M.
Isabel M. Stewart recalls the early years. *American Journal of Nursing*, Oct. 1960, p. 1426-30.

STILL, ALICIA LLOYD
Dame Alicia Lloyd Still, D.B.E., R.R.C., 1869-1944, a memoir, by Lucy Ridgely Seymer. The Nightingale Fellowship, St. Thomas's Hospital, 1953.
[For private circulation only.]

STOREY, MARGARET
Matron, Victoria Hospital, Keighley. *British Journal of Nursing*, June 23, 1906, p. 496.

STRONG, REBECCA
Rebecca Strong, pioneer of preliminary training schools, by R. M. Hallowes. *Nursing Mirror*, Nov. 25, 1955, p. xi-xii.

STRONG, REBECCA
Reminiscences. Edinburgh, Douglas & Foulis, 1935.

TERROT, SARAH A.
Crimean nurse. *Nursing Times*, Sept. 11, 1909, p. 741.

THOMAS, MARION
Matron, Birmingham Infirmary. *British Journal of Nursing*, July 18, 1914, p. 59.

THURSTON, MABEL
Lady Superintendent, Christchurch Hospital, New Zealand. *British Journal of Nursing*, Oct. 1, 1910, p. 266.

THURSTON, VIOLETTA
Matron, Civil Hospital, Spezia, Italy. *British Journal of Nursing*, Feb. 15, 1913, p. 130.

TINDALL, S. GRACE
Matron of the Cama and Allbless Hospitals, Bombay.
British Journal of Nursing, July 16, 1910, p. 47.

TIPPETTS, LILIAN M.
President of the Association of Nursing Superintendents
of India. *British Journal of Nursing*, June 24, 1911, p. 493.

TODD, ANNIE BURLAND
Matron, West Norfolk and Lynn Hospital, King's Lynn.
British Journal of Nursing, April 4, 1903, p. 265.

TRAIFOROS, ELENE
Matron, General Infirmary, Macclesfield. *Nursing Record*,
Sept. 7, 1901, p. 187.

TREACY, KILDARE
President, Irish Nurses' Association. *British Journal of
Nursing*, April 6, 1907, p. 249.

TURNER, E. M. CARPENTER
Matron, Royal Hants County Hospital, Winchester.
British Journal of Nursing, Nov. 24, 1906, p. 416.

TURTON, M. AMY
A nursing pioneer. *British Journal of Nursing*, Jan. 25,
1913, p. 69.

VINCENT DE PAUL, SAINT
Apostle of charity: the life of St. Vincent de Paul, by
Theodore Maynard. Allen & Unwin, 1940.

VINCENT DE PAUL, SAINT
Vincent de Paul, priest and philanthropist, 1576-1660, by
E. K. Sanders. Heath, Cranton & Ouseley, 1913.

VINCENT DE PAUL, SAINT
Saint Vincent de Paul, by Jean Calvet, translated by
Lancelot C. Sheppard. Burns Oates, 1952.

VINCENT DE PAUL, SAINT
Saint Vincent de Paul, by M. V. Woodgate. Dublin,
Browne & Nolan, 1958.

WADE, JANE
Lady Superintendent, Scottish Branch, Queen Victoria's
Jubilee Institute for Nurses. *Nursing Record*, Jan. 1, 1898,
p. 4.

WALD, LILLIAN D.
Lillian D. Wald, by G. W. Alger. *American Journal of
Nursing*, Mar. 1960, p. 354.

WALD, LILLIAN D.
Lillian Wald, neighbour and crusader, by R. L. Duffus.
New York, Macmillan, 1938.

WALD, LILLIAN D.
Lillian Wald, angel of Henry Street, by Beryl W. Epstein.
New York, Messner, 1948.

WALKER, LUCY
Matron, Pennsylvania Hospital, Philadelphia. *Nursing
Record*, July 1, 1899, p. 8.

WALLACE, ROSE E.
Matron of the Southwark Infirmary, East Dulwich. *British
Journal of Nursing*, Feb. 18, 1911, p. 132.

WARDROPER, SARAH
Mrs. Sarah Wardroper, Matron, St. Thomas's Hospital,
1854-87, first superintendent of the Nightingale Training
School, by various authors. *Nightingale Fellowship Journal*,
June 1957, p. 10-18.

WARDROPER, SARAH
Sarah Wardroper, Matron, St. Thomas's Hospital, London,
1854-1887, by R. Hallowes. *Nursing Mirror*, Mar. 8, 1957,
p. vii and vi.

WHITE, JEANETTE V.
Jeanette V. White, 1908-1957. *American Journal of Nursing*,
April 1957, p. 461.

WILLIAMSON, ANNA M.
Fifty years in starch. Culver City, Calif., Murray & Gee,
1948.

WINMILL, MARY
Matron, Children's Infirmary, Carshalton. *British Journal
of Nursing*, Dec. 17, 1910, p. 488.

WINSLOW, CHARLES-EDWARD AMORY
We pay tribute to Charles-Edward Amory Winslow, by
M. M. Roberts. *Nursing Outlook*, Mar. 1957, p. 155-6.
[Dr. Winslow was largely responsible for the founding of
Yale University School of Nursing.]

XAVIER BERKELEY
Sister Xavier Berkeley (1861-1944), Sister of Charity of
St. Vincent de Paul, fifty-four years a missionary in China,
by M.L.H. Burns Oates, 1949.

YOULDEN, E. F.
Matron, Brentford Union Infirmary, Isleworth. *British
Journal of Nursing*, Jan. 6, 1912, p. 11.

YOUNG, ESTHER HARRIET
Matron of Guy's Hospital. *Nursing Record*, April 7, 1900,
p. 272.

NURSING AS A PROFESSION

GENERAL WORKS

ARNOLD, VIRGINIA
Nursing around the world. *Public Health Reports*, May 1958, p. 412-7.

BACALA, JESUS C.
The professionalization of nursing. [Manila, P.I.], Novel Publishing Co., [c. 1959].

BAGGALLAY, O.
The nurse and the community. *Nursing Times*, July 26, 1957, p. 828-9.

BENNE, KENNETH D., *and* BENNIS, WARREN
Role confusion and conflict in nursing; the role of the professional nurse. *American Journal of Nursing*, Feb. 1959, p. 196-8.

BENNE, KENNETH D., *and* BENNIS, WARREN
What is real nursing? *American Journal of Nursing*, Mar. 1959, p. 380-3.

BENTLEY, R. S.
The male potential. *Canadian Nurse*, April 1959, p. 344 and 346.

BISHOP, W. J.
Dr. Thomas Fuller's ideal nurse. *Nursing Mirror*, June 18, 1954, p. 759.

BIXLER, G. K. *and* R. W.
The professional status of nursing. *American Journal of Nursing*, Aug. 1959, p. 1142-7.

BRIDGES, DAISY C.
Nursing—an international service. *American Journal of Nursing*, Oct. 1956, p. 1273.

BRIDGES, DAISY C.
Nursing—a world-wide social activity. *Nursing Times*, Dec. 23, 1955, p. 1448-9.

BROTHERSTON, J. H. F.
Nursing responsibilities to meet changing health needs. *Nursing Mirror*, July 6, 1956, p. 1009-10.

CARD, W. I.
What is the purpose of the nurse? *Nursing Mirror*, Dec. 9, 1955, p. 685-6.

CHAMBERLIN, R.
Are nurses meeting their responsibilities? *Hospitals*, Oct. 16, 1960, p. 75-78.

CREELMAN, LYLE
Nursing in the world. *Canadian Nurse*, Sept. 1958, p. 814-9.

CREELMAN, LYLE
Relationship between the W.H.O. and professional nursing. *Nursing Times*, Oct. 24, 1953, p. 1085-7.

CURRAN, J. A.
Challenge to nursing—1959. *Journal of the Maine Medical Association*, Nov. 1959, p. 389-93.

DALZELL-WARD, A. J.
The reason and need for professional organisations. *Nursing Mirror*, Nov. 8, 1957, p. 431-2.

DE PLEDGE, JOSEPHINE L.
Nursing as a profession. *Nursing Record*, July 6, 1893, p. 336-9.

DOCK, LAVINIA L.
Short papers on nursing subjects. New York, no pub., 1900.

DOCK, LAVINIA L.
Status of the nurse in the working world. *British Journal of Nursing*, Jan. 3, 1914, p. 4-6.

ELLIOTT, F. E.
Concepts of nursing. *Canadian Nurse*, Nov. 1960, p. 999-1003.

FENWICK, ETHEL GORDON
The better organisation of the nursing profession. *Nursing Record*, Nov. 6, 1897, p. 369-71, and Nov. 13, 1897, p. 689-91.

FENWICK, ETHEL GORDON
The development of the art of nursing. *Nursing Record*, Oct. 11, 1888, p. 379-83, and Oct. 18, 1888, p. 395-8.

FENWICK, ETHEL GORDON
The matron: being a paper read before the British Nurses' Association on February 15, 1889. *Nursing Record*, Feb. 21, 1889, p. 117-9, and Feb. 28, 1889, p. 135-8.

FENWICK, ETHEL GORDON
The necessity for union amongst nurses. *Nursing Record*, July 5, 1888, p. 159-61.

FENWICK, ETHEL GORDON
The organisation of the nursing profession; by its members: by the State. *British Journal of Nursing*, May 2, 1908, p. 350-1.

FENWICK, ETHEL GORDON
Trained nursing as a profession for women, from an educational, economic and social aspect. *British Journal of Nursing*, June 18, 1904, p. 491-4.

FRANK, CHARLES MARIE, SISTER
The professional nurse—yesterday, today, and tomorrow. *Nursing World*, Dec. 1959, p. 19, 20 and 34.

FROST, HARRIET
Nursing in sickness and health: the social aspects of nursing. New York, Macmillan, 1939.

GEISTER, J. M.
Organic unity or professional solidarity? *Nursing Outlook*, April 1958, p. 215-7.

HALL, W.
Nursing is now a great profession. *South African Nursing Journal*, Feb. 1960, p. 29.

HAMILTON, T. S.
The future nurse; her place and preparation. *Hospitals*, Mar. 1, 1959, p. 32-6.

HEIDGERKEN, LORETTA
Some problems in modern nursing. *Nursing Outlook*, July 1959, p. 394-7.

HICKMAN, W. H.
The other three R's: some aspects of professionalism. *Canadian Nurse*, June 1959, p. 516-20.

INGLES, T.
The nurse today. *Maryland State Medical Journal*, Jan. 1959, p. 38-41.

INTERNATIONAL COUNCIL OF NURSES
International congress of nurses. 1901-[in progress].

JAMES, J. T.
Men in nursing. *Hospital Progress*, June 1958, p. 78-9.

JATON, RENÉE
The Red Cross and the future of nursing. Geneva, League of Red Cross Societies, 1954.

JOHNSON, DOROTHY E.
The nature of a science of nursing. *Nursing Outlook*, May 1959, p. 291-4.

JOHNSON, DOROTHY E.
A philosophy of nursing. *Nursing Outlook*, April 1959, p. 198-200.

JOHNSON, MIRIAM M., *and* MARTIN, HARRY W.
A sociological analysis of the nurse role. *American Journal of Nursing*, Mar. 1958, p. 373-7.

JONES, H.
An essay on nursing. Reprinted from "Holiday Papers" by the same author. London, 1864.

KANE, J. J.
The spirit of nursing. *Hospital Progress*, Sept. 1957, p. 94-5.

KOONTZ, A. R.
On nursing disciplines. *Maryland State Medical Journal*, May 1960, p. 255-7.

LAWSON, M. G.
The modern outlook on nursing. *Nursing Mirror*, Oct. 7, 1955, p. 45-6; Oct. 14, 1955, p. 125-6; Oct. 21, 1955, p. x and xii.

LEONE, LUCILE PETRY
The art of nursing. *Journal of the American Medical Association*, April 16, 1955, p. 1381-3.

LEONE, LUCILE PETRY
What is nursing's major challenge? *Nursing World*, Jan. 1959, p. 18-20.

MACANDREW, C., *and* ELLIOTT, J. E.
Varying images of the professional nurse: a case study. *Nursing Research*, Winter 1959, p. 33-5.

McCONNELL, RAYMOND A.
What makes a good nurse. *Nursing World*, July 1956, p. 13-30.

McKINNEY, J. C., *and* INGLES, T.
The professionalization of nurses. *Nursing Outlook*, June 1959, p. 365-6.

MacLEOD, A. ISOBEL
A nurse views the problems. *Canadian Nurse*, Jan. 1958, p. 27-31.

McMANUS, R. L.
Nurses want a chance to be professional. *Modern Hospital*, Oct. 1958, p. 88-91.

MALLORY, E.
Whither we are tending. *Canadian Nurse*, June 1960, p. 521-38.

MEAD, MARGARET
Nursing—primitive and civilized. *Nursing Times*, Nov. 9, 1956, p. 1132-4.

MERCIER, C. A.
The ideal nurse—address to nurses. London, 1917.

MERTON, R. K.
The search for professional status. *American Journal of Nursing*, May 1960, p. 662-4.

MOLLETT, M.
The duty of the matron to her profession. *Nursing Record*, Sept. 17, 1898, p. 255-7.

MULLANE, M. K.
Has nursing changed? *Nursing Outlook*, June 1958, p. 323.

NAHM, H.
A decade of change. *American Journal of Nursing*, Nov. 1959, p. 1588-90.

NELSON, ROY C.
The nurse speaks. Philadelphia, Davis, 1958.

NIGHTINGALE, FLORENCE
Address from Florence Nightingale to the probationer nurses in the "Nightingale Fund" school at St. Thomas' Hospital and the nurses trained there, July 23, 1874. Spottiswoode, 1874.

NIGHTINGALE, FLORENCE
Talks to pupils: a selection of addresses to probationers and nurses. New York, Macmillan, 1914.

NURSING OUTLOOK
What is professionalism? *Nursing Outlook*, Mar. 1958, p. 143.

AN OLD WOMAN, *pseud.*
The nurse. Houliston & Stoneman, [1850].

OSLER, WILLIAM
Medicine and nursing. New York, 1919.

PARSONS, SARA E.
Nursing problems and obligations. Boston, Whitcomb & Burrows, 1916.
2nd edn., 1917/18?
3rd edn., 1919.

PRINGLE, ANGELIQUE LUCILLE
A study in nursing. Macmillan, 1905.

RAVITZ, M. J.
Occupational values and occupational selection. *Nursing Research*, June 1957, p. 35-40.

REED, C. A. L.
The relations of the nursing profession to that of medicine and to society. Cincinnati Lancet Clinic, 1908.

RICE, FLORENCE FRANCES
Hospitals and nurses . . . read before the Worcester Women's Club, December 23, 1891. Published by request, Boston, Dawrell & Upham, 1892.

ROSS, A. D.
The nursing profession and social change. *Canadian Nurse*, Sept. 1958, p. 824-32.

ROSS, R. I.
Assuming responsibilities. *Canadian Nurse*, Oct. 1957, p. 895-6.

RUNELL, E. S.
The present status of nursing. *Nursing Record*, Sept. 15, 1892, p. 765-9.

RUSSELL, E. K.
Changes in the patterns of nursing. *Canadian Nurse*, June 1958, p. 529-30.

SANDERS, B. H.
Are we equal to our future? *Canadian Nurse*, Oct. 1956, p. 781-5.

SAUNDERS, LYLE
Permanence and change. *American Journal of Nursing*, July 1958, p. 969-72.

SCHULZ, CECILIA
What's right with the modern nurse? *American Journal of Nursing*, Aug. 1956, p. 1011-13.

SEVERINGHAUS, A. E.
Education for professional responsibility. *Canadian Nurse*, June 1955, p. 439-44.

SINCLAIR, A.
The bifocal approach. *Canadian Nurse*, Nov. 1956, p. 880-4.
[Co-operation of nursing profession in the solution of world-wide health problems.]

SPALDING, EUGENIA K.
The forward look in nursing. *Hospital Progress*, Dec. 1957, p. 74-7.

STORER, HORATIO ROBINSON
On nurses and nursing, 1868.

THORNU, ISIDOR
Nursing: the functional significance of an institutional pattern. *American Sociological Review*, Oct. 1955, p. 531-8.

UPRICHARD, MURIEL
Black cats, dark rooms and blind men—(being a short essay on why nurses need a philosophy). *Canadian Nurse*, Aug. 1957, p. 711-4.

WATKIN, B. V.
Present position of male nurses in hospital. *Nursing Mirror*, May 1, 1959, p. 353-4, and May 15, 1959, p. 519-20.

WATKIN, B .V.
The professional status of hospital nurses. 1 and 2. *Nursing Times*, June 15, 1956, p. 545-6, and June 29, 1956, p. 600-1.

WEDGERY, A.
A new deal for male nurses. *Canadian Nurse*, Aug. 1956, p. 636-8.

WILLIAMS, T. R., *and* WILLIAMS, M. M.
The socialization of the student nurse. *Nursing Research*, Winter 1959, p. 18-25.

WILLIS, L. D.
The scope of professional nursing. *Canadian Nurse*, July 1960, p. 624-32.

WITNEY, F.
Is nursing meeting its obligation to society? *American Journal of Nursing*, Sept. 1956, p. 1127-31.

WOLF, L. K.
The nurse as a person. *American Journal of Nursing*, Mar. 1951, p. 176-8.

WOOD, CATHERINE JANE
The wants of the nursing profession. *Nursing Times*, June 29, 1918, p. 689.

WORCESTER, A.
Is nursing really a profession? *British Journal of Nursing*, Aug. 30, 1902, p. 173-5, and Sept. 6, 1902, p. 193-5.

WORLD HEALTH ORGANIZATION
Guide for national studies of nursing resources, by Margaret G. Arnstein. Geneva, W.H.O., 1953.

WORLD HEALTH ORGANIZATION. EXPERT COMMITTEE ON NURSING
First report. Technical Report Series No. 24. Geneva, W.H.O., 1950.

WORLD HEALTH ORGANIZATION. EXPERT COMMITTEE ON NURSING
Second report. Technical Report Series No. 49. Geneva, W.H.O., 1952.

WORLD HEALTH ORGANIZATION. EXPERT COMMITTEE ON NURSING
Third report. Technical Report Series No. 91. Geneva, W.H.O., 1954.

WORLD HEALTH ORGANIZATION. REGIONAL OFFICE FOR EUROPE
European conference of nurses, Mont-Pelerin/Vevey, [Switzerland], 4-17 October, 1953. Geneva, W.H.O., 1954.

WORLD HEALTH ORGANIZATION. REGIONAL OFFICE FOR EUROPE
Seminar on team-work in nursing services, Istanbul, 17-30 October, 1954. Geneva, W.H.O., 1955.

WRIGHT, W. R.
Present-day problems in nursing. *Canadian Journal of Public Health*, Mar. 1957, p. 109-14.

YOUNG, VIOLET
Talks to probationers. Stockwell, 1932.

ZERNAY, JOHN, *and* OSMOND, HUMPHREY
In defence of nursing. I. *Canadian Medical Association Journal*, Nov. 1, 1956, p. 752-6.
II, by Rae Chittick and Moyra Allen. *Canadian Medical Association Journal*, Feb. 1, 1957, p. 228-9.

NURSING IN INDIVIDUAL COUNTRIES

AUSTRALIA

AVERY, L. M.
Student nurses' associations in Australia. *American Journal of Nursing*, Feb. 1957, p. 182-3.

BOWE, E. J., *and* McRAE, C.
Nursing in the Australian military services. *American Journal of Nursing*, Mar. 1958, p. 378-80.

"COLONIAL"
Nursing in Brisbane. *Nursing Record*, Mar. 28, 1889, p. 199-200.

GARTRELL, MARJORIE
Dear primitive: a nurse among the Aborigines. Sydney, Angus & Robertson, 1957.

McGAHEY, SUSAN B.
The nursing organisation in the Australasian Commonwealth. *Nursing Record*, Dec. 21, 1901, p. 494-7.

MORRIS, E. E.
Suggestions for the improvement of nursing in Victoria. *Nursing Record*, Mar. 26, 1891, p. 147-50.

"TASMANIA", *pseud.*
Nursing in Tasmania. *Nursing Record*, Nov. 7, 1889, p. 262-3.

BALUCHISTAN

MORRIS, J. M.
A nursing sister in Baluchistan. Zenith Press, [19?].

BELGIUM

D'URSEL, LOUISE
Nursing in Belgium. *British Journal of Nursing*, Aug. 26, 1922, p. 134-6, and Sept. 2, 1922, p. 150-2.

BRAZIL

JACKSON, JANE A.
Nursing in Brazil. *Nursing Record*, Jan. 18, 1902, p. 49.

CANADA

BANFILL, B. J.
Labrador nurse. Robert Hale, 1954.

CANADIAN NURSES' ASSOCIATION
Information on nurses and nursing in Canada. Ottawa, Canadian Nurses' Association, 1952.

CANADIAN NURSES' ASSOCIATION
Public relations guide. Ottawa, Canadian Nurses' Association, 1956.

HOPE, MARY E.
Lamp on the snow. Angus & Robertson, 1955.
[Experiences as a nurse in Labrador.]

LIPSETT, G. E. A.
The trained nurse in Western Canada. *British Journal of Nursing*, Jan. 13, 1912, p. 23-4.
[Training School for Nurses, Winnipeg.]

McARTHUR, HELEN G.
A College of Nurses for Ontario? *Canadian Nurse*, June 1960, p. 515-8.

McARTHUR, HELEN G.
The world at your finger tips. *Canadian Nurse*, Oct. 1958, p. 919-22.

MacGREGOR, J. E.
Education, then service. *Canadian Nurse*, Feb. 1958, p. 110-3.

MONTEITH, J. W.
Nursing and National Health Program. *Canadian Nurse*, Sept. 1958, p. 820-3.

SMITH, L. O.
Nursing in New Brunswick. *Canadian Nurse*, Mar. 1959, p. 199-200.

TRAINING SCHOOL FOR NURSES, GENERAL HOSPITAL, TORONTO, CANADA
Nursing in Toronto. *Nursing Record*, Dec. 26, 1889, p. 343-4.

WOOD, CATHERINE J.
The nursing profession in Canada. *Nursing Times*, Aug. 29, 1908, p. 674-5.

YOUNG, M. A.
This is Canada. *Canadian Nurse*, July 1959, p. 601-10.

CHINA

TOMLINSON, SADA C.
Opportunities for nursing in China. *British Journal of Nursing*, Oct. 8, 1910, p. 284-6.

CUBA

NUNEZ, MARGUERITA
Nursing in Cuba. *British Journal of Nursing*, Sept. 25, 1909, p. 261-3.

DENMARK

NORRIE, CHARLOTTE, pseud.
Nursing in Denmark. *Nursing Record*, Mar. 8, 1902, p. 189-90.

NORRIE, CHARLOTTE, *pseud.*
A plan for a nursing school in Denmark. *Nursing Record*, Jan. 17, 1889, p. 36-9.

NORRIE, CHARLOTTE, pseud.
Sick nursing in Denmark. *Nursing Record*, Jan. 12, 1893, p. 27-9.

EGYPT

WATKINS, J. G.
Nursing in Egypt. *Nursing Record*, Nov. 16, 1901, p. 393-4.

EIRE

CUNNINGHAM, R.
Our place in the changing scenes of nursing. *Irish Nurses' Magazine*, Feb. 1959, p. 9-10.

FALKINER, NINIAN M.
The nurse and the state: paper with discussion. Dublin, Statistical and Social Enquiry Society of Ireland, [1920].

MATHESON, VERA
A plea for Irish nurses. Dublin, Thom, [19?].

FIJI

ANDERSON, MAY C.
Nursing in Fiji. *British Journal of Nursing*, Oct. 11, 1902, p. 301-3.

FINLAND

PASANEN, ULLA
A Finnish nursing school. *Nursing Outlook*, Oct. 1959, p. 594-5.
[Tampere School of Nursing.]

FORMOSA

SMITH, EMILY MYRTLE
Taiwan nursing report. Feb. 1952-Feb. 1954. Washington, U.S. Public Health Service, [1955].

FRANCE

HAMILTON, ANNA
The position of nursing in France. *British Journal of Nursing*, Aug. 22, 1903, p. 156-8, and Aug. 29, 1903, p. 176.

HAMILTON, ANNA
The progress of the Nightingale system of nursing in France. *British Journal of Nursing*, Dec. 4, 1909, p. 466-7.

JACQUES, —
Training of hospital nurses at Paris. *British Journal of Nursing*, Dec. 11, 1909, p. 475-7.

GERMANY

KARLL, AGNES
The future training of the German nurse. *British Journal of Nursing*, Aug. 27, 1904, p. 166-8.

KARLL, AGNES
The professional co-operation of the sick nurses of Germany. *British Journal of Nursing*, Aug. 8, 1903, p. 108-110.

KARLL, AGNES
The progress of nursing in Germany. *British Journal of Nursing*, Aug. 3, 1907, p. 84-5.

KARLL, AGNES
Training nurses in Germany. *British Journal of Nursing*, Oct. 2, 1909, p. 273-5.

GREECE

FENWICK, ETHEL GORDON
Nursing in Greece. *Nursing Record*, Nov. 23, 1901, p. 422-3.

GORMAN, MARIE ROSANA
The nurse in Greek life. Boston, 1917.

HAWAII

CAMARA, A.
Progress of practical nursing in Hawaii. *Hawaii Medical Journal and Inter-Island Nurses' Bulletin*, Jan.-Feb. 1957, p. 308-10.

TERRITORIAL COMMISSION ON NURSING EDUCATION AND NURSING SERVICES
The nurse of tomorrow: a report on nursing in Hawaii, based on the survey for the Nursing Study Committee by Ruth I. Gillan. Honolulu, The Commission, 1952.

HOLLAND

BAARSLAG, C. A. LA BASTIDE
Sick nursing in Holland. *Nursing Record*, Oct. 26, 1901, p. 334-7.

INDIA

ANON.
Some experiences of an English nurse in India. *Nursing Record*, Feb. 14, 1889, p. 100-3.

KLOSZ, W. H.
The need for state registration in India. *British Journal of Nursing*, June 10, 1911, p. 453-5.

MITCHISON, E. L.
District nursing in India. *Nursing Record*, Aug. 29, 1889, p. 132-5.

ISRAEL

DRUCKMAN-FRANKENSTEIN, R.
Nursing in an Israeli family health service. *American Journal of Nursing*, Nov. 1957, p. 1436-8.

GOULD, ETTA M.
A pilot study in modern Israel. *Canadian Nurse*, Mar. 1957, p. 214-7.

ISRAEL, MINISTRY OF HEALTH
Nursing in Israel: a survey prepared for the Ninth World Health Assembly by the Nursing Division, Ministry of Health. Jerusalem, The Ministry, 1956.

LYONS-BERGMAN, R.
Elderly citizens—novice nurses. *Nursing Outlook*, Dec. 1957, p. 716-8.

ITALY
DOCK, LAVINIA L.
The nursing system of Italian hospitals. *British Journal of Nursing*, April 30, 1904, p. 354-6; May 21, 1904, p. 416-7; Aug. 6, 1904, p. 105-7.

SGARRA, A.
The nursing profession in Italy. *Nursing Mirror*, May 24, 1957, p. v-vii.

TURTON, AMY
Report on hospital training in Italy. *British Journal of Nursing*, Oct. 2, 1909, p. 282-4.

TURTON, AMY
Report on nursing in Italy. *Nursing Record*, Oct. 19, 1901, p. 313-4.

JORDAN
MUSALLAM, A.
Nursing in Jordan. *American Journal of Nursing*, Sept. 1958, p. 1249-51.

LIBERIA
YERGAN, L. H.
Mission in Liberia. *Nursing Outlook*, Oct. 1956, p. 564-6.

MALAYA
KARIM, R. B.
Missi Ubat: the Malayan medicine miss. *Nursing Outlook*, April 1959, p. 224-6.

MOROCCO
HERZ-HABER, ZIPPORAH G.
Moroccan adventure in staff education. *American Journal of Nursing*, Feb. 1960, p. 219-22.

NEWFOUNDLAND
STORY, J.
Five years of progress. *Canadian Nurse*, July 1959, p. 599-600.

NEW ZEALAND
WALKER, R. E.
Nursing on the waterfront. *American Journal of Nursing*, Aug. 1959, p. 1139-41.

WOOD, CATHERINE J.
Conditions of nursing in New Zealand. *Nursing Times*, April 18, 1908, p. 304-5.

NORWAY
ØRN, E.
Norway and points East and South. *American Journal of Nursing*, April 1959, p. 516-7.
[Men nurse-deacons in Norway.]

PAKISTAN
MOWLA, K.
Progress in Pakistan. *American Journal of Nursing*, Feb. 1958, p. 237-9.

PANAMA
DUNCAN, SILVIA, *and* RICHARDSON, GENEVIEVE
Going forward in Panama. *American Journal of Nursing*, Oct. 1959, p. 1422-5.

SOUTH AFRICA
GROBBELAAR, A.
South African experiments with the basic collegiate program. *American Journal of Nursing*, Oct. 1958, p. 1401-2.

SWEDEN
KROG, GINA
Nursing in Sweden. *Nursing Record*, Feb. 1, 1902, p. 89-91.

SWITZERLAND
KRAFFT, C.
The trained nurse. *Nursing Times*, June 30, 1906, p. 534-6.
The nursing profession in Switzerland. *Nursing Times*, Aug. 24, 1907, p. 732-5.

SYRIA
WORTABET, EDLA
A history of nursing in Syria. *Nursing Times*, May 19, 1906, p. 407-9, and May 26, 1906, p. 426-8.

THAILAND
BUCKOKE, LILLIAN
Thailand's hospital and nursing services. *Nursing Mirror*, July 22, 1960, p. xii-xiii.

UNITED KINGDOM OF GREAT BRITAIN AND NORTHERN IRELAND
BENNETT, BETHINA A.
A guide to professional nursing: nursing, midwifery and the allied professions. Faber, 1951.

BENNETT, BETHINA A.
Nursing and the National Health Service. *American Journal of Nursing*, Dec. 1957, p. 1561-4.

BERKELEY, COMYNS, *ed.*
A guide to the profession of nursing before and after state registration. Newnes, [1931].

BEVINGTON, SHEILA M.
Nursing life and discipline: a study based on over 500 interviews. Lewis, 1943.

BRIGHT, PAMELA
Breakfast at night. MacGibbon & Kee, 1956.
[An autobiographical account of life as a hospital nurse.]

BRIGHT, PAMELA
Life in our hands. MacGibbon & Kee, 1955.

BURDEN, JOY
What about nursing? S.P.C.K., 1959.

Burdett's official Nursing Directory: containing an outline of the principal laws affecting nurses—particulars of nurse-training schools in the United Kingdom and abroad, nursing institutions, etc., and a directory of nurses ... compiled and edited by Sir Henry Burdett, 1898. London, 1898.

BURDETT, HENRY
Nursing profession: how and where to train. Scientific Press, 1899.

BURDETT, HENRY, *ed.*
How to succeed as a trained nurse, being a guide to her remunerative employment, with particulars of the various openings in the United Kingdom and abroad, government and municipal departments, associations and co-operations where the services of private nurses are in demand. Scientific Press, 1913.

CARTER, G. B.
A new deal for nurses. Gollancz, 1939.

CARTER, G. B., *and* PEARCE, EVELYN C.
Reconsideration of nursing: its fundamentals, purpose and place in the community. *Nursing Mirror*, 1946.

COCHRANE, MARY S.
Nursing. Geoffrey Bles, 1930.

COCKAYNE, E.
Ten years of nursing in the National Health Service. *Nursing Times*, July 4, 1958, p. 762-3.

DARNELL, LILLIAN M.
Nursing. Robert Hale, 1959.

DRYBOROUGH-SMITH, E.
Do you want to be a nurse? Bristol, Wright, 1941.

GANT, FREDERICK JAMES
Mock-nurses of the latest fashion, A.D. 1901. Professional experiences in short stories and the nursing question; with a short memoir of the author. Bailliere, Tindall & Cox, 1900.
2nd edn., 1901.

GODDEN, G. M.
Careers in nursing, 1960, edited by John Callaghan. Classic Pub., 1960.

GRANT, JANE
Come hither nurse. Hale, 1957.

GREAT BRITAIN. PARLIAMENT, SELECT COMMITTEE ON THE G.N.C.
Report from the Select Committee on the General Nursing Council, together with proceedings of the committee and the minutes of evidence. London, 1925.

GREY, MONA E.
Progressive professional nursing. Edinburgh, Livingstone, 1950.

HALDANE, ELIZABETH SANDERSON
Nursing as a profession, 1922. The Nineteenth Century, Sept. 1922, p. 442-8.

HARDY, GLADYS M.
Nursing as a career and livelihood. Beck, 1954.

HAWKINS-AMBLER, G. A.
Gentle art of nursing the sick. Scott, 1895.

HOLLAND, D. SYDNEY
Two talks to the nurses of the London Hospital, Dec. 1897. 2 parts in 1. [Whitehead, n.d.]

HOSPITAL ASSOCIATION, LONDON
Registration of trained nurses. Report of the Joint Sectional Committee on Registration. Adopted by the Council, 25 March, 1888. London, 1888.

INTERDEPARTMENTAL COMMITTEE ON NURSING SERVICES
Interim report. H.M.S.O., 1939.
[Set up by the Ministry of Health and the Board of Education. Chairman: The Earl of Athlone.]

LABOUR PARTY
The Labour Party and the nursing profession: a statement of policy with regard to nursing. Labour Party, [1927].

MACKENZIE, NORAH
Needs and resources in the nursing profession. *Nursing Times*, [1954].
[A series of five articles, reprinted from the *Nursing Times*, Dec. 1953 and Jan. 1954.]

MACKENZIE, NORAH
The nurse and the modern community: a series of five lectures given as part of a refresher course for sister tutors organized by the Education Department, Royal College of Nursing. *Nursing Times*, 1949.
[Reprinted from the *Nursing Times*, Oct. and Nov. 1949.]

"MIDLAND DOCTOR", *pseud.*
Letters to a nurse. John Bale, 1921.

MOLES, CHARLOTTE L.
Nursing as a career. Pitman, 1933.

MONCRIEFF, ALAN, *and* FOWLER, KATHLEEN A. B., *editors*
Progress in nursing: a survey of recent developments in medicine and surgery. Arnold, 1954.

MORTEN, HONNOR
How to become a nurse. 3rd edn. Scientific Press, 1895

MORWYN, JOAN
How I became a nursing sister. Nelson, 1954.

NATIONAL ASSOCIATION OF LOCAL GOVERNMENT OFFICERS
A woman's calling. N.A.L.G.O., [193?].

NIGHTINGALE, FLORENCE
Florence Nightingale to her nurses: a selection from Miss Nightingale's addresses to probationers and nurses of the Nightingale School at St. Thomas's Hospital. Macmillan, 1914.

Nursing Directory—including the directory of nurses in London . . . the provinces . . . in Scotland . . . in Ireland, a directory of nurses resident abroad. Also statistical and general information of the training schools for nurses, the nursing services, institutes, societies, insurance offices, etc., in the United Kingdom. London, 1892.

NUTTALL, PEGGY
Nursing as a career. Batsford, 1960.

PRINGLE, ANGELIQUE LUCILLE
A study in nursing. Macmillan, 1905.

ROYAL COLLEGE OF NURSING
Memorandum relating to conditions in the nursing profession, for submission to the Interdepartmental Committee on the Nursing Services. The College, 1938.

ROYAL COLLEGE OF NURSING
Observations and objectives: a statement on nursing policy. Royal College of Nursing, 1956.

ROYAL COLLEGE OF NURSING
NURSING RECONSTRUCTION COMMITTEE
Report. Section 1, The assistant nurse. Royal College of Nursing, [1942].
[Chairman: Lord Horder.]

ROYAL COLLEGE OF NURSING.
NURSING RECONSTRUCTION COMMITTEE
Report. Section 2, Education and training. Section 3, Recruitment. Royal College of Nursing, [1943].
[Chairman: Lord Horder.]

ROYAL COLLEGE OF NURSING.
NURSING RECONSTRUCTION COMMITTEE
Report. Section 4, The social and economic conditions of the nurse. Royal College of Nursing, [1949].
[Chairman: Lord Horder.]

ROYAL COLLEGE OF NURSING.
NURSING RECONSTRUCTION COMMITTEE
Supplements to the Report on Education and Training of the Nursing Reconstruction Committee. A. Minimum standards for nurse training schools. Royal College of Nursing, [1945].
[Chairman: Lord Horder.]

ROYAL COLLEGE OF NURSING.
NURSING RECONSTRUCTION COMMITTEE
Supplements to the Report on Education and Training of the Nursing Reconstruction Committee. B. Post registration nursing education, 1, The training of public health nurses. Royal College of Nursing, [194?].
[Chairman: Lord Horder.]

ROYAL COLLEGE OF NURSING.
NURSING RECONSTRUCTION COMMITTEE
Supplements to the Report on Education and Training of the Nursing Reconstruction Committee. B. Post-registration nursing education, 2, Advanced nursing studies: an aspect of modern adult education. Royal College of Nursing, [1946].
[Chairman: Lord Horder.]

ROYAL COLLEGE OF NURSING AND BRITISH HOSPITALS ASSOCIATION
Nurses' representative councils: introductory note and suggested form of constitution, prepared jointly by the Royal College of Nursing and the British Hospitals Association, on the advice of their liaison committee. The College *and* The Association, 1944.

SMYTH, M. J.
Functions of the Standing Nursing Advisory Committee of the Central Health Services Council. *Nursing Times*, June 21, 1952, p. 607-8.

TATHAM, —
Nursing as a career for women. Newnes, 1919.

WARTIME SOCIAL SURVEY
The attitudes of women towards nursing, by Kathleen Box, assisted by Enid Croft-White. The Survey, 1943.

WHITE, A. M. W.
Planning in Ulster. *Nursing Times*, Jan. 29, 1960, p. 138.

UNITED STATES OF AMERICA

AMERICAN NURSES' ASSOCIATION
Issues in the growth of a profession: presented at the 41st convention of the American Nurses' Association, Atlantic City, N.J., June 10, 1958. [New York, The Association, 1958.]

AMERICAN NURSES' ASSOCIATION
Nursing: a profession for college women. New York, Nursing Information Bureau of A.N.A. and N.L.N.E. and N.O.P.H.N., 1945.

AMERICAN NURSES' ASSOCIATION
Nursing—as it is defined in nursing practice acts. New York, the Association, 1957.

AMERICAN NURSES' ASSOCIATION
Today and tomorrow: report to the members from the President. New York, American Nurses' Association, 1957.

AMERICAN NURSES' ASSOCIATION
Toward one organization? A discussion on the desirability of one organization meeting the needs of the nursing profession. The A.N.A. *vis-á-vis* the N.L.N. *American Journal of Nursing*, April 1959, p. 540-3.

AMERICAN NURSES' ASSOCIATION.
INTER-GROUP RELATIONS PROGRAM
Progress in inter-group relations in nursing: Annual Report, May 20, 1955-May 1, 1956. New York, A.N.A., [1956].

AMERICAN NURSES' FOUNDATION
Becoming a nurse: a study of changing values in nursing students; a research report . . . January 1959. New York, The Foundation, 1959.

AMERICAN NURSES' FOUNDATION
Formal education and the process of professionalization: a study of student nurses, by Thomas S. McPartland. Kansas City, Missouri, Community Studies, 1957.

AMIDON, BEULAH
Better nursing for America. New York, Public Affairs Committee, 1941.

ANDERSON, BERNICE E.
The facilitation of interstate movement of registered nurses. Philadelphia, Lippincott, 1950.

ANDERSON, BERNICE
Functions, standards and qualifications; legal aspects. *American Journal of Nursing*, June 1957, p. 749-50.

BRESSLER, MARVIN, *and* KEPHART, WILLIAM
Career dynamics: a survey of selected aspects of the nursing profession. Study conducted for the Pennsylvania Nurses' Association. Harrisburg, Penn., The Association, 1955.

BROWN, ESTHER LUCILE
Nursing as a profession. New York, Russell Sage Foundation, 1936.

BROWN, ESTHER LUCILE
Nursing for the future: a report prepared for the National Nursing Council. New York, Russell Sage Foundation, 1948.

BULLOCK, ROBERT P.
What do nurses think of their profession? Occupational role and function as related to job satisfaction among registered nurses. Final report to the Ohio State Nurses' Association. Columbus, Ohio, Ohio State University, Research Foundation, 1954.

CHAYER, MARY ELLA
Nursing in modern society. New York, Putnam, 1947.

COMMITTEE ON THE FUNCTION OF NURSING
A program for the nursing profession. New York, Macmillan, 1949.
[Chairman: Eli Ginzberg.]

COMMITTEE ON THE GRADING OF NURSING SCHOOLS
Nurses: production, education, distribution and pay. New York, The Committee, 1930.

COMMITTEE ON THE STRUCTURE OF NATIONAL NURSING
ORGANIZATIONS
Handbook on the structure of organized nursing. New York, The Committee, 1949.

COMMITTEE ON THE STRUCTURE OF NATIONAL NURSING
ORGANIZATIONS AND STRUCTURE STEERING COMMITTEE
New horizons in nursing: the story of a profession's search for better ways through which its members may co-operate with each other and with the people served by the profession; compiled by Josephine Nelson. New York, Macmillan, 1950.

CULVER, V. M.
Some facts about nursing in North Carolina. *North Carolina Medical Journal*, July 1960, p. 279-81.

DEMING, DOROTHY
Careers for nurses. New York, McGraw-Hill, 1947.
2nd edn., 1952.

DEUTSCHER, IRWIN
The graduate nurse and her professional organizations. *Nursing World*, March 1958, p. 23-9.

DEUTSCHER, IRWIN
Public images of the nurse. Part II. A study of the registered nurse in a metropolitan community. Kansas City, Community Studies, 1955.

DEVEREUX, GEORGE, *and* WEINER, FLORENCE R.
The occupational status of nurses. *American Sociological Review*, Oct. 1950.

DOCK, LAVINIA L.
Report on the status of nursing in the United States. *Nursing Record*, Oct. 19, 1901, p. 315-7.

FRUMKIN, ROBERT M.
Hospital nursing: a sociological interpretation. Buffalo, University of Buffalo, 1956.

FRUMKIN, ROBERT M.
The nurse as a human being. Buffalo, University of Buffalo, [1956].

FRUMKIN, ROBERT M.
Nursing students' attitudes towards civil liberties. *Nursing Outlook*, Mar. 1956, p. 162-3.

GELINAS, AGNES
Nursing and nursing education. New York, Commonwealth Fund, 1946.

GOLDSTEIN, RHODA L.
Negro nurses in hospitals. *American Journal of Nursing*, Feb. 1960, p. 215-7.

HODSON, JANE, *ed.*
How to become a trained nurse—a manual of information in detail with a complete list of the various training schools in the U.S.A. and Canada. New York, Abbott, 1898.

HUGHES, EVERETT C., *and others*
Twenty thousand nurses tell their story, by Everett C. Hughes, Helen MacGill Hughes [and] Irwin Deutscher. Philadelphia, Lippincott, 1958.
[A report on studies of nursing functions sponsored by the American Nurses' Association.]

INTERNATIONAL CONGRESS OF CHARITIES, CORRECTION AND PHILANTHROPY, CHICAGO, 1893.
Hospitals, dispensaries and nursing—papers and discussions in the International Congress of Charities Correction and Philanthropy, sect. iii, Chicago, June 12-17, 1893, ed. by John S. Billings and Henry M. Hurd. Baltimore, 1894.

JONES, WALTER B., *and* IFFERT, R. E.
Fitness for nursing. Pittsburgh, Pa., Bureau of Educational Records and Research, 1933.

KENEALY, ANNESLEY
Hospital life in America. *Nursing Record*, May 9, 1889, p. 296-7.

McBRIDE, MARGUERITE
Nursing on an Indian reservation. *American Journal of Nursing*, Sept. 1957, p. 1168-9.

McIVER, P.
Functions, standards and qualifications: next steps. *American Journal of Nursing*, June 1957, p. 748-50.

McKENNA, FRANCES M.
Thresholds to professional nursing practice. Philadelphia, Saunders, 1955.
2nd edn., 1960.

McMANUS, R. LOUISE
The effect of experience on nursing achievement. New York, Teachers' College, Columbia University, 1949.

MERRICK, ELLIOTT
Northern nurse. New York, Charles Scribner, 1942.

MINNESOTA NURSES' ASSOCIATION *and* MINNESOTA BOARD OF NURSING
Nursing in Minnesota: a statistical review. St. Paul, The Association, 1957.

MITCHELL, SILAS WEIR
... address delivered ... to the graduating class of New York Hospital Training School for Nurses, Feb. 28, 1908. New York, Society of the New York Hospital, 1908.

MORGAN, KATHRYN
Tired feet: the story of a registered nurse. New York, Vantage Press, 1952.

MORISON, LUELLA J.
Stepping-stones to professional nursing: text and workbook for student nurses. St. Louis, Mosby, 1954.
2nd edn., 1957.
3rd edn., 1960.

MOSBY'S COMPREHENSIVE REVIEW OF NURSING
St. Louis, Mosby, 1949. [In progress.]

MOSES, E. B.
The profile of a professional nurse. Some facts and figures about the nursing force in America today. *American Journal of Nursing*, Mar. 1960, p. 368-70.

MUNRO, AENEAS
Science and the art of nursing the sick. Hamilton, 1873.

NATIONAL LEAGUE FOR NURSING EDUCATION
Committee on vocational guidance: handbook for career counselors on the profession of nursing. New York, The League, 1948.

NATIONAL LEAGUE FOR NURSING. COMMITTEE ON CAREERS
Look to your future in hospital nursing. New York, The League, n.d.

NATIONAL LEAGUE FOR NURSING. COMMITTEE ON CAREERS
Men working: for a career in nursing. New York, The League, n.d.

NATIONAL LEAGUE FOR NURSING. COMMITTEE ON CAREERS
Team mates. New York, The League, 1958.

NATIONAL LEAGUE FOR NURSING. COMMITTEE ON THE FUTURE
Nurses for a growing nation. New York, The League, 1957.

NURSING OUTLOOK
Do we need a league for nursing? *Nursing Outlook*, April 1959, p. 197.

REINHARDT, JAMES M.
Society and the nursing profession, with contributions by Paul Meadows. Philadelphia, Saunders, 1953.

RUSSELL, SHEILA MACKAY
A lamp is heavy. Angus & Robertson, 1954.

SCHULZ, CECILIA L.
Your career in nursing. New York, McGraw-Hill, 1941.

SENN, NICHOLAS
Address to the graduating class of the Mary Thompson Hospital Training School for Nurses. [Chicago], 1905.

SPALDING, H. S.
Talks to nurses. New York, 1920.

STORER, HORATIO ROBINSON
Our nurses and nursing: with a special reference to the management of sick women. Boston, Lee & Shepard, 1868.

SUTHERLAND, DOROTHY GERTRUDE
Do you want to be a nurse? New York, Doubleday, Doran, 1942.

UNITED STATES DEPARTMENT OF THE ARMY. OFFICE OF THE SURGEON GENERAL. TECHNICAL LIAISON OFFICE
Background information on the Army Nurse Corps. Washington, Govt. Printing Office, 1953.

UNITED STATES PUBLIC HEALTH SERVICE
Nursing careers among the American Indians. Washington, Government Printing Office, 1955.

UNITED STATES PUBLIC HEALTH SERVICE. DIVISION OF NURSING RESOURCES
Nursing resources: a progress report of the program of the Division of Nursing Resources, prepared ... by Apollonia O. Adams. Washington, Govt. Printing Office, [1958].

WOLF, L. K.
Nursing. New York, Appleton-Century, 1947.

WORCESTER, ALFRED
Modern nursing. An address at the graduation of nurses, St. Luke's Hospital, New Bedford, Massachusetts, May 15, 1931. *New England Journal of Medicine*, Aug. 13, 1931, p. 334-6.

UNION OF SOVIET SOCIALIST REPUBLICS

ARCHER, P.
The Piroquov Hospital, Moscow. *Nursing Times*, Feb. 20, 1959, p. 231-2.

BLAIR-FISH, HILARY M.
A nurse looks at Russia; some notes of the College of Nursing study tour to Leningrad and Moscow, July 1935. *Nursing Times*, [1935].
[Reprint of a series of articles in the *Nursing Times*.]

HOLLIDAY, J.
Glimpses of nursing in Russia. *Nursing Outlook*, Sept. 1958, p. 496-7.

PARK, P. M.
In search of a sluice: Botkin Hospital, Moscow. *Nursing Times*, Nov. 1, 1957, p. 1247-9.

WORTHINGTON, G.
Visit to Russia. *Nursing Times*, Nov. 1, 1957, p. 1245-7.

VIETNAM

LESTER, M. R.
A salute to nursing in Vietnam. *Nursing Outlook*, Sept. 1957, p. 528-31.

YERGEN, LAURA
The "new look" in Vietnamese nursing. *American Journal of Nursing*, Sept. 1956, p. 1132-4.

ORGANIZATIONS AND ASSOCIATIONS AND THEIR HISTORY

ALTSCHUL, A.
Professional organisations and the mental nurse. *Nursing Mirror*, Oct. 4, 1957, p. 43.

AMERICAN JOURNAL OF NURSING
Toward one organization? *American Journal of Nursing*, April 1959, p. 540-2.

AMERICAN NURSES' ASSOCIATION
The head nurse: her section membership; a historical review, by A. Logsdon. *American Journal of Nursing*, June 1959, p. 825-7.

AMERICAN NURSES' ASSOCIATION
Historical sketch of the American Nurses' Association, prepared by Virginia McCormick. New York, American Nurses' Association, 1929.

AMERICAN NURSES' FOUNDATION INTERNATIONAL NURSING PROJECT
Knowing our exchange visitors, by Jeanne Broadhurst. *Nursing Outlook*, April 1958, p. 198-201.
[An account of the work of the American Nurses' Foundation International Nursing Project.]

AMERICAN SOCIETY OF SUPERINTENDENTS OF TRAINING SCHOOLS FOR NURSES
Constitution. *Nursing Record*, Jan. 12, 1895, p. 23-4.

AUSTRALIAN NURSES' ASSOCIATION
Note of its foundation, together with its objects and bye-laws. *Nursing Record*, Sept. 22, 1892, p. 779-80.

BRITISH NURSES' ASSOCIATION
Policy statement. *Nursing Record*, June 21, 1888, p. 135-7.

BRITISH NURSES' ASSOCIATION
Report of its foundation. *Nursing Record*, April 5, 1888, p. 2.

BRITISH NURSES' ASSOCIATION
Report of meeting on 10th January, 1890, at which a resolution changing the conditions of membership was passed. *Nursing Record*, Jan. 16, 1890, p. 28-9.

CANADIAN NURSES' ASSOCIATION
A brief history of the Canadian Nurses' Association. Winnipeg, The Association, 1925.

CANADIAN NURSES' ASSOCIATION
The first ten years, by E. Johns. *Canadian Nurse*, June 1958, p. 520-4.

CANADIAN NURSES' ASSOCIATION
Yesterday; today; tomorrow: an appreciation, by A. E. Reid. *Canadian Nurse*, June 1958, p. 511-2.

CANADIAN NURSES' ASSOCIATION
Historical sketch of C.N.A., by M. Pearl Stiver. *Canadian Nurse*, Mar. 1955, p. 188-9.

CENTRAL COUNCIL FOR DISTRICT NURSING IN LONDON
History of the Central Council for District Nursing, London, 1914-44. The Council, [194?].

COLLEGE OF NURSING
Circular letter from the Hon. Arthur Stanley to chairmen of hospitals and infirmaries on the aims of the College. *British Journal of Nursing*, April 29, 1916, p. 383-4.

COLLEGE OF NURSING
Details of the scheme at a representative meeting. *Nursing Times*, Mar. 4, 1916, p. 262-6.

COLLEGE OF NURSING
Formation of the Consultative Board [report of a meeting]. *Nursing Times*, June 24, 1916, p. 755-7.

COLLEGE OF NURSING
Meeting to discuss the formation of a consultative committee. *British Journal of Nursing*, April 15, 1916, p. 340-2.

COLLEGE OF NURSING
Meeting with Hon. Arthur Stanley about the proposed College of Nursing. *British Journal of Nursing*, Mar. 18, 1916, p. 250-5.

COLLEGE OF NURSING
Memorandum on the College of Nursing by the Chairman and Matron of the London Hospital. *British Journal of Nursing*, Mar. 17, 1917, p. 191-2.

COLLEGE OF NURSING
Report of a meeting in support of the formation of a College of Nursing. *British Journal of Nursing*, Mar. 4, 1916, p. 204-10.
See also
[ROYAL COLLEGE OF NURSING]

CONNECTICUT STATE NURSE ASSOCIATION
Five decades—historical sketch, 1904-1954. Helen W. Munson, compiler. Hartford, Conn., The Association, 1954.

DISTRICT NURSING ASSOCIATION OF NORTHERN WESTCHESTER COUNTY (N.Y.)
The District Nursing Association for Northern Westchester County, 1898-1948. Mount Kisco, N.Y., 1948.

DUTCH NURSES' ASSOCIATION
Objects and rules. *Nursing Record*, June 22, 1893, p. 308-10.

FLORENCE NIGHTINGALE INTERNATIONAL FOUNDATION
The Florence Nightingale International Foundation. The Foundation, 1947.

FLORENCE NIGHTINGALE INTERNATIONAL FOUNDATION
The lamp radiant: the story of an association of nurses from many lands, by two of its members, N. L. Dorsey and M. M. Killby. [The Florence Nightingale International Foundation, 195?.]
[The story of the Old Internationals' Association of Scholars and Fellows of the Florence Nightingale International Foundation.]

FLORENCE NIGHTINGALE INTERNATIONAL FOUNDATION
A study of the Florence Nightingale International Foundation, by H. R. Hamley and Muriel Uprichard. The Foundation, 1948.

FLORENCE NIGHTINGALE INTERNATIONAL FOUNDATION
Towards the Florence Nightingale International Foundation. Paris, League of Red Cross Societies, 1934.

GEISTER, J.
One organization—why? *American Association of Industrial Nurses' Journal*, Mar. 1959, p. 21-3.
[The pros and cons of one organization for nurses.]

GENERAL NURSING COUNCIL FOR ENGLAND AND WALES
The General Nursing Council, by Ethel Gordon Fenwick. *British Journal of Nursing*, Jan. 31, 1920, p. 67-8.

GENERAL NURSING COUNCIL FOR ENGLAND AND WALES
The General Nursing Council for England and Wales; its history and functions. 1. Its constitution and structure, by M. Henry. *Nursing Mirror*, Jan. 3, 1958, p. v-vi.

GENERAL NURSING COUNCIL FOR ENGLAND AND WALES
The General Nursing Council for England and Wales; its history and functions. 2. The training of nurses, by M. Henry. *Nursing Mirror*, Jan. 10, 1958, p. v-vi.

GENERAL NURSING COUNCIL FOR ENGLAND AND WALES
The General Nursing Council for England and Wales; its history and functions. 3. Examinations and assessments, by M. Henry. *Nursing Mirror*, Jan. 17, 1958, p. xi-xii.

GENERAL NURSING COUNCIL FOR ENGLAND AND WALES
The General Nursing Council for England and Wales; its history and functions. 4. Registration and enrolment, by M. Henry. *Nursing Mirror*, Jan. 24, 1958, p. 1221-2.

GENERAL NURSING COUNCIL FOR ENGLAND AND WALES
The General Nursing Council for England and Wales; its history and functions. 5. Miscellaneous duties, by M. Henry. *Nursing Mirror*, Jan. 31, 1958, p. xi-xii.

GENERAL NURSING COUNCIL FOR ENGLAND AND WALES
The General Nursing Council for England and Wales, by D. M. Smith. *Nursing Times*, April 15, 1955, p. 398-9.

GILHOOLY, M. A. N., *and* ELLIOTT, F. E.
The status of organizations in schools of nursing. *American Journal of Nursing*, May 1958, p. 703-5.

HUNTER, T. G.
Our professional association. *Canadian Nurse*, Sept. 1958, p. 807-9.

ILLINOIS STATE NURSES' ASSOCIATION
A history of the Illinois State Nurses' Association, 1901-1935, by Mary Dunwiddie. Chicago, The Association, 1937.

INCORPORATED SOCIETY FOR PROMOTING THE HIGHER EDUCATION AND TRAINING OF NURSES
Memorandum of Association. *British Journal of Nursing*, Feb. 11, 1905, p. 105-14. Editorial comment, Feb. 11, 1905, p. 114-5.

INTERNATIONAL COUNCIL OF NURSES
Brief history of the Council, and description of new headquarters. *Nursing Times*, May 4, 1956, p. 370-6.

INTERNATIONAL COUNCIL OF NURSES
Constitution and list of Councillors. *Nursing Record*, Aug. 18, 1900, p. 129-30.

INTERNATIONAL COUNCIL OF NURSES
History of the International Council of Nurses, 1899-1925, by Margaret Breay and Ethel Gordon Fenwick. Geneva, I.C.N., 1931.

INTERNATIONAL COUNCIL OF NURSES
The International Council of Nurses, by Agnes Ohlson. *Canadian Nurse*, Sept. 1958, p. 810-3.

IOWA STATE ASSOCIATION OF REGISTERED NURSES
Historical outline of the Iowa State Association of Registered Nurses and related organizations, by Emma C. Wilson. 1931?

IRISH NURSES' ASSOCIATION
Inaugural meeting. *British Journal of Nursing*, Jan. 23, 1904, p. 70.

KANSAS STATE NURSES' ASSOCIATION
Lamps on the prairie, a history of nursing in Kansas, compiled by the Works Project Administrator. Emporia, Kansas, Gazette Press, 1942.

LEAGUE OF ST. BARTHOLOMEW'S NURSES
Inaugural meeting and constitution. *Nursing Record*, Dec. 9, 1899, p. 473-5.

LEAGUE OF SCHOOL NURSES
Account of meeting held to form the League. *British Journal of Nursing*, Feb. 1, 1908, p. 87-8.

LOUISIANA STATE NURSES' ASSOCIATION
History of the Louisiana State Nurses' Association, Silver Jubilee, 1904-1929, by Geneva A. Peters. 1929?

MARSH, H. N.
The Visiting Nurse Association celebrates 60 years. *Medical Annals of the District of Columbia*, April 1960, p. 239-41.

MARYLAND STATE NURSES' ASSOCIATION
Twenty-fifth anniversary of the Maryland State Nurses' Association: an historical sketch 1903-1928, with a prologue of nursing history in Maryland prior to 1903, by Helen C. Bartlett. Baltimore, Furst, 1928.

MASSACHUSETTS MEMORIAL HOSPITAL
The Massachusetts Memorial Hospitals School of Nursing, by F. Flores. *Boston Medical Quarterly*, Dec. 1956, p. 108-12.

MASSACHUSETTS STATE NURSES' ASSOCIATION
Massachusetts State Nurses' Association: A review of the first fifty years, 1903-53, by Anna Roth. Boston, The Association, n.d.

MASSACHUSETTS STATE NURSES' ASSOCIATION
Thirty-five years of the Massachusetts State Nurses' Association, by Anna Roth. Boston, The Association, 1938.

MATRONS' COUNCIL
Account of business at the meeting to bring the Council into being, held at St. Bartholomew's Hospital. *Nursing Record*, July 21, 1894, p. 49-52. Editorial comment, July 21, 1894, p. 41-2.

MATRONS' COUNCIL *and* SOCIETY FOR THE STATE REGISTRATION OF TRAINED NURSES
Meeting held to protest against the formation of the Incorporated Society for Promoting the Higher Education and Training of Nurses. *British Journal of Nursing*, Feb. 25, 1905, p. 145-7.

MENTAL HOSPITAL AND INSTITUTIONAL WORKERS' UNION
The history of the Mental Hospital and Institutional Workers' Union from infancy to its 21st year: a record of endeavour and accomplishment. Manchester, The Union, [1931].

NATIONAL COUNCIL OF NURSES FOR GREAT BRITAIN AND IRELAND
Constitution. *British Journal of Nursing*, Feb. 8, 1908, p. 106-7.

NATIONAL COUNCIL OF TRAINED NURSES OF GREAT BRITAIN AND IRELAND
Meeting held to discuss Mr. Arthur Stanley's proposal to form a College of Nursing. *British Journal of Nursing*, Feb. 19, 1916, p. 153-62.

NATIONAL LEAGUE FOR NURSING
Our first five years, by Anna Filimore. *Nursing Outlook*, Jan. 1958, p. 14-17.

NATIONAL LEAGUE OF CERTIFICATED NURSES OF GREAT BRITAIN AND IRELAND
Constitution. *Nursing Record*, Jan. 19, 1901, p. 47.

NATIONAL LEAGUE OF NURSING EDUCATION
The story of the National League of Nursing Education, by Helen W. Munson and Katharine Stevens. Philadelphia, Saunders, 1934.

NATIONAL NURSING COUNCIL. HISTORY COMMITTEE
The history of the National Nursing Council, by Hope Newell. [New York], National Nursing Council, [1948].

NATIONAL PENSION FUND
Foundation and prospectus, with editorial comment. *Nursing Record*, April 12, 1888, p. 16; April 19, 1888, p. 27-30; April 26, 1888, p. 38-39; May 17, 1888, p. 75-6.

NATIONAL UNION OF TRAINED NURSES
A history of the National Union of Trained Nurses. N.U.T.N., 1927.

NEBRASKA STATE NURSES' ASSOCIATION
The first fifty years, 1906-1956; edited by Lona L. Trott. [Omaha], Nebraska State Nurses' Association, 1956.

NEW SOUTH WALES TRAINED NURSES' ASSOCIATION
Constitution. *Nursing Record*, Dec. 2, 1899, p. 459-60.

NEWSTEAD, W. K.
Professional organizations and the trained mental nurse. *Nursing Times*, Nov. 8, 1957, p. 1271-2.

NURSES' ASSOCIATED ALUMNAE OF THE UNITED STATES AND CANADA
Constitution and bye-laws. *Nursing Record*, Aug. 21, 1897, p. 146-8, and Aug. 28, 1897, p. 167-9.

NURSES' ASSOCIATION OF CHINA
Constitution. *British Journal of Nursing*, Sept. 9, 1922, p. 166-8; Sept. 16, 1922, p. 186; Sept. 23, 1922, p. 200-1.

OKLAHOMA STATE NURSES' ASSOCIATION
History of the Oklahoma State Nurses' Association, n.d.

PROFESSIONAL UNION OF TRAINED NURSES
Inaugural meeting. *British Journal of Nursing*, Nov. 1, 1919, p. 263-70.

REGISTERED NURSES' PARLIAMENTARY COUNCIL
Constitution and articles. *British Journal of Nursing*, May 6, 1922, p. 282-3.

ROBB, ISABEL HAMPTON
The possibilities of alumnae associations. *Nursing Record*, Jan. 30, 1897, p. 90-1, and Feb. 6, 1897, p. 111-2.

ROYAL BRITISH NURSES' ASSOCIATION
Case in opposition to the petition [for a Royal Charter] of the R.B.N.A., by R. B. Finlay and L. S. Bristowe. *Nursing Record*, Dec. 15, 1892, p. 1020-7.

ROYAL BRITISH NURSES' ASSOCIATION
Draft charter. *Nursing Record*, Mar. 17, 1892, p. 221-6.

ROYAL BRITISH NURSES' ASSOCIATION
Editorial commemorating the change of name. *Nursing Record*, Feb. 12, 1891, p. 73-5.

ROYAL BRITISH NURSES' ASSOCIATION
Existing bye-laws and proposed new bye-laws with comments by the Members Rights Defence Committee. *Nursing Record*, Feb. 5, 1898, p. 114-5; Feb. 12, 1898, p. 134; Feb. 19, 1898, p. 154-5; Feb. 26, 1898, p. 174-6; Mar. 5, 1898, p. 195-6.

ROYAL BRITISH NURSES' ASSOCIATION
1. From the point of view of Her Royal Highness the President, by H.R.H. Princess Christian. *Nursing Record*, Oct. 7, 1893, p. 151-2.
2. From the point of view of a medical man, by W. Bezly Thorne. *Nursing Record*, Oct. 14, 1893, p. 171-2.
3. From the point of view of a hospital matron, by Ethel Gordon Fenwick. *Nursing Record*, Oct. 21, 1893, p. 187-8.
4. From the point of view of a trained nurse, by Henrietta Kenealy. *Nursing Record*, Oct. 28, 1893, p. 203-5.
5. From the point of view of a hospital manager, by W. H. Cross. *Nursing Record*, Nov. 4, 1893, p. 219-20.
6. From the point of view of a member, by Marian Humfrey. *Nursing Record*, Nov. 11, 1893, p. 235-6.
7. From the point of view of one of the public, by Mary Jeune. *Nursing Record*, Nov. 18, 1893, p. 251-2.

ROYAL BRITISH NURSES' ASSOCIATION
The latest attempt to stifle free speech. Correspondence between Margaret Breay and the Secretary. *Nursing Record*, Aug. 1, 1896, p. 84-6. Further correspondence, *Nursing Record*, Aug. 29, 1896, p. 178.

ROYAL BRITISH NURSES' ASSOCIATION
Petition of a charter, and account of the proceedings before the Privy Council. *Nursing Record*, Nov. 24, 1892, p. 942-63; Dec. 1, 1892, p. 966-88.

ROYAL BRITISH NURSES' ASSOCIATION
Petition to the Privy Council against the mismanagement of the R.B.N.A., by the Incorporated Medical Practitioners' Association. *Nursing Record*, April 9, 1898, p. 294-5.

ROYAL BRITISH NURSES' ASSOCIATION
Royal Charter. *Nursing Record*, June 15, 1893, p. 295-8.

ROYAL BRITISH NURSES' ASSOCIATION
A short history of the Association: prepared as a memento for the members of the Festival of Britain Study Tour for Nurses, Sept. 12th, 1951.

ROYAL BRITISH NURSES' ASSOCIATION
Special general meeting to discuss a report on the negotiations between the Association and the College of Nursing. *British Journal of Nursing*, Dec. 22, 1917, p. 413-6.

ROYAL BRITISH NURSES' ASSOCIATION *and* COLLEGE OF NURSING
Draft supplemental charter, and as amended by the Lords of the Privy Council, and correspondence between the Solicitors of the Corporation and the Clerk of the Council. *British Journal of Nursing*, Nov. 10, 1917, p. 302-4.

ROYAL COLLEGE OF NURSING
The College and the future. *Nursing Times*, May 22, 1959, p. 595 and 605-6.

ROYAL COLLEGE OF NURSING
The College of Nursing and Cowdray Club. The College, [1927].

ROYAL COLLEGE OF NURSING
The College of Nursing, its history and progress. The College, [193?].

ROYAL COLLEGE OF NURSING
The Council: its Standing Committees, Scottish Board and Northern Ireland Committee. *Nursing Times*, June 22, 1956, p. 569-75.
[*see also* COLLEGE OF NURSING].

ROYAL NATIONAL PENSION FUND FOR NURSES
Stream of time: the story of the Royal National Pension Fund for Nurses, 1887-1937. The Fund, [1937].

ROYAL NATIONAL PENSION FUND FOR NURSES
Ministering women: the story of the Royal National Pension Fund for Nurses, by George William Potter. The Hospital, 1891.

SMITH, F. C.
The International Council of Nurses, the American Nurses' Association and the United Nations. *American Journal of Nursing*, Jan. 1959, p. 83.

SOCIETY FOR THE STATE REGISTRATION OF TRAINED NURSES
The humble petition of the nurses to the King in Council re the petition of the Royal British Nurses' Association for a supplemental charter and new bye-laws. *British Journal of Nursing*, Oct. 6, 1917, p. 216-9.

SOCIETY FOR THE STATE REGISTRATION OF TRAINED NURSES
Inauguration and constitution. *Nursing Record*, June 7, 1902, p. 452-3.

SOCIETY OF CHARTERED NURSES
Circumstances of its formation. *Nursing Record*, April 11, 1896, p. 292-3.

"SPECTATOR", *pseud*.
Nursing organizations. 1. The past. 2. The future? *Nursing Times*, Feb. 26, 1960, p. 241-2, and Mar. 4, 1960, p. 279-80.

TENNESSEE STATE NURSES' ASSOCIATION
A history of the Tennessee State Nurses' Association, by Nina E. Wootton and Golden Williams. Nashville, Tenn., Trained Nurses' Assn., 1955.

TEXAS GRADUATE NURSES' ASSOCIATION
History of the Texas Graduate Nurses' Association organised at Fort Worth, Texas, Feb. 22, 1907. Fort Worth, Texas, The Association, 1931.

VERMONT STATE NURSES' ASSOCIATION
We who serve: a story of nursing in Vermont. Vermont, The Association, 1941.

VICTORIAN ORDER OF NURSES FOR CANADA
The Victorian Order of Nurses for Canada: 50th anniversary, 1897-1947, by John Murray Gibbon.

VICTORIAN ORDER OF NURSES FOR CANADA
The Victorian Order of Nurses for Canada, by M. C. Livingston. *Nursing Outlook*, Jan. 1958, p. 42-4.

VICTORIAN TRAINED NURSES' ASSOCIATION
Constitution. *British Journal of Nursing*, Sept. 20, 1902, p. 234-6.

VISITING NURSE ASSOCIATION OF DETROIT
Thirty-fifth anniversary of the Visiting Nurse Association of Detroit, 1898-1933. 1934?

WASHINGTON STATE NURSES' ASSOCIATION
Fifty years of progress, 1908-1958; written by Noreen Salvino Kimerer. Seattle, Washington State Nurses' Association, [1958].

WEST VIRGINIA STATE NURSES' ASSOCIATION
A half-century of nursing in West Virginia: the history of the West Virginia State Nurses' Association, 1907-1957, by Donovan H. Bond. Charleston?, West Virginia State Nurses' Assn., [1957].

WEST VIRGINIA STATE NURSES' ASSOCIATION
Thirty-five years of the West Virginia State Nurses' Association: a history of nursing in West Virginia. Material compiled by M. E. Reid and ed. by M. J. Steele. Charleston, West Virginia State Nurses' Assn., 1941.

WISCONSIN STATE NURSES' ASSOCIATION
An historical sketch. [Madison], The Association, 1935.

NURSING JOURNALS AND THEIR HISTORY

ALFORD, BARBARA L.
Nursing journals in Norway, Sweden and Denmark. *South African Nursing Journal*, June 1959, p. 6-7 and 9.

AMERICAN JOURNAL OF NURSING
The story of the American Journal of Nursing. New York, *American Journal of Nursing*, 1940.

BEATTY, W. K.
Needed: an index to nursing journals. *Nursing Outlook*, Oct. 1959, p. 569.

BEEBY, N. V.
The world's nursing journals. *International Nursing Review*, July 1958, p. 57-67.

NURSING LEGISLATION

GENERAL WORKS

CARROLL, M. F.
Planning for nursing legislation. *International Nursing Review*, Feb. 1960, p. 29-31.

WORLD HEALTH ORGANIZATION
Nursing, a survey of recent legislation. Geneva, W.H.O., 1953.

AUSTRALIA

QUEENSLAND
The Nurses and Masseurs Registration Act, 1928 to 1948, and Regulations. Brisbane, Tucker, Govt. Printer, 1957. [Compiled to June 30, 1957.]

SOUTH AUSTRALIA, PARLIAMENT
Nurses' Registration Act, 1920. Adelaide, Govt. Printer, 1920.

TASMANIA
Mothercraft Nurses' Registration Act, 1947.
Mothercraft Nurses' Registration Regulations, 1948.
Hobart, Tasmania, Pimblett, Govt. Printer.

TASMANIA
Regulations under the Nurses' Registration Act, 1927. Tasmania, 1951.
Nurses' Registration (No. 10 of 1952).
Nurses' Registration (No. 73 of 1954).
Nurses' Registration (No. 3 of 1958).
Tasmania, Shea, Govt. Printer.

TASMANIA
Tasmanian Auxiliary Nursing Service (No. 37 of 1949) and Amendment (No. 74 of 1954).
Tasmanian Auxiliary Nursing Service Regulations, 1950, and Amendments.
Tasmanian Auxiliary Nursing Service Amendment Regulations, 1957.
Tasmanian Auxiliary Nursing Service, No. 5 of 1957.
Tasmanian Auxiliary Nursing Service (No. 2), No. 49 of 1957.

VICTORIA [AUSTRALIA] PARLIAMENT
Nurses Act, 1956.

WESTERN AUSTRALIA
Nurses' registration; an act to provide for the registration of trained nurses and for other relative purposes. [Perth, 1922.]
Amendments to Act: (No. 61 of 1953), 1921-52.
(No. 33 of 1956), 1921-53.
(No. 19 of 1957), 1921-56.
(No. 64 of 1957), 1921-56.

CANADA

FIDLER, N. D., *and* GRAY, K. G.
Law and the practice of nursing. Toronto, Ryerson Press, 1947.

WAHN, E. V.
Some legal obligations of the professional nurse. *Canadian Hospital*, July 1960, p. 56-8, and Aug. 1960, p. 45-6.

LATIN AMERICA

CHAGAS, A. W.
Notes on nursing legislation in Latin America. *International Nursing Review*, Feb. 1960, p. 32-5.

NEW ZEALAND

NEW ZEALAND. PARLIAMENT
Hospital Employment Regulations, 1957.
Hospital Employment (Nurses) Regulations, 1957.
Hospital Employment (Nurses) Regulations, 1957, Amendment No. 1.
Wellington, Owen, Govt. Printer, 1957.

NEW ZEALAND. PARLIAMENT
The Nurses' Registration Regulations, 1958. Wellington, Owen, Govt. Printer, 1958.

NEW ZEALAND. PARLIAMENT
Regulations under the Nurses and Midwives Registration Act, 1925. Wellington, Govt. Printer, 1926.

SOUTH AFRICA

BORCHERDS, M. G.
The South African Nursing Act. *International Nursing Review*, July 1958, p. 33-43.

LANCET
Apartheid in nursing. *The Lancet*, June 8, 1957, p. 1182.

PRICE, T. W.
Law notes for nurses and midwives in South Africa. Pretoria, The South African Nursing Association, 1958. [Afrikaans translation at end of pamphlet.]

SOUTH AFRICAN NURSING COUNCIL
Comparison between the 1944 and 1957 (South African) Nursing Acts, indicating the major changes which have taken place. *South African Nursing Journal*, Aug. 1957, p. 10-14.

SOUTH AFRICAN NURSING COUNCIL
Main differences between Nursing Acts of 1944 and 1957 (excluding parts dealing with South African Nursing Association). *South African Nursing Journal*, Jan. 1958, p. 10 and 12.

UNION OF SOUTH AFRICA. SENATE AND HOUSE OF ASSEMBLY
Act to consolidate and amend the laws in force in the Union relating to medical practitioners, dentists, chemists and druggists, nurses, midwives, masseurs and other classes of persons; the keeping and sale of poisons. . . . No. 13, 1928.
[Text in English and Afrikaans.]

UNION OF SOUTH AFRICA. SENATE AND HOUSE OF ASSEMBLY
Act to consolidate and amend the law relating to the exercise of the calling of a nurse or midwife and other incidental matters. No. 69, 1957.
[Called "The Nursing Act 1957". Text in English and Afrikaans.]

UNION OF SOUTH AFRICA. SENATE AND HOUSE OF ASSEMBLY
The Nursing Act, No. 45 of 1944, as amended by Act
No. 12 of 1946, together with extracts from Act No. 13 of
1928. South African Nursing Council, 1946.

UNION OF SOUTH AFRICA. SENATE AND HOUSE OF ASSEMBLY,
SELECT COMMITTEE ON THE SUBJECT OF THE NURSING
AMENDMENT BILL Report. Parow, Cape, Cape
Times, 1957.

UNITED KINGDOM OF GREAT BRITAIN AND NORTHERN IRELAND

EDDY, J. P.
Professional negligence. Stevens, 1955.

EVANS, S. J. H.
The legal liability of nurses in the course of professional
duties. *Nursing Times*, Feb. 20, 1954, p. 201-2.

FORBES, R.
Professional responsibility.
1. The student nurse. *Nursing Times*, Feb. 2, 1952, p.
105-6.
2. Registered nurse. *Nursing Times*, Mar. 8, 1952, p.
232-3.
3. Preventing burns. *Nursing Times*, April 12, 1952, p.
371-2.
4. Injection therapy. *Nursing Times*, May 10, 1952, p.
463-4.
5. Professional confidence. *Nursing Times*, June 14, 1952,
p. 590-1.
6. Theatre duties. *Nursing Times*, July 12, 1952, p. 681-3.
7. Terms and conditions of employment. *Nursing Times*,
Aug. 16, 1952, p. 798-9.
8. Infection. *Nursing Times*, Sept. 13, 1952, p. 901-2.
9. Employer and employee. *Nursing Times*, Oct. 11, 1952,
p. 1001-2.
10. In the witness box. *Nursing Times*, Nov. 8, 1952, p.
1102-4.

FRIEDMAN, G. A.
The nurse and the law. *Medical Times*, June 1958, p.
788-94.

GORSKY, J. A.
Some medico-legal aspects of district nursing practice—1.
Nursing Mirror, Oct. 25, 1957, p. 281-2.

GORSKY, J. A.
Some medico-legal aspects of district nursing practice—2.
Nursing Mirror, Nov. 1, 1957, p. 355-6.

GORSKY, J. A.
Some medico-legal aspects of district nursing practice—3.
Nursing Mirror, Nov. 8, 1957, p. 443-4.

THE HOSPITAL
Nursing or medicine (delegation of duties and the nurse's
responsibility). *Hospital*, Nov. 1958, p. 779-81.

NORTHERN IRELAND. PARLIAMENT
Joint Nursing and Midwives Council Act (Northern
Ireland), 1922. Belfast, Govt. Printer, [1922].

NORTHERN IRELAND. PARLIAMENT
Nurses and Midwives Act (Northern Ireland), 1959.
Belfast, H.M.S.O., 1959.

PARLIAMENT
Nurses Registration Act, 1919. H.M.S.O., 1919.

PARLIAMENT
Nurses Act, 1943. H.M.S.O., 1943.

PARLIAMENT
Nurses Act, 1945. H.M.S.O., 1945.

PARLIAMENT
Nurses Act, 1949. H.M.S.O., 1949.

PARLIAMENT
Nurses Act, 1957. H.M.S.O., 1957.

PARLIAMENT
Nurses Agencies Act, 1957. H.M.S.O., 1957.

PARLIAMENT
Nurses' Registration (Ireland) Act, 1919. H.M.S.O., 1919.

PARLIAMENT
Nurses' Registration (Scotland) Act, 1919. H.M.S.O.,
1919.

PARLIAMENT
Nurses (Scotland) Act, 1943. H.M.S.O., 1943.

PARLIAMENT
Nurses (Scotland) Act, 1949. H.M.S.O., 1949.

PARLIAMENT
Nurses (Scotland) Act, 1951. H.M.S.O., 1951.

SELECT COMMITTEE ON REGISTRATION OF NURSES
Report. H.M.S.O., 1905.

SPELLER, S. R.
Injections by nurses. *Hospital*, Feb. 1954, p. 97-9.

SPELLER, S. R.
Law for nurses and nurse-administrators. Lewis, 1940.

SPELLER, S. R.
Law notes for nurses. Royal College of Nursing, 1954.
2nd edn., 1956, with a supplement for Scotland, by R. A.
Bennett.

SPELLER, S. R.
The nurse and the law. *International Nursing Review*,
April 1955, p. 20-4.

UNITED STATES OF AMERICA

AMERICAN ASSOCIATION OF NURSE ANAESTHETISTS
Notes on legal aspects of anaesthesia by nurses. Chicago,
The Association, 1950.

AMERICAN MEDICAL ASSOCIATION—COUNCIL ON
INDUSTRIAL HEALTH
The legal scope of industrial nursing practice. *J.A.M.A.*,
Mar. 7, 1959, p. 1072-5.

BARBEE, G. C.
Changing nurse patterns produce changing professional
liability patterns. I. *Hospital Management*, Aug. 1958,
p. 110. II. *Hospital Management*, Sept. 1958, p. 108-10.

CREIGHTON, HELEN
Law every nurse should know. Philadelphia, Saunders,
1957.

CREIGHTON, HELEN
Your liability in off-duty first aid. *R.N.*, May 1959, p. 36.

DESPRES, L. M.
What is a contract? *American Journal of Nursing*, Oct.
1958, p. 1403-4.

HARRISON, GENE
The nurse and the law. . . . Philadelphia, Davis, 1945.
2nd edn., 1948.

HAYT, EMANUEL, *and* HAYT, L. R.
Law of hospital and nurse. New York, Hospital Textbook
Co., 1947.
2nd edn., 1952.
3rd edn., 1958.

JACOBSEN, MARGUERITE, ANDERSON, BERNICE E., *and*
GIVEN, LELIA I.
Legislation manual for committees on legislation of State
Nurses' Associations of the American Nurses' Association.
New York, The Association, 1950.

LESNICK, MILTON J., *and* ANDERSON, BERNICE E.
Legal aspects of nursing. Philadelphia, Lippincott, 1947.

LESNICK, MILTON J., *and* ANDERSON, BERNICE E.
Nursing practice and the law. Philadelphia, Lippincott,
1955.
[Previously called "Legal aspects of nursing", pub. 1947.]

REGAN, W. A.
Nurses and the law. *Hospital Progress*, Dec. 1959, p. 77-8.

SCHEFFEL, CARL
Jurisprudence for nurses: legal knowledge bearing upon
Acts, and relationships involved in the practice of nursing.
New York, Lakeside Publishing Co., 1931.
2nd edn., 1938.
3rd edn., 1945, by C. Scheffel and Eleanor McGarvan.

SCOTT, WILLIAM C., and SMITH, DONALD W.
The Taft-Hartley Act and the nurse. *American Journal of Nursing*, Dec. 1956, p. 1556-8.

TERENZIO, J. V.
The O.R. nurse and the law. 1. *Hospitals*, Oct. 16, 1956, p. 34-6. 2. *Hospitals*, Nov. 1, 1956, p. 52-3.

TERENZIO, J. V.
Some legal aspects of evening and night nursing supervision. *Nursing Outlook*, Nov. 1956, p. 606-9.

SALARIES AND CONDITIONS OF WORK

GENERAL WORKS

AKESTER, J. M.
Student or apprentice? *Nursing Times*, June 12, 1959, p. 681-2.

ANDERSON, B. E.
The question of student employment. *American Journal of Nursing*, Nov. 1959, p. 1575-9.

COLLEGE OF NURSING
Scale of minimum salaries recommended by the College of Nursing, with editorial comment. *British Journal of Nursing*, Jan. 15, 1921, p. 29.

CONTA, A. LIONNE
What happens at the bargaining table? *American Journal of Nursing*, Oct. 1959, p. 1436-8.

DEVEREUX, GEORGE, and WEINER, F. R.
The occupational status of nurses. *American Sociological Review*, vol. 15, 1950, p. 628-34.

GARDNER, MARY
"State aid" as it would affect nurses. *British Journal of Nursing*, Nov. 25, 1911, p. 429-30.

GRIFFITH, O.
Hours of duty for mental nurses. *Nursing Times*, Dec. 27, 1957, p. 1477-8.

HOLLAND, SYDNEY
A charter of liberty for nurses: hours of hospital nurses. *Nursing Record*, Nov. 21, 1896, p. 414-5.

INTERNATIONAL COUNCIL OF NURSES
Report of the Economic Consultant to the President and Members of the Board of Directors and Grand Council of the International Council of Nurses, Rome, May 1957. [The Council, 1957?].

INTERNATIONAL COUNCIL OF NURSES. ECONOMIC WELFARE COMMITTEE
Report of the Economic Welfare Committee to the President and Members of the Board of Directors and Grand Council of the International Council of Nurses, Sao Paulo, Brazil, July 1953. The Council, 1953.

INTERNATIONAL LABOUR ORGANIZATION
Employment and conditions of work of nurses. Geneva, I.L.O., 1960.

MACANDREW, CRAIG
The nurse's image of just and equitable wages. *Nursing Research*, Summer 1960, p. 156-7.

MASTERMAN, C.
A new approach to nurses' accommodation. *Hospital and Health Management*, Aug. 1956, p. 212.

MASTERMAN, C.
Nurses' accommodation. Experiment in conversion. *Nursing Times*, Oct. 19, 1956, p. 1053-4 and 1059.

NETHERLANDS CONSULTING CENTRE FOR HOSPITAL PLANNING
New type of residential building for nurses and hospital domestic staff. *Nursing Mirror*, Feb. 14, 1958, p. 1463-4.

NURSING TIMES
Student nurses' opinions. *Nursing Times*, Feb. 22, 1957, p. 203-4.

ROSSITER, E.
A statement regarding labor relations. *Canadian Nurse*, Sept. 1957, p. 799.

UDELL, F.
The economic status of nurses. *International Nursing Review*, July 1958, p. 8-11.

WHITNEY, F.
Is nursing meeting its obligation to society. *American Journal of Nursing*, Sept. 1956, p. 1127-31.

AUSTRALIA

AUSTRALIA
Deputation to the Premier of Victoria, Australia, on the hours of hospital nurses. *Nursing Record*, Sept. 12, 1896, p. 213-5.

NEW SOUTH WALES ASSEMBLY
Debate on eight-hour day for nurses, report from the *Sydney Telegraph*. *Nursing Record*, Oct. 16, 1897, p. 313-5.

CANADA

BALL, RITA M.
Our nurses plan their time. *Canadian Nurse*, Dec. 1960, p. 1086-7.

BEAUDIN, N. R.
The C.N.A. retirement plan becomes a reality. *Canadian Nurse*, April 1959, p. 329-30.

INDIA

INDIA. MINISTRY OF HEALTH. COMMITTEE TO REVIEW CONDITIONS OF SERVICE, EMOLUMENTS, ETC., OF THE NURSING PROFESSION
Report. New Delhi, Government of India Press, 1955.

UNITED KINGDOM OF GREAT BRITAIN AND NORTHERN IRELAND

AUSTEN, A.
The 44-hour week. [Mayday Hospital, Croydon.] *Nursing Times*, Sept. 5, 1958, p. 1044.

DAVIES, M. E.
Nurses' and Midwives' Whitley Council: how it works. *Nursing Times*, July 4, 1958, p. 778-80, and July 25, 1958, p. 867-8.

FEDERATED SUPERANNUATION SCHEME FOR NURSES AND HOSPITAL OFFICERS (CONTRIBUTORY)
A scheme providing pensions or other similar benefits for nurses, hospital officers and the eligible employees of voluntary hospitals and kindred charitable institutions. *The Scheme*, 1931.

HARDMAN, E.
Royal Free Hospital Scheme. (The 44-hour week.) *Nursing Times*, Sept. 25, 1959, p. 902-3.

KING, V. G.
Introducing the 44-hour week. [Whiteabbey Hospital, Co. Antrim.] *Nursing Mirror*, Nov. 18, 1960, p. 629 and 632.

LEWIS, IVOR
Nurses' hours: an experiment with the 48-hour week and 8-hour day in a large general hospital. *The Hospital*, 1938. [Reprinted from *The Hospital*, Feb. 1938.]

MERRITT, W.
Why not a 38-hour week for nurses? *Health Services Journal*, Jan.-Feb. 1959, p. 5.

MINISTRY OF HEALTH. NURSES' SALARIES COMMITTEE
First report: salaries and emoluments of female nurses in hospitals. H.M.S.O., 1943.
[Chairman: Lord Rushcliffe.]

MINISTRY OF HEALTH. NURSES' SALARIES COMMITTEE
Second report: salaries and emoluments of male nurses, public health nurses and state registered nurses in nurseries. H.M.S.O., 1943.
[Chairman: Lord Rushcliffe.]

MINISTRY OF HEALTH. NURSES' SALARIES COMMITTEE
Points of interpretation arising from the recommendations made by the Committee and revised recommendations regarding certain grades of nurses. H.M.S.O., 1943-48.
[S.C. Notes Nos. 1, 2, 3, 4, 5, 6, 7, 8, 9, 10, 11, 12, 13, 14, 15, 16, 17, 18. (No. 15 consolidated recommendations.)]

MINISTRY OF HEALTH. NURSES' SALARIES COMMITTEE
Supplement to first report . . . notes on application of scales of salary (with examples) for the guidance of hospital authorities. H.M.S.O., 1943.

MINISTRY OF HEALTH. NURSES' SALARIES COMMITTEE.
MENTAL NURSES' SUB-COMMITTEE.
Report. H.M.S.O., 1944.
[Chairman: Lord Rushcliffe.]

MINISTRY OF HEALTH. NURSES' SALARIES COMMITTEE.
MENTAL NURSES' SUB-COMMITTEE
Further recommendations. Notes Nos. 1-10. H.M.S.O., 1945-48.

MINISTRY OF LABOUR
Inquiry to discuss the inclusion of various grades of nurses in hospitals in the Unemployment Insurance Act. *British Journal of Nursing*, Jan. 15, 1921, p. 36-7.

NATIONAL COUNCIL OF WOMEN OF GREAT BRITAIN AND IRELAND
Report of the special committee on the economic position of nurses. *British Journal of Nursing*, Sept. 27, 1919, p. 189-94.

NORBURY, F.
Forty-four-hour week modified shift system. Holloway Sanatorium, Virginia Water. *Nursing Mirror*, Nov. 21, 1958, p. 589-90.

NORTHERN IRELAND. PARLIAMENT
Report of the General Nurses' Committee for Northern Ireland on salaries and conditions of service of nurses and midwives in hospitals (other than mental hospitals). Belfast, H.M.S.O., 1947.

ROBINSON, M.
The 44-hour week. (Maudsley Hospital.) *Nursing Times*, Sept. 12, 1958, p. 1064.

ROYAL COLLEGE OF NURSING. PUBLIC HEALTH SECTION
The Nurses' and Midwives' Whitley Council. Royal College of Nursing, [1948].

SCOTLAND. DEPARTMENT OF HEALTH
NURSES' SALARIES COMMITTEE
Interim report. Edinburgh, H.M.S.O., 1943.
[Chairman: Professor T. M. Taylor.]

SCOTLAND. DEPARTMENT OF HEALTH.
NURSES' SALARIES COMMITTEE
Second report. Edinburgh, H.M.S.O., 1943.
[Chairman: Professor T. M. Taylor.]

SCOTLAND. DEPARTMENT OF HEALTH.
NURSES' SALARIES COMMITTEE
Third report (supplement to the second report). Edinburgh, H.M.S.O., 1944.
[Chairman: Professor T. M. Taylor.]

STAMP, M.
The 44-hour week: trial scheme at Torbay Hospital. *Nursing Times*, Nov. 14, 1958, p. 1335.

THOMPSON, P. M.
Night duty. Harrogate & District Hospital. *Nursing Times*, Nov. 7, 1958, p. 1316-8.

TOLMON, J.
Forty-four-hour week. Straight shift system at Sefton General Hospital, Liverpool. *Nursing Times*, Dec. 5, 1958, p. 1424-5.

WALTON, A. M.
Forty-four-hour week. Scheme at Brompton Hospital, London. *Nursing Times*, Dec. 12, 1958, p. 1460.

WATKIN, B.
British nurses plan a shorter work week. *Nursing Outlook*, Oct. 1959, p. 588-90.

UNITED STATES OF AMERICA

AMERICAN NURSES' ASSOCIATION
Study of incomes, salaries and employment conditions affecting nurses (exclusive of those engaged in public health nursing). New York, American Nurses' Association, 1938.

COMMITTEE ON THE GRADING OF NURSING SCHOOLS
Nurses, patients and pocketbooks: a report of a study of the economics of nursing; May Ayres Burges, director. New York, The Committee, 1928.

COMMITTEE ON THE GRADING OF NURSING SCHOOLS
Nurses' production, education, distribution and pay. New York, The Committee, 1930.

COMMUNITY COUNCIL OF GREATER NEW YORK.
RESEARCH DEPARTMENT
Salaries and related personnel practices in voluntary social and health agencies in New York City, September 1958. New York, The Council, 1959.

LEOPOLD, ALICE K., *and* GLAGUE, EWAN
The B.L.S. survey of nurses' salaries and supplementary benefits, made in co-operation with the Women's Bureau of the U.S. Dept. of Labor. New York, *American Journal of Nursing*, 1958.
[Reprinted from *A.J.N.*, vol. 58, Sept. 1958.]

NATIONAL LEAGUE OF NURSING EDUCATION.
DEPARTMENT OF STUDIES
Annual salaries and salary increases and allowance paid to general staff nurses: a study. New York, American Nurses' Association, 1943.

UNITED STATES. WOMEN'S BUREAU
Nurses and other hospital personnel: their earnings and employment conditions. U.S. Dept. of Labor, 1958.

UNITED STATES DEPARTMENT OF LABOR.
BUREAU OF LABOR STATISTICS
The economic status of registered professional nurses, 1946-47. Washington, Govt. Printing Office, [1948].

WOLFSON, T.
Another look at the A.N.A. economic security program. *American Journal of Nursing*, Oct. 1957, p. 1287-9.

HEALTH AND WELFARE

GENERAL WORKS

AMERICAN HOSPITAL ASSOCIATION *and others*
A study of the incidence and costs of illness amongst nurses: [a report by] a Joint Committee of Nursing Service and Nursing Education of the American Hospital Association, National League of Nursing Education and the American Nurses' Association. New York, The Joint Committee, 1938.

ANDREWES, F. W.
The health of nurses. *Nursing Times*, Aug. 12, 1905, p. 262-4.

BARR, A.
Hospital size and staff sickness rates. *British Journal of Preventive and Social Medicine*, July 1958, p. 156-8.

BARR, A.
Sickness absence among hospital nurses. *British Journal of Preventive and Social Medicine*, April 1960, p. 89-98.

BELL, D.
When a nurse has diabetes. *Canadian Nurse*, Aug. 1956, p. 627-30.

BRANSON, H. K.
The physically handicapped nurse. *Hospital Management*, June 1959, p. 102 *passim*.

BREAY, MARGARET
The overstrain of nurses. *British Journal of Nursing*, Oct. 26, 1912, p. 330-2.

BURDETT, HENRY C.
Nurses' food, work and hours of recreation. Hospital Association, 1890.
[Appendix D to 2nd report of the Select Committee of the House of Lords Committee on Metropolitan Hospitals, 1891.]

COUNIHAN, H. E.
BCG vaccination and student nurses. *Industrial Medicine and Surgery*, Oct. 1956, p. 496-7.

COWEN, E. D. H.
An account of the health of nurses at Westminster Hospital from July 1943 to July 1946. *Journal of Hygiene*, 1947.
[Reprinted from the *Journal of Hygiene*, vol. 45, no. 4, Dec. 1947.]

DAVIES, J. O., *and* BARR, A.
Sickness and non-sickness absence among nurses. *Monthly Bulletin of the Ministry of Health and the Public Health Laboratory Service*, Aug. 1956, p. 158-94.

ELLENBERG, M.
Diabetic applicants to nursing schools. *Nursing Outlook*, Nov. 1958, p. 626-7.

FARRELL, M.
Hospital employees get sick too. Nurses, interns, technicians—all personnel benefit from a service which includes health maintenance and pre-employment measures. *American Journal of Nursing*, Nov. 1960, p. 1622-5.

HATHAWAY, J. S., BROWN, M. L., *and* MEIGS, J. W.
The role of the nurse in the preventive services of a student health clinic. 1. A preliminary report. *Student Medicine*, Dec. 1960, p. 137-41.

HECKER, H.
The overstrain of nurses: an address delivered . . . to the International Council of Nurses, Cologne 1912. Translated from the German by Caius Praetorius and Anita Becker. [I.C.N., 1912.]

HICKS, W. J.
Sickness in nursing staff. *Nursing Mirror*, May 15, 1959, p. 517-8.

INTERNATIONAL COUNCIL OF NURSES
Report of the Health Statistics Committee presented at the Congress in London, July 1937. International Council of Nurses, [1937].

JOINT COMMITTEE OF NURSING SERVICE AND NURSING EDUCATION
A study of the incidence and costs of illness amongst nurses. New York, The Committee, 1938.

KING EDWARD'S HOSPITAL FUND FOR LONDON
Memorandum on the supervision of nurses' health for consideration by hospitals. The Fund, 1943.
2nd edn., 1950.

LABECKI, G., *and* MERROW, S.
How wisely do students select their diets? *Nursing Outlook*, Aug. 1959, p. 471-3.

LANCET
The unvaccinated nurse. *Lancet*, April 7, 1956, p. 372-3.

LEVY, L., LEVIN, D., SARWER-FONER, G. J., *and* DANCEY, T. E.
A technique for lessening tension among general hospital nurses. *Medical Services Journal*, April 1959, p. 264-8.

LIPTON, M. B., ROCKBERGER, H., *and* EFRON, H. Y.
The screening of student psychiatric nurses by means of a group projective inventory. *Psychiatric Quarterly Supplement*, 1955, p. 197-208.

MELLOR, M. D.
The medical care of the student nurse. *Canadian Nurse*, April 1958, p. 305-6.

MUSSON, E. M.
The feeding of nurses in hospitals. *Nursing Times*, Nov. 12, 1910, p. 947-54.

NURSING MIRROR. COMMITTEE ON OVERTAXED NURSES
Overtaxed nurses: report of a committee set up by the Nursing Mirror to consider correspondence appearing in that journal between September and November 1954. *Nursing Mirror*, 1957.

OXFORD REGIONAL HOSPITAL BOARD
The health of the hospital nurse: final report on the sickness absence among hospital nurses during the year ending 31st March, 1957. Oxford, The Board, 1959.

PERRY, H.
Nurses' Health Service. *Canadian Nurse*, April 1958, p. 306-9.

TOBIN, M. J.
Health and sickness of nursing staff. *Nursing Times*, July 18, 1958, p. 827-30.

ACCOMMODATION FOR NURSES

ASHBY, LUCY E.
The "living-in" controversy. *Nursing Times*, Nov. 7, 1908, p. 881.

BRYAN, MARY DE GARMO
Furnishings and equipment for residence halls, by M. de G. Bryan and Etta M. Hardy. New York, Columbia University Teachers' College, 1933.

GOLDFINCH, D. A.
Design of a nurses' home. *Hospital*, Jan. 1952, p. 13-17.

MARKUS, F. E.
Swiss nurses' residence was designed with the residents in mind. *Hospitals*, Feb. 16, 1960, p. 47-9.

NURSES' HOUSE, INC.
The story of Nurses' House at Babylon, Long Island. New York, 1954.

STEPHEN, SISTER
Residence living—necessity or tradition? *Hospital Progress*, April 1960, p. 86-8.

DERMATITIS IN NURSES

DANTO, JULIUS L., STEWART, WILLIAM D., *and*
MADDIN, STUART
Bed-pan hands. *Canadian Nurse*, June 1960, p. 510-1.

HOWELLS, G.
Prevention of streptomycin dermatitis in nurses. *Lancet*, May 26, 1956, p. 780-1.

HOWELLS, G.
Streptomycin dermatitis—its prevention in nurses and the desensitization of the sensitized. *Nursing Times*, Mar. 22, 1957, p. 318-20.

MARTIN-SCOTT, I.
The care of the nurse's skin. *Nursing Mirror*, Mar. 15, 1957, p. 1741-2.

SCHWEISHEIMER, W.
Dermatitis among nurses. *Canadian Nurse*, Sept. 1951, p. 661-3.

WILSON, H. T. H.
Streptomycin dermatitis in nurses. *British Medical Journal*, June 14, 1958, p. 1378-82.

INFECTIONS IN NURSES

BRODIE, J., and others
Coagulese-positive staphylococci: a serial survey for nasal carriers during the first six months of nursing training. *British Medical Journal*, Mar. 24, 1956, p. 667-9.

DAIKOS, G. K., and others
Benign myalgic encephalomyelitis: an outbreak in a nurses' school in Athens. *Lancet*, April 4, 1959, p. 693-6.

DAVIES, D. M.
Staphylococcal infection in nurses. *Lancet*, Mar. 19, 1960, p. 644-5.

GREEN, D., and TRACY, S. M.
An outbreak of acute infective encephalomyelitis in a residential home for nurses. *British Medical Journal*, Oct. 19, 1957, p. 904-6.

GREENBERG, A. J.
Communicability of infectious hepatitis: with special reference to its incidence in student nurses. *Minnesota Medicine*, Dec. 1956, p. 768-70.

MACRAE, A. D., and GALPINE, J. F.
An illness resembling poliomyelitis observed in nurses. *Lancet*, Aug. 21, 1954, p. 350-2.

TUBERCULOSIS IN NURSES

FERGUSON, R. G.
Tuberculosis among nurses. *Canadian Nurse*, Jan. 1953, p. 20-2.

HARLOW, M. J., and STEWART, C. B.
The prevention of tuberculosis in nurses. *Canadian Nurse*, April 1955, p. 285-9.

JOINT TUBERCULOSIS COUNCIL
Tuberculosis among nurses. The Council, 1937.

LANCET
Tuberculosis in Nurses. *Lancet*, Aug. 15, 1959, p. 121.

NATIONAL LEAGUE FOR NURSING.
TUBERCULOSIS NURSING ADVISORY SERVICE
A guide to precautions in the care of patients; safer ways in nursing to protect against tuberculosis. [New York], National Tuberculosis Association, 1948. 2nd edn., 1955.

RILEY, F.
Tuberculosis in hospital nurses—five years' figures. *Monthly Bulletin of M.O.H.*, Mar. 1959, p. 38-44.

SIMMONDS, F. A. H.
The protection of the nurse against tuberculosis. N.A.P.T., 1952.
2nd edn., 1960.

STOKES, K. R.
Protecting the nurse. *N.A.P.T. Bulletin*, Feb. 1955, p. 5.

THEODORE, ANDREW, and others
A follow-up study of tuberculosis in student nurses. *Journal of Chronic Diseases*, Aug. 1956, p. 111-30.

VERNEY, R. E.
Tuberculosis in students and nurses. *British Medical Journal*, Oct. 15, 1955, p. 929-34.

WHITNEY, JESSAMINE S., and STACER, HELEN JANE
Tuberculosis among nurses. New York, National Tuberculosis Association, 1941.

YOUNG, HENRY
Three phases of a tuberculosis control program for student nurses. *American Review of Tuberculosis*, June 1956, p. 868-81.

RECRUITMENT AND WASTAGE

GENERAL WORKS IN CONTENTS

AMERICAN HOSPITAL ASSOCIATION
A study of the nursing problem with reference to the need for more nurses trained to care for certain specific diseases ... to the need of standards, and to the care of the sick in the home. Philadelphia, The Association, 1916.

AMERICAN NURSES' ASSOCIATION.
PROFESSIONAL COUNSELING AND PLACEMENT SERVICE
The older nurse. New York, The Association, 1954.

BALL, F. E.
The present shortage of hospital nursing personnel and the responsibility of the doctor. *Journal of the American Geriatrics Society*, Feb. 1957, p. 141-5.

BARCLAY, JAMES
Why no nurses: the nursing recruitment problem; its history, terms and solution. Faber, 1946.

BENNETT, B. A.
Facing the facts about womanpower in relation to nursing. *Nursing Mirror*, Sept. 21, 1956, p. 1781-2.

BENNETT, B. A.
Some causes of wastage among nurses. *Nursing Mirror*, Jan. 10, 1958, p. 1061-2.

BENNETT, B. A.
Why student nurses leave. *Nursing Mirror*, May 10, 1957, p. 403.

BENNETT, SAMUEL V.
A study of the nursing shortage in Kalamazoo. Kalamazoo, Mich., The W. E. Upjohn Institute for Community Research, 1956.

BIRD, A. H. K.
The student nurse. *Nursing Times*, April 26, 1957, p. 463-4.

BURNS, M. G.
The shift system as a means of recruiting and retaining staff. *Nursing Mirror*, July 25, 1958, p. 1273-4.

CLIFFORD, S. C. A.
Powers of prediction: a top management method of dealing with trends in nursing recruitment. *Hospital and Social Service Journal*, Oct. 23, 1959, p. 1099.

COOPER, P. S.
A successful venture in day nursery care. *American Journal of Nursing*, Mar. 1959, p. 364-5.

CROSS, K. W., and HALL, DORIS L. A.
Survey of entrants to nurse training schools, and of student nurse wastage in the Birmingham region. British Medical Association, 1954.
[Reprinted from *British Journal of Preventive and Social Medicine*, vol. 8, April 1954.]

CUTHBERT, T. M.
Recruitment and retention of psychiatric nursing staff. *Nursing Times*, Oct. 11, 1952, p. 996-9.

DARLEY, V. E.
Tackling the problem of staff shortage. *Nursing Mirror*, June 3, 1955, p. iii-v.

DEUTSCHER, I.
The identification of the complement of graduate nurses in a metropolitan area. *Nursing Research*, Oct. 1956, p. 65-70.

DIAMOND, L. K., and FOX, D. J.
Turnover among hospital staff nurses. *Nursing Outlook*, July 1958, p. 388-91.

DODGE, J. S.
Why nurses leave: and what to do about it. *Modern Hospital*, May 1960, p. 116-20.

DONNELLY, P. R.
Students recruit students. *Hospital Progress*, July 1960, p. 96-7.

EGSTROM, L.
A gimmick to promote nurse recruitment. *Hospital Management*, Aug. 1957, p. 48-50.

GUINEE, K. K.
What explains student withdrawal from the general nursing program on college level? *Nursing World*, Nov. 1959, p. 9-12 and 33.

HALE, T.
The five sides of the nursing problem. *Modern Hospital*, July 1957, p. 71-6.

HALE, T.
Why the nursing supply is failing to meet the demand. *Modern Hospital*, Sept. 1960, p. 100-4.

HOSPITAL AND HEALTH MANAGEMENT
Why nurses leave. *Hospital and Health Management*, Mar. 1958, p. 69-70.

JARRETT, R. F., *and others*
The shortage of mental deficiency nurses: a challenge to society. *Lancet*, Jan. 16, 1954, p. 147-8.

JEPHCOTT, P.
Why I wouldn't become a nurse. *Nursing Mirror*, Sept. 24, 1949, p. 411-2.

KAKOSH, M.
Shortages: nurses or nursing? *Canadian Nurse*, Feb. 1960, p. 131-2.

KEEZER, D. M., *and* LEONE, LUCILE PETRY
Our future patients and their nursing needs. *American Journal of Nursing*, Jan. 1957, p. 50-1.

KELLY, P. W.
One solution to the shortage of registered nurses: nurse sampling. *Hospital Management*, Nov. 1957, p. 106-8.

KING EDWARD'S HOSPITAL FUND FOR LONDON.
NURSING RECRUITMENT SERVICE
Loss of trained nursing staff from hospitals: report on a survey made by the Nursing Recruitment Service, King Edward's Hospital Fund for London. *The Lancet*, 1948.
[Reprinted from *The Lancet*, Aug. 14, 1948.]

LANCET COMMISSION ON NURSING
The Lancet Commission on Nursing, first interim report: with statistical analysis of the shorter questionnaire (questions 1 to 12) issued to hospitals by the Commission, by A. Bradford Hill. *The Lancet*, 1931.
[Reprinted from *The Lancet*, Feb. 28, 1931.]

LANCET COMMISSION ON NURSING
The Lancet Commission on Nursing, second interim report: with statistical analysis of the questionnaire issued to hospitals by the Commission, by A. Bradford Hill. *The Lancet*, 1931.
[Supplement to *The Lancet*, Aug. 15, 1931.]

LANCET COMMISSION ON NURSING
Final report. *The Lancet*, 1932.

LEONE, LUCILE PETRY
Some recent steps in meeting our nursing needs. *Military Medicine*, Nov. 1956, p. 289-91.

LINDBERG, S. M.
Scholarships help them recruit nurses. *Modern Hospital*, Sept. 1957, p. 81-4.

LORENTZ, M.
Where nursing standards are high, so are applications for schools of nursing. *Modern Hospital*, Nov. 1957, p. 60-2.

MARY STEPHEN, SISTER
Impact; acute shortage. *Hospital Progress*, Mar. 1957, p. 82-4.

METROPOLITAN ASYLUMS BOARD
The shortage of nurses. *British Journal of Nursing*, April 11, 1914, p. 324-5.

MINISTRY OF HEALTH, *and others*
Staffing the hospitals, an urgent national need, by the Minister of Health, Secretary of State for Scotland and Minister of Labour and National Service. H.M.S.O., 1945.

MINISTRY OF HEALTH, *and others*
Working Party on the Recruitment and Training of Nurses. Report. H.M.S.O., 1947.

MINISTRY OF HEALTH, *and others*
Working Party on the Recruitment and Training of Nurses. Minority report, by John Cohen. H.M.S.O., 1948.

GENERAL NURSING COUNCIL FOR ENGLAND AND WALES
Memorandum on the Report of the Working Party on the Recruitment and Training of Nurses submitted to the Minister of Health. The Council, 1948.

KING EDWARD'S HOSPITAL FUND FOR LONDON
Comments on the Report of the Working Party on the Recruitment and Training of Nurses submitted to the Minister. The Fund, 1947.

NUFFIELD PROVINCIAL HOSPITALS TRUST
Observations submitted to the Ministry's Working Party Report on the Recruitment and Training of Nurses. O.U.P., 1948.

ROYAL COLLEGE OF NURSING
Memorandum on the Report of the Working Party on the Recruitment and Training of Nurses. The College, 1948.

TEN GROUP
Working Party Report on the Recruitment and Training of Nurses: comments submitted to the Minister of Health. Croydon, Ten Group, 1948.

MOAK, F. L.
Report of field counsellor on careers in nursing in Mississippi. *Mississippi Doctor*, Sept. 1956, p. 103-4.

MOLGREN, R.
We increased our nursing staff. *Hospital Management*, June 1958, p. 64-5.

MURRAY, MARGUERITE
Nursing needs and resources for $4\frac{1}{2}$ million people: the Detroit and Tri-county Community, 1965: a forecast for Wayne, Oakland and Macomb Counties in Michigan. Detroit and Tri-county League for Nursing, 1959.

NATIONAL LEAGUE FOR NURSING. COMMITTEE ON CAREERS
Manual for student nurse recruiters. New York, The League, 1955.

NATIONAL LEAGUE OF NURSING EDUCATION
Manual of information on the pre-nursing and guidance tests. New York, The League, 1944.

NATIONAL LEAGUE OF NURSING EDUCATION
Withdrawal of students: a three-year study of withdrawal of students from schools of nursing, prepared by Ella A. Taylor. New York, The League, 1951.

NEW, P. K., NITE, G., *and* CALLAHAN, J.
Too many nurses may be worse than too few. *Modern Hospital*, Oct. 1959, p. 104-8.

NURSING MIRROR
Change-over in recruitment. *Nursing Mirror*, April 12, 1957, p. 116.

PATMORE, E.
Recruitment and retention of nursing staff. *Hospital*, Dec. 1958, p. 887-9.

RAYNER, C. B.
Closing the gap. A solution to the staff shortage problem? *Hospital*, Sept. 1958, p. 682-4.

REID, L. D.
The trouble with nursing? No nurses. *Modern Hospital*, Jan. 1957, p. 58-60.

REIDY, JOHN P.
Scholarships as recruiting aids. *Nursing Outlook*, Dec. 1960, p. 670-1.

REVANS, R. W.
Twin myths—abundance and authority. *Nursing Times*, May 16, 1958, p. 562-3.

RIPPINGTON, A. E.
Recruitment and training. *Hospital*, April 1955, p. 238-43.

SHEE, W. A.
Do we want the part-time nurse? *Nursing Mirror*, Mar. 4, 1960, p. 1954-5.

SHERRER, Q. M.
This nursery brings nurses back to work. *Modern Hospital*, Dec. 1957, p. 59-61.

SIBLEY, H.
In Connecticut they all work together to find a solution to nursing shortage. *Modern Hospital*, Oct. 1956, p. 65-7.

SMITH, N., *and* SILVERMAN, S.
A plan to help break the nursing shortage: a high school pre-nursing program to develop professional nurses. *New York Journal of Medicine*, Sept. 1, 1960, p. 2708-11.

SNOKE, A. W.
The responsibility of hospitals for nursing service. *Hospitals*, Aug. 1, 1958, part I, p. 28-32.

SOCIAL SURVEY
The recruitment of hospital nursing staff by advertisement, by Geoffrey Thomas; an inquiry carried out for the Ministry of Labour and National Service in April 1949. Central Office of Information, 1949.

SOCIALIST MEDICAL ASSOCIATION
Nursing in the post-war world: a memorandum on the shortage of nurses, with constructive proposals. Socialist Medical Association, 1945.

SUPPLY OF NURSES COMMITTEE
Report of the Supply of Nurses Committee. The main recommendations. *British Journal of Nursing*, May 26, 1917, p. 303. Editorial comment, June 2, 1917, p. 384, and June 9, 1917, p. 401.

UNITED STATES OFFICE OF EDUCATION
Professional nurses are needed. Washington, Govt. Printing Office, 1942.

WARTIME SOCIAL SURVEY
Recruitment to nursing: an inquiry into the attitudes of student nurses to their profession with special reference to the present recruiting campaign, by Kathleen Box assisted by Enid Croft-White. The Survey, 1943.

WEIL, T. P., *and* WARMAN, G. A.
The nursing shortage; a review of the literature and possible solutions.
I. *Hospital Management*, Feb. 1959, p. 98-. *passim.*
II *Hospital Management*, Mar. 1959, p. 104 *passim.*

APTITUDE AND PERSONALITY TESTS (SELECTION)

BEYERL, M. C.
Selection procedures—why and when. Suggested methods. *Nursing Outlook*, Jan. 1959, p. 36-7, and Feb. 1959, p. 94-7.

BRITISH MEDICAL JOURNAL
Selection and training of student nurses. *British Medical Journal*, April 9, 1960, p. 1120-1.

BROWN, AMY FRANCES
Ability grouping. *Nursing Outlook*, Mar. 1957, p. 168-9.

DORFFELD, M. E., RAY, T. S., *and* BAUMBERGER, T. S.
A study of selection criteria for nursing school applicants. *Nursing Research*, June 1958, p. 67-70.

FAIR, E.
Selection for promotion. *Nursing Mirror*, July 15, 1960, p. 1387-8.

FLORENTINE, H. G.
Assets unlimited. *Nursing Outlook*, Jan. 1958, p. 48-50.

GARSIDE, R. F.
Assessment for vocational selection. *Nursing Times*, Mar. 14, 1958, p. 296-7.

GRYGIER, P.
Personality and the selection of nurses. *Nursing Times*, Aug. 16, 1957, p. 910-2.

HAWARD, L. R. C.
The selection of nurses: a new approach. *Occupational Psychology*, Jan. 1960, p. 31-7.

INTERNATIONAL COUNCIL OF NURSES.
ELEVENTH QUADRENNIAL CONGRESS
Responsibility for the selection of nurses. 2. From the point of view of the needs of the community, by Mrs. R. A. Ordiz. *Nursing Times*, Oct. 11, 1957, p. 1145-7.

INTERNATIONAL COUNCIL OF NURSES.
ELEVENTH QUADRENNIAL CONGRESS
Responsibility for the selection of nurses. 2. From the point of view of the needs of the community, by Eli Magnussen. *Nursing Times*, Aug. 30, 1957, p. 972 and 977-8.

JONES, WALTER BENTON, *and* IFFERT, R. E.
Fitness for nursing: a study of student selection in schools of nursing, under the auspices of a committee appointed by the Pennsylvania League of Nursing Education. Pittsburgh, Bureau of Educational Records and Research, 1933.

KULLMANN, G.
Some important questions on the selection of nurses. *Nursing Mirror*, July 12, 1957, p. xii.

LEAHY, K. M.
Selecting the dean of a nursing school. *Nursing Outlook*, Dec. 1958, p. 705.

LEE, T.
Predicting the successful nurse. (A survey made at the Royal Devon and Exeter Hospital.) *Nursing Times*, April 29, 1960, p. 538-40.

LEE, T.
The selection of student nurses: a revised procedure. *Occupational Psychology*, Oct. 1959, p. 209-16.

LOANE, M.
The selection of hospital probationers. *British Journal of Nursing*, Oct. 20, 1906, p. 310-1.

MINDESS, H.
Psychological indices in the selection of student nurses. *Journal of Protective Techniques*, Mar. 1957, p. 37-9.

NATIONAL LEAGUE FOR NURSING
The use of tests in schools of nursing. New York, The League, 1954.

NATIONAL LEAGUE OF NURSING EDUCATION
Suggested minimum qualifications of personnel for nursing schools and hospital nursing services. New York, The League, 1943.

PETRIE, ASENETH, *and* POWELL, MURIEL B.
The selection of nurses in England. The American Psychological Association Inc., [1951].
[Reprinted from the *Journal of Applied Psychology*, vol. 35, no. 4, Aug. 1951.]

SAWERS, JEAN
Psychological tests as an aid to the selection of nursing candidates: a survey of their development and use in the United States; report submitted to the Education Committee of the Florence Nightingale International Foundation. . . . [F.N.I.F.], 1949.

SCHOTT, G.
Responsibility for the selection of nurses. *Nursing Times*, Aug. 16, 1957, p. 915-6 and 920-2.

VAN ALLYN, K.
Sound selection procedures: a psychological approach. *Hospital Progress*, July 1958, p. 60-2.

EDUCATION AND TRAINING

BASIC TRAINING—GENERAL WORKS

ANDERSON, JAMES WALLACE
Lectures on nursing delivered in the Royal Infirmary Glasgow. 2nd edn. New York, Macmillan, 1893.

ADRANVALA, T. K.
Trends in nursing education. *Journal of the Christian Medical Association of India*, Sept. 1957, p. 255-8.

AKESTER, J. M.
The education of the nurse. *Nursing Times*, Aug. 19, 1955, p. 918-20, and Oct. 14, 1955, p. 1163-5.

ALINQUIST, —
The professional training and status of nurses in Sweden. *Nursing Record*, Sept. 2, 1899, p. 185-7.

AMERICAN ASSOCIATION OF MEDICAL SOCIAL WORKERS
Medical social work looks at nursing education: a report prepared under the auspices of a sub-committee of the Education Committee of the American Association of Social Workers, 1954, by Eckka Gordon.... Washington, The Association, 1954.

AMERICAN MEDICAL ASSOCIATION
Report of the Committee on the Training of Nurses. Philadelphia, 1869.
[Transactions of the American Medical Assn., vol. 22, no. 161, p. 174.]

AMERICAN NURSES' FOUNDATION
Formal education and the process of professionalization: a study of student nurses, by Thomas S. McPartland. Kansas City, Missouri, Community Studies, 1957.

ARMIGER, SISTER BERNADETTE
Objectives of nursing education. *Maryland State Medical Journal*, April 1959, p. 152-4.

ARNSTEIN, M.
Balance in nursing. *American Journal of Nursing*, Dec. 1958, p. 1690-2.

ATLEE, H. B.
The farce of nursing education. *Canadian Nurse*, Sept. 1957, p. 791-4.

AYNES, E. A.
Are nurses holding back nursing education? *Modern Hospital*, July 1960, p. 57-60.

AYNES, E. A.
Nurses' training must fit the nurses' jobs. *Modern Hospital*, Sept. 1958, p. 89-92.

BALME, HAROLD
A criticism of nursing education, with suggestions for constructive reform. O.U.P., 1937.

BARR, A.
Some results of training student nurses in general hospitals. *Ministry of Health Monthly Bulletin*, June 1957, p. 94-106.

BARR, A.
Training of student nurses. *British Journal of Preventive and Social Medicine*, July 1959, p. 149-55.

BELCHER, H. C., *and* BROER, M. R.
General education and the student nurse: physical education in the nursing curriculum. *Nursing Outlook*, Mar. 1957, p. 149-51.

BELL, H. G.
Nursing education and the shortage of nurses. *American Journal of Surgery*, Aug. 1958, p. 133-6.

BENNETT, B. A.
Modern trends in nurse training and nursing practice....
In
INTERNATIONAL HOSPITAL FEDERATION
Report of first post-war congress. [1950.]

BERKOWITZ, JOANNE E., *and* BERKOWITZ, NORMAN H.
Nursing education and role conception. *Nursing Research*, Fall 1960, p. 218-9.

BERTHIAUME, A. B.
Observing is more than watching. *Nursing Outlook*, May 1957, p. 290-3.

BERTRANDE, SISTER
Today's student, tomorrow's leader. *Catholic Nurse*, December 1956, p. 44-52.

BONE, A. I. C.
Combined training scheme at Ayr hospitals. *Nursing Times*, Aug. 3, 1956, p. 739-43.

BRACKETT, MARY E.
Hospital nursing service—a practice field for nursing students. *Nursing Outlook*, Oct. 1960, p. 556-9.

BRIDGMAN, MARGARET
On types of programs. *American Journal of Nursing*, Oct. 1960, p. 1465-8.

BROE, E.
New trends in nursing education. *New Zealand Nursing Journal*, Aug. 1959, p. 125-7 and 129.

BROWN, CHARLOTTE AMBROSE
The junior nurse. Philadelphia, Lea and Febiger, 1914.

BURR, MARY
The training of nurses in Switzerland. *British Journal of Nursing*, Feb. 20, 1904, p. 144-7.

CATHCART, H. R.
A hospital school experiment. *Hospitals*, Mar. 1, 1956, p. 28, 31-2 and 91-2.

CHARLES MARIE, SISTER
Nursing education. The way ahead. *Hospital Progress*, Oct. 1960, p. 84-92.

CHARLES MARIE, SISTER
On continuing growth. *American Journal of Nursing*, Oct. 1960, p. 1488-90.

CIVIL SERVICE CHRONICLE, NEW YORK
Nurse instruction for civil service examinations covering nurse, trained nurse, hospital nurse, visiting nurse, field nurse, tuberculosis nurse, school nurse and nurse's assistant. Answers to examination questions and 250 specimen questions. New York City, New York State, New Jersey, Chicago, and Federal Services. New York, 1916.

CLARK, HENRY E.
On the training of sick nurses. *Nursing Record*, Nov. 25, 1893, p. 266-7; Dec. 2, 1893, p. 283-4; Dec. 9, 1893, p. 299-300.

CLARKE, F.
Life, profession and school.
1. Philosophy and theory of nursing training. *Canadian Nurse*, Aug. 1956, p. 640-6.
2. Apprenticeship and graduate education. *Canadian Nurse*, Sept. 1956, p. 715-22.

CLEMENCE, M.
How successful in nursing school are graduates from a commercial high school course. *Nursing Research*, Oct. 1956, p. 82-4.

CLINE, D. S.
An analysis of spelling errors made by professional nurses. *Nursing Outlook*, July 1959, p. 400-2.

CLYNE, DOUGLAS G. WILSON
Final examination questions for nurses: selected questions from the General Nursing Council's examination papers for the final examination for the General Part of the Register in England and Wales. Faber, 1959.

CLYNE, DOUGLAS G. WILSON
Preliminary examination questions for nurses: selected questions from the General Nursing Council's examination papers for the Preliminary Examination in England and Wales. Faber, 1959.

COCKAYNE, E.
The education of the nurse to meet the needs of today. *Nursing Mirror*, May 22, 1959, p. vii-x and 604.

COLADARCI, A. P.
The nurse's stake in general education. *American Journal of Nursing*, Sept 1957, p. 1151-2.

COLUMBIA UNIVERSITY DEPARTMENT OF NURSING,
FACULTY OF MEDICINE
Nursing student responses to the clinical field. New York,
The University, 1958.

COLUMBIA UNIVERSITY. TEACHERS' COLLEGE.
Education for nursing; past, present and future: papers
presented at the anniversary celebration. New York,
National League for Nursing, 1959.

COLUMBIA UNIVERSITY. TEACHERS' COLLEGE
The future of nursing education: proceedings of the fiftieth
anniversary celebration of nursing education in Teachers'
College, Columbia University. Columbia University,
Bureau of Publications, 1950.

COLUMBIA UNIVERSITY. TEACHERS' COLLEGE
Improvements in education practice which have been
brought about through research in nursing: a study done
by a group of students in educational research. New York,
Columbia University, 1955.

COLUMBIA UNIVERSITY. TEACHERS' COLLEGE
International aspects of nursing education—a series of
addresses provided through the Annie W. Goodrich
Lectureship Fund. New York, Columbia University, 1931.

COLUMBIA UNIVERSITY. TEACHERS' COLLEGE
Nursing education, twenty-five years of nursing education
in Teachers' College, 1899-1925. Teachers' College Bulletin,
17th series, no. 3, Feb. 1926.

COLUMBIA UNIVERSITY. TEACHERS' COLLEGE.
Regional planning for nursing and nursing education:
report of work conference held at Plymouth, New Hamp-
shire, June 12 to June 23, 1950. New York, Columbia
University, 1950.

COMMITTEE FOR THE STUDY OF NURSING EDUCATION
Nursing and nursing education in the United States:
report of the Committee . . . ; and report of a survey, by
Josephine Goldmark. New York, Macmillan, 1923.
[Chairman: C. E. A. Winslow.]

COWLIN, GERTRUDE
Training and position of the British hospital nurse.
Stuttgart, Kohlhammer, 1931.
[Reprinted from the journal Nosokomeion, April 1931,
p. 326-39. There is a resumé in English, French and
German.]

CUNNINGHAM, M. R.
Face the future. Hospital Progress, Sept. 1960, p. 78-81.

CUNNINGHAM, P. J., and COUSENS, H. M.
Public health for the nursing student. Faber, 1953.

CURRAN, JEAN A., and BUNGE, HELEN L.
Better nursing: a study of nursing care and education in
Washington. Seattle, University of Washington Press,
1951.

CUTBUSH, R. E.
Secondary modern schools and nursing. Nursing Times,
May 22, 1959, p. 602-5.

DEUTSCHER, IRWIN
Educational characteristics of the nurse. Nursing World,
April 1958, p. 17-24, and May 1958, p. 11-17.

DRUMMOND, E. E.
International studies in nursing education. Nursing
Research, June 1958, p. 88-90.

DUFF-GRANT, L.
The nursing profession and its main issues today. The
preparation of the nurse. Nursing Mirror, July 29, 1955,
p. 1201; Aug. 5th 1955 p. 1268.

ENARSON, HAROLD L.
Systematic innovation in nursing education. Nursing
Outlook, July 1960, p. 368-70.

ENRIQUES, B.
Professional nurses and their training in Italy. International
Nursing Review, May 1957, p. 19-21.

FAGAN, EDNA A.
Accreditation as I see it. Nursing Outlook, Jan. 1960, p.
41-3.

FIELDHOUSE, A. E.
The future of basic nursing education in New Zealand.
New Zealand Nursing Journal, June 1959, p. 101-3.

FOLCK, MARILYN MELCHER, and NIE, PHYLLIS J.
Nursing students learn to face death. Nursing Outlook,
Sept. 1959, p. 510-3.

FOLEY, M. M.
Catholic nursing education: basic degree and diploma,
practical; graduate. Hospital Progress, Feb. 1957, part II,
p. 161-9.

FOLEY, M. M.
Nursing education facilities: United States and Canada.
Hospital Progress, Feb. 1958, part II, p. 157-203.

FOOTE, JOHN, editor
State Board questions and answers for nurses: being the
actual questions submitted at the examinations of 31
state examining boards for nurses, with answers. Philadelphia, Lippincott, 1917.
2nd edn., 1919.
3rd edn., 1924.
4th edn., 1926.
5th edn., 1927.
6th edn., 1928.
7th edn., 1929.
8th edn., 1930.
13th edn., 1935.

FOX, D. J., and DIAMOND, L. K.
The identification of satisfying and stressful situations in
basic programs in nursing education: a progress report.
Nursing Research, Winter 1959, p. 4-12.

FUERST, ELINOR V., and WOLFF, LU VERNE
Fundamentals of nursing: the humanities and the sciences
in nursing. Philadelphia, Lippincott, 1956.
2nd edn., 1959.

FUERST, ELINOR, V., and WOLFF, LU VERNE
Teaching fundamentals of nursing: method, content and
evaluation. Philadelphia, Lippincott, 1956.
2nd edn., 1958.
3rd edn., 1960.

GABIG, M. G.
The place of nursing education and nursing service in
Catholic hospitals. Hospital Progress, April 1959, p. 67-9.

GELINAS, A.
Progress in nursing education. Nursing World, Dec. 1956,
p. 8-11.

GENERAL NURSING COUNCIL FOR ENGLAND AND WALES
Conditions under which hospitals are approved as training
schools for student nurses for admission to the Register
of Nurses . . . and for pupil assistant nurses, The Council,
1960.

GENERAL NURSING COUNCIL FOR ENGLAND AND WALES
Conference on nursing education. British Journal of
Nursing, May 7, 1921, p. 266-72, and May 14, 1921, p.
283-9.

GENERAL NURSING COUNCIL FOR ENGLAND AND WALES
Guide to the training scheme for nurses for mental
diseases. The Council, [1957].

GENERAL NURSING COUNCIL FOR ENGLAND AND WALES
Secondment of student nurses for special experience.
Nursing Mirror, Nov. 13, 1959, p. 559-60.

GLASGOW ROYAL INFIRMARY
Assessing an assessment. [Nursing Mirror assessment of
the experimental scheme of nurse training at Glasgow
R.I.] Nursing Mirror, Dec. 16, 1960, p. 997-1000 and 1003.

GLASGOW ROYAL INFIRMARY
Glasgow's comprehensive two-year training. Survey of
Royal Infirmary "Alternative Course". Nursing Mirror,
Aug. 29, 1958, p. vii-x and 1637.

GLASGOW ROYAL INFIRMARY
Glasgow experiment. Great Britain, like the United States, is taking a critical look at nurse education and trying new methods, by Winifred Morgan. *American Journal of Nursing*, Dec. 1960, p. 1758-60.

GLASGOW ROYAL INFIRMARY
Important experiment in Glasgow. *Nursing Times*, June 7, 1957, p. 627.

GLASGOW ROYAL INFIRMARY
Scotland's experimental training scheme, by Scottish Health Services Council and General Nursing Council for Scotland. *Nursing Times*, Feb. 10, 1956, p. 136-8.

GODDEN, G. M.
Nursing education and the future. *Nursing Times*, Feb. 8, 1957, p. 153-4.

GOODRICH, ANNIE WARBURTON
Some international aspects of nursing education and service. New York, Columbia University Teachers' College, 1936.

GORDON, A. KNYVETT
The position of the isolation hospital in the training of a nurse. *British Journal of Nursing*, Jan. 26, 1907, p. 63-5.

GREAT BRITAIN. COLONIAL OFFICE
Committee on the Training of Nurses for the Colonies. Report. H.M.S.O., 1945.

GREENHOUGH-SMITH, MAUD
The training of male nurses. *Nursing Record*, Oct. 1, 1898, p. 265-7.

GROSS, SAMUEL DAVID
Remarks on the training of nurses. Philadelphia, Collins, 1869.

HADLEY, ERNEST C.
Some practical points in the future training of nurses. *The Medical Press and Circular*, June 20, 1945, p. 388-91.

HAMILTON, D. I. W.
Behind the screens. Melbourne and Sydney, Lothran Pub. Co., 1925.
[The training of nurses in Australia.]

HAMPTON, ISABEL A.
Educational standards for nurses.
In
HAMPTON, ISABEL A., *and others*
Nursing of the sick, 1893.

HARVEY, S.
Trained or educated. *Nursing Times*, Aug. 14, 1959, p. 731-2.

HASSENPLUG, L. W.
Continuity in nursing education. *Nursing Outlook*, April 1957, p. 200-3.

HAWKINS-DEMPSTER, H.
Explanatory lectures for nurses and their teachers. Bristol, John Wright, 1913.

HEATON, HILARY M.
Nursing education in England. New York, Rockefeller Foundation, 1932.
[Reprinted from "*Methods and problems of medical education*," 21st series].

HEIDGERKEN, LORETTA
Some problems in modern nursing: nursing practice and education. *Nursing Outlook*, July 1959, p. 394-7.

HORNER, HARLAN H.
Nursing education and practice in New York State. Albany, University of the State of New York Press, 1934.

HOSPITAL FOR SICK CHILDREN *and* MIDDLESEX HOSPITAL
General training based on a children's hospital: experimental scheme. *Nursing Times*, Dec. 4, 1959, p. 1221-4.

INGLES, THELMA
On developing skilled practitioners. *American Journal of Nursing*, Oct. 1960, p. 1482-4.

INGLES, THELMA
The patient, the student and the teacher. *Nursing World*, Sept. 1959, p. 9-11.

INTERNATIONAL COUNCIL OF NURSES.
EDUCATION COMMITTEE
The educational program of the school of nursing, prepared by Isabel M. Stewart. Geneva, I.C.N., 1934. 1952 edn., entitled "The basic education of the professional nurse".

INTERNATIONAL COUNCIL OF NURSES.
FLORENCE NIGHTINGALE INTERNATIONAL FOUNDATION
Basic nursing education; principles and practices of nursing education. A report prepared under the auspices of the Florence Nightingale International Foundation, by Frances Beck, assisted by the Staff of the Foundation. International Council of Nurses, 1958.

INTERNATIONAL COUNCIL OF NURSES.
FLORENCE NIGHTINGALE INTERNATIONAL FOUNDATION
International conference on the planning of nursing studies, held at ... Sevres, France, 12th-24th November, 1956; report prepared by Margaret G. Arnstein and Ellen Broe. [Geneva], I.C.N., 1956.

ISRAEL, EUGENE
The future education of the German nurse; translated by Miss L. L. Dock. *British Journal of Nursing*, Dec. 10, 1904, p. 471-4.

IZYCKA, J.
Nursing education in Poland. *Nursing Outlook*, June 1960, p. 304-7.

JESSEE, R. W.
A comparative study of fully accredited basic nursing programs. *Nursing Research*, Oct. 1958, p. 100-12.

JOHNSTON, RUTH V.
Personnel program guide for nursing education and nursing service agencies. Philadelphia, Saunders, 1958.

KEEFE, A. E.
Is nursing overlooking its intellectuals. *Nursing World*, Dec. 1958, p. 11-12 and 31.

KNAPP, LOUISE
The out-patient department in the education of the nurse. New York, National League for Nursing Education, 1932.

KOLLEN, DR.
The training of male and female nurses in Catholic Orders.
In
HAMPTON, ISABEL A., *and others*
Nursing of the sick, 1893.

KRAKOWER, HYMAN
Tests and measurements applied to nursing education. New York, Putnam, 1949.

LA CROIX, M. A.
The power of enthusiasm. *Canadian Nurse*, Feb. 1957, p. 101-3.

LAKE, VERA M.
New preliminary questions and answers: answers to questions set in the Preliminary state examinations in nursing. Faber, 1956.

LAMB, M. C. N.
The future preparation of the British nurse. *Nursing Times*, Oct. 28, 1955, p. 1217-9.

LAMBERTSEN, E. C.
Nursing service and education. *Hospitals*, April 16, 1959, p. 92-9.

LANDALE, E. J. R.
How is the standard of training in small hospitals to be raised? *Nursing Record*, April 7, 1892, p. 281-4.

LANDALE, E. J. R.
Three factors in the training of probationers. *Nursing Record*, Feb. 23, 1893, p. 104-6.

LIPELES, J. C.
Case material: a meeting ground for nurses and social workers. *Nursing Outlook*, June 1959, p. 343-5.

LOCKERBY, FLORENCE K.
Communication for nurses. St. Louis, Mosby, 1958.

LONG, JAMES
Lectures to the nurses of the Liverpool Royal Infirmary. Liverpool, privately printed, 1878.

LONIE, T. C.
The social implications of nursing training in developing communities. Roumea, New Caledonia, South Pacific Commission, 1958.

LORD, A. R.
Report of the evaluation of the Metropolitan School of Nursing, Windsor, Ontario. [Canadian Nurses' Association], 1952.

LOUCKS, PHYLLIS M.
The training function in nursing service. New York, National League for Nursing, 1956.

LUCOW, W. H.
Test construction in nursing education. *Canadian Nurse*, Jan. 1960, p. 23-33.

MACGREGOR, F. C.
Social sciences and nursing education. *American Journal of Nursing*, July 1957, p. 899-902.

MACLAGGAN, K.
A crisis in nursing education. *Canadian Nurse*, June 1957, p. 517-9.

MCMANUS, R. LOUISE
Society's demands on nurses that influence nursing education: analyst's report at work conference on problems of graduate nurse education. New York, Columbia University, 1951.

MACPHAIL, HECTOR
Model answers for the preliminary nursing examination. Faber, 1940.
2nd edn., 1944.
3rd edn., 1953.

MCQUARRIE, F.
The evolution of nursing education. *Canadian Nurse*, Mar. 1955, p. 194-9.

MALLORY, EVELYN
Whither we are tending. *Canadian Nurse*, June 1960, p. 521-38.

MARTIN, HARRY W.
Education and service: division and unity. *Nursing Outlook*, Nov. 1959, p. 650-3.

MARY CAROLYN, SISTER
What courses should precede or parallel nutrition in the basic curriculum? *Journal of the American Dietetic Association*, April 1957, p. 380-1.

MARY FELICITAS, SISTER
Better utilization of the student's time in the clinical field. *Canadian Nurse*, April 1959, p. 321-5.

METZGER, M. E.
Why professional education? Preservice baccalaureate program. *Hospital Progress*, July 1960, p. 74-7.

MILLER, H.
Is nursing education broad enough? *Nursing Outlook*, Oct. 1960, p. 553-5.

MITCHELL, RUTH J.
Training hospital corpsmen in the Navy. *Nursing Outlook*, May 1955, p. 281-3.

MOLLETT, M.
The twentieth-century probationer. *British Journal of Nursing*, April 27, 1907, p. 307-8, and May 4, 1907, p. 323-4.

MONTAG, MILDRED L.
Experimental programs in nursing. *American Journal of Nursing*, Jan. 1955, p. 45-6.

MORIARTY, HONORA R.
Educating the nurse in Norway. Oslo, Academisk Forlag, 1954.

MURRAY, R.
Looking ahead—the education of the student nurse. *Nursing Times*, May 4, 1956, p. 362-6.

MUSE, MAUDE BLANCHE
Guiding learning experience: principles of progressive education applied to nursing education. New York, Macmillan, 1950.

MUSE, MAUDE BLANCHE
A study outline designed to assist students of nursing who are taking an introductory course in educational psychology. Philadelphia, Saunders, 1928.

NAHM, HELEN
Continuity and progression in nursing education. *American Journal of Nursing*, June 1958, p. 845-7.

NAHM, HELEN
A decade of change. *American Journal of Nursing*, Nov. 1959, p. 1588-90.

NAHM, HELEN
Planning for the future of education in nursing. *Canadian Nurse*, Dec. 1960, p. 1073-8.

NATIONAL LEAGUE FOR NURSING
Criteria for the evaluation of educational programs in nursing leading to a diploma. New York, The League, 1958.

NATIONAL LEAGUE FOR NURSING
Opportunities for education in nursing. *Nursing Outlook*, Sept. 1960, p. 482-6.

NATIONAL LEAGUE FOR NURSING
Preparing tomorrow's nurses, by Elizabeth Ogg. New York, The League, 1952.

NATIONAL LEAGUE FOR NURSING
A report on progress in nursing education.
  I. Undergraduate education. *Nursing Outlook*, June 1958, p. 336-41.
  II. Graduate education. *Nursing Outlook*, July 1958, p. 397-401.

NATIONAL LEAGUE FOR NURSING
Roles and relationships in nursing education: viewpoints expressed at the 1959 Regional Conferences of Representatives of Nursing Service and Nursing Education. New York, The League, 1959.

NATIONAL LEAGUE FOR NURSING. COMMITTEE ON CAREERS
Look to your future in nursing education. New York, The League, n.d.

NATIONAL LEAGUE FOR NURSING. COMMITTEE ON CAREERS
A preliminary report on state-wide scholarships for nursing education: from official and voluntary sources. New York, The League, 1958.

NATIONAL LEAGUE FOR NURSING. DEPARTMENT OF BACCALAUREATE AND HIGHER DEGREE PROGRAMS
Articulation between graduate and undergraduate education in nursing: report of the conference of the Council of Member Agencies of the N.L.N. Department of Baccalaureate and Higher Degree Programs, Chicago, February 19-21, 1958. New York, The League, 1958.

NATIONAL LEAGUE FOR NURSING. DIVISION OF NURSING EDUCATION
Objectives of educational programs in nursing. New York, The League, 1955.

NATIONAL LEAGUE OF NURSING EDUCATION
The contribution of physical therapy to nursing education, prepared by the sub-committee on the utilization of special therapists in the teaching of student nurses of the Committee on Curriculum. New York, The League, 1948.

NATIONAL LEAGUE OF NURSING EDUCATION.
COMMITTEE ON DISPENSARY DEVELOPMENT
The pupil nurse in the out-patient department. New York, The League, 1925.

NAYER, D. D.
On American Nurses' Association's responsibilities: how the professional organization concerns itself with the education of practitioners. *American Journal of Nursing*, Oct. 1960, p. 1469-71.

NEW BRUNSWICK UNIVERSITY
The report of a study of nursing education in New Brunswick, by Edith Kathleen Russell; conducted at the University of New Brunswick. Frederickton, Canada, The University, 1956.

NEW YORK STATE INTERDEPARTMENTAL HEALTH COUNCIL.
ADVISORY COMMITTEE ON NURSING SERVICES
Proposals for the improvement of nursing education and service. Albany, The Council, 1950.

NEW YORK STATE UNIVERSITY. STATE EDUCATION
DEPARTMENT. DIVISION OF PROFESSIONAL EDUCATION
Experimental programs in nursing curriculums—New York State. Albany, The University, 1957.

NEW YORK STATE UNIVERSITY. STATE EDUCATION
DEPARTMENT. NURSE RESOURCES STUDY GROUP
Needs and facilities in professional nursing education in New York State. Albany, The University, 1959.

NIGHTINGALE, FLORENCE
Proposed plan for the training and employment of women in hospital, district and private nursing, 1861. Letter from Miss Nightingale to the Chairman of the Liverpool Training School for Nurses, November 30th, 1861.
In
LIVERPOOL NURSES' TRAINING SCHOOL
Organization for nursing. . . . 1865.

NORDMARK, MADELYN TITUS, *and* ROHWEDER, ANNE E.
Science principles applied to nursing: a reference for nurse educators. Philadelphia, Lippincott, 1959.

NURSING OUTLOOK
Educational resources for the preparation of nurses. *Nursing Outlook*, Jan. 1958, p. 32-8.

NUTTING, MARY ADELAIDE
Educational status of nursing. Washington, U.S. Bureau of Education, 1912.

NUTTING, MARY ADELAIDE
Some results of preparatory instruction. *British Journal of Nursing*, June 24, 1905, p. 488-91; July 1, 1905, p. 5-6; July 8, 1905, p. 28-30.

NUTTING, MARY ADELAIDE
Suggestions for educational standard for state registration. *British Journal of Nursing*, Feb. 16, 1904, p. 45-51.

OWEN, SISTER MARY RUTH
Philosophy, a basic factor in the curriculum. Proceedings of the symposium on philosophy, religion, ethics, history, sociology, psychology and integration of public health. Principles in the basic professional curriculum of a school of nursing. Washington, Catholic University of America, 1939.

OXFORD REGIONAL HOSPITAL BOARD
Training of nurses in general hospitals: a report of a survey of four training schools. Oxford Regional Hospital Board, 1956.

PACKARD, JOHN H.
Training of nurses for the sick, read before the Association, Jan. 20, 1876. Philadelphia, Social Science Association of Philadelphia, 1876.

PEARSE, HELEN L.
The necessity for an international standard of nursing education. *British Journal of Nursing*, June 10, 1922, p. 365-7.

POOLE, DRUSILLA
Searching for know-how toward progress in nursing service through in-service education. *Military Medicine*, June 1957, p. 426-9.

PRANGLEY, R. R., *and* DE YOUNG, L.
Nursing education changes to meet service needs of patient care. *Rocky Mountain Medical Journal*, Jan. 1959, p. 48-52.

REESE, D. E., *and* SIEGAL, S. E.
Educational preparation of nurses employed in non-federal hospitals. *Hospital Management*, April 1960, p. 108-12.

RIDDELL, MARGARET S.
A first-year nursing manual. Faber, 1931.

RIDDELL, MARGARET S.
Lectures to nurses. Faber, 1928.

ROBB, ISABEL HAMPTON
Educational standards for nurses. Cleveland, Ohio, Koeckert, 1907.

ROBB, ISABEL HAMPTON
An international educational standard for nurses. *British Journal of Nursing*, Sept. 18, 1909, p. 231-3.

ROBB, ISABEL HAMPTON
The three years' course of training in connection with the eight-hour system. *Nursing Record*, June 1, 1895, p. 375-7, and June 8, 1895, p. 395-6.

ROCKEFELLER FOUNDATION
Methods and problems of medical education (twenty-first series). New York, The Foundation, 1932.
[This volume is entirely concerned with nursing education.]

RUSSELL, CHARLES H.
Liberal education and nursing. New York, Columbia University Teachers' College, 1959.

RUSSELL, CHARLES H.
Liberal education and nursing. *Nursing Research*, Oct. 1958, p. 116-26.

RUSSELL, CHARLES H.
On a liberal background. *American Journal of Nursing*, Oct. 1960, p. 1485-7.

RUSSELL, EDITH KATHLEEN
An evaluation of the centralized lecture program for the Schools of Nursing in Saskatchewan. Regina, Board of Administration of the Centralized Teaching Program, 1954.

SAND, OLE
Nursing education in the forefront. *Nursing Outlook*, Jan. 1957, p. 15.

SAND, OLE, *and* BELCHER, HELEN C.
An experience in basic nursing education. New York, Putnam, 1958.

SCHMITT, LOUISE M.
Basic nursing education study; report of the status of basic nursing education programs in Saskatchewan, prepared for the Steering Committee of the Board of Administration of the Centralized Teaching Program for Nursing Students in Saskatchewan. Regina, Saskatchewan Registered Nurses' Association, 1957.

SCHWIER, M. E., *and* HEIM, E. M.
The general educator and education for nursing. *Teachers' College Record*, Jan. 1956, p. 428-56.

SCOTLAND. DEPARTMENT OF HEALTH
Report of the Scottish Departmental Committee on the Training of Nurses. Edinburgh, H.M.S.O., 1936.

SHEEN, D.
The introductory lecture to a course of lectures on nursing given to the probationer nurses at the Cardiff Infirmary. *Nursing Record*, Mar. 20, 1890, p. 139-42, and Mar. 27, 1890, p. 149-50.

SMITH, KATHRYN M.
The new tomorrow in nursing. *Nursing Outlook*, Oct. 1960, p. 547-9.

SPALDING, EUGENIA KENNEDY
Current problems of nurse educators. *Teachers' College Record*, Oct. 1955, p. 38-46.

SPEER, THEODORE V.
The training of male nurses [at the Mills School, Bellevue Hospital, New York]. *Nursing Record*, Jan. 6, 1900, p. 10-11.

SQUIBBS, A. E. A.
Correlation of theoretical and practical work in nurse training. *Nursing Mirror*, Dec. 16, 1955, p. vii-x.

STEWART, ISABEL MAITLAND
Developments in nursing education since 1918. Washington, U.S. Govt. Printing Office, 1921.

STEWART, ISABEL MAITLAND
The education of nurses: historical foundations and modern trends. New York, Macmillan, 1944.

STEWART, ISLA
The education of nurses. *British Journal of Nursing*, Aug. 20, 1904, p. 147-8.

STEWART, ISLA
The training school. *Nursing Record*, June 20, 1896, p. 492-5.

STICHT, V.
How shall we prepare the professional nurse. *Nursing World*, Feb. 1957, p. 7-9.

STONSBY, E. V.
An 8-year plan for nursing education. (A description of the programme in nursing at Rutgers University, New Jersey, U.S.A.). *Nursing Outlook*, Oct. 1959, p. 596-8.

STRONG, REBECCA
Education in nursing: an address given in London in 1895. Glasgow, James Maclehose, 1916.
[Also facsimile privately printed in Edinburgh by Douglas & Foulis, 1927.]

STRONG, REBECCA
Introductory remarks to practical classes on ward work, held by Mrs. Strong, Matron, Royal Infirmary, Glasgow, 1893. Edinburgh, Douglas & Foulis, 1929.
[Syllabus of the first and second course included].

STRONG, REBECCA
A plea for uniformity of education in nursing. Paper read before the 1st Conference of the Matrons' Council. *Nursing Record*, Nov. 10, 1894, p. 307-10.

STRONG, REBECCA
Preparatory instruction for nurses. *Nursing Record*, Jan. 4, 1902, p. 5-11.

SYMONDS, P. M.
Evaluation in professional education. *Nursing Outlook*, Mar. 1957, p. 166-8.

TAYLER, DORIS
General nursing questions and answers: model answers, written and oral, to questions for the final state examination in nursing. Faber & Gwyer, 1925.
2nd edn., 1928.
3rd edn., 1931.
5th edn., 1940.
6th edn., 1945.
7th edn., 1950.

TODD, HELEN
The affiliation of the smaller and special hospitals for training purposes. *British Journal of Nursing*, July 8, 1905, p. 30-2.

TSCHUDIN, MARY S., *and others*
Evaluation in basic nursing education, by Mary S. Tschudin, Helen C. Belcher [and] Leo Nedelsky. New York, Putnam, 1958.

UNITED STATES. PUBLIC HEALTH SERVICE
Professional nurse traineeships, part II. Facts about the nurse supply and educational needs of nurses based on data compiled for the national conference to evaluate two years' of training grants for professional nurses, prepared under the direction of Apollonia O. Adams. Washington, Govt. Printing Office, 1959.

URBANIC, D.
Nursing in Yugoslavia. *American Journal of Nursing*, May 1956, p. 585-7.

WALKER, LUCY
The progress made in establishing a three years' course in training schools for nurses [in America]. *Nursing Record*, Aug. 14, 1897, p. 127-9.

WALLACE, W. STEWART
Report on the experiment in nursing education of the Atkinson School of Nursing, the Toronto Western Hospital, 1950-55. Toronto, University of Toronto Press, 1956.

WAR OFFICE
The training of male nurses. *British Journal of Nursing*, Feb. 27, 1904, p. 166.

WATERER, J.
Man nurse educator in WHO. *American Journal of Nursing*, July 1959, p. 985-7.

WATKIN, B.
Is a comprehensive training for nurses in this country desirable and practicable. *Male Nurses' Journal*, Jan.-Feb. 1957, p. 5-13.

WEDDELL, D.
The education of the nurse: plea for a particular experiment. *Nursing Times*, Sept. 16, 1955, p. 1039-40.

WEIR, G. M.
Survey of nursing education in Canada. Toronto, University of Toronto Press, 1932.

WELCH, JANET
Nursing education related to the cultural background in East and South-East African colonies. New York, Columbia University Press, [1941].

WESTERN INTERSTATE COMMISSION FOR HIGHER EDUCATION
Professional training for western nurses: a plan of action. Boulder, Colorado, The Commission, 1956.

WILLIAMS, T. R., *and* WILLIAMS, M. M.
The socialization of the student nurse. *Nursing Research*, Winter 1959, p. 18-25.

WORCESTER, ALFRED
The education of nurses. Chicago University, University Press, 1903.

WORCESTER, ALFRED
A new way of training nurses. Boston, Cupples & Hurd, 1888.

WORLD HEALTH ORGANIZATION
African conference on the development of nursing education in countries south of the Sahara. Kampala, Uganda, 28th September to 7th October, 1953. Geneva, W.H.O., [1953].

WORLD HEALTH ORGANIZATION
Basic nursing curriculum. Recommendations of W.H.O. study group held in Brussels, November 1955. *Nursing Times*, Feb. 10, 1956, p. 151.

WORLD HEALTH ORGANIZATION
Nurses: their education and their role in health programmes; report of the technical discussions at the Ninth World Health Assembly, 1956.
[Reprint from *Chronicle of the World Health Organization*, vol. 10, no. 7, July 1956.]

WORLD HEALTH ORGANIZATION. REGIONAL OFFICE FOR EUROPE
Basic nursing curriculum in Europe: report of a study group ... Brussels, 17-26 November, 1955. Geneva, W.H.O., 1956.

WORLD HEALTH ORGANIZATION. WESTERN PACIFIC REGION
Second nursing education seminar, Central Nursing School, Suva, Fiji. Geneva, W.H.O., 1955.

WORLD HEALTH ORGANIZATION. WORKING CONFERENCE ON NURSING EDUCATION
Report. Geneva, W.H.O., 1953.

Administration

BIXLER, ROY W., and BIXLER, GENEVIEVE K.
Administration for nursing education in a period of transition. New York, Putnam, 1954.

BUECHEL, J. F. MARVIN
Principles of administration in junior and community college education for nursing. New York, Putnam, 1956.

BURR, MARY
Should nurses pay for their training? *Nursing Record*, Feb. 9, 1901, p. 108-11.

FINETTE, FLORENCE
The administration of faculty. *Nursing Outlook*, Aug. 1960, p. 432-5.

GOOCH, M.
The director of nursing education looks at costs. *Nursing Outlook*, May 1958, p. 282-4.

HEALY, SISTER FRANCES
A study of the cost of educating a student in a basic professional degree curriculum in nursing. Washington, Catholic University of America Press, 1946.

HEIDGERKEN, LORETTA
Meeting the teacher shortage. *Nursing Outlook*, Sept. 1956, p. 514-6.

THE HOSPITAL
Area nurse training committees. *Hospital*, Nov. 1959, p. 956-8.

HUNGATE, T. L.
Use of cost studies of nursing education. New York, Columbia University, 1951.

KNOTT, LESLIE K., VREELAND, ELLWYNNE M., and GOOCH, MARJORIE
Cost analysis for collegiate programs in nursing: Part 1. Analysis of expenditures. New York, National League for Nursing, 1956.

KNOTT, LESLIE K., VREELAND, ELLWYNNE M., and GOOCH, MARJORIE
Cost analysis for collegiate programs in nursing: Part 2. Current income and other resources. New York, National League for Nursing, 1957.

LINDBERG, S. M., and CORBIN, M.
Financing nursing education: schools must face financial facts of life. *Hospitals*, Oct. 1, 1959, p. 51-4.

MILLS, H. C.
Financing nursing education: N.L.N. study seeks base for future planning. *Hospitals*, Oct. 1, 1959, p. 48-50.

MULLANE, MARY KELLY
Education for nursing service administration; an experience in program development by fourteen universities. Michigan, W. K. Kellogg Foundation, 1959.

NATIONAL LEAGUE OF NURSING EDUCATION. EDUCATION COMMITTEE
The nursing school faculty: duties, qualifications and preparation. New York, National League of Nursing Education, 1933.

NURSING RECORD
Matrons in Council [or whether probationers should pay for their training]. *Nursing Record*, Nov. 25, 1893, p. 265-6.

NUTTING, MARY ADELAIDE
A sound economic basis for schools of nursing, and other addresses. New York, Putnam, 1926.

PETRY, LUCILE, and BLOCK, LOUIS
Cost analysis for schools of nursing: a manual of methods and procedures. Washington, Govt. Printing Office, 1946.

STEINER, E.
Administrators' responsibility and obligation to nursing education. *Hospital Progress*, Jan. 1959, p. 78-81.

STERN, W. E.
The responsibility of the doctor of medicine in the training of nursing personnel and the governing of nursing care policy in the modern hospital. *Surgery*, Aug. 1959, p. 444-6.

WILLIAMS, DOROTHY ROGERS
Administration of schools of nursing, edited by Isabel M. Stewart. New York, Macmillan, 1950.

WILSON, LOLA
Cost study of basic nursing education programs in Saskatchewan, prepared under the direction of the Steering Committee for the Board of Administration of the centralized teaching program for nursing students in Saskatchewan. Regina, Saskatchewan Registered Nurses' Association, 1958.

Bibliographies

NATIONAL LEAGUE FOR NURSING
Bibliographies on nursing. Vol. I. Anatomy and physiology; chemistry; microbiology; physics. New York, The League, 1952.

NATIONAL LEAGUE FOR NURSING
Bibliographies on nursing. Vol. II. Ethics; group process; history; psychology and mental health; health and social aspects of nursing; sociology and anthropology. New York, The League, 1952.

NATIONAL LEAGUE FOR NURSING
Bibliographies on nursing. Vol. III. Nursing art and science; nutrition and diet therapy; pharmacology. New York, The League, 1952.

NATIONAL LEAGUE FOR NURSING
Bibliographies on nursing. Vol. IV. Medical and surgical nursing. New York, The League, 1952.

NATIONAL LEAGUE FOR NURSING
Bibliographies on nursing. Vol. VI. Communicable disease nursing; poliomyelitis nursing; tuberculosis nursing; venereal disease nursing. New York, The League, 1952.

NATIONAL LEAGUE FOR NURSING
Bibliographies on nursing. Vol. VII. Psychiatric nursing and mental health nursing. New York, The League, 1952.

NATIONAL LEAGUE FOR NURSING
Bibliographies on nursing. Vol. VIII. Cancer nursing; nursing in diseases of the eye, ear, nose and throat; neurologic and neurosurgical nursing; orthopedic nursing; urologic nursing; occupational health nursing; tropical disease nursing. New York, The League, 1952.

NATIONAL LEAGUE FOR NURSING
Bibliographies on nursing. Vol. IX. Professional adjustments; economic background and economic security; legislation and legal aspects of nursing. New York, The League, 1952.

NATIONAL LEAGUE FOR NURSING
Bibliographies on nursing. Vol. X. Curriculum; in-service education; library science; methods of instruction; research; student selection, evaluation and guidance; administration in schools of nursing; administration and supervision in nursing services. New York, The League, 1952.

NATIONAL LEAGUE FOR NURSING
Supplements to the bibliographies on nursing. Vol. II. Ethics; group process; history; psychology and mental health; health and social aspects of nursing; sociology and anthropology. New York, The League, 1954.

NATIONAL LEAGUE FOR NURSING
Supplements to the bibliographies on nursing. Vol. IV. Medical and surgical nursing. New York, The League, 1954.

NATIONAL LEAGUE FOR NURSING
Bibliographies on nursing. Vol. II. Nutrition and diet; pharmacology. New York, The League, 1957.

NATIONAL LEAGUE FOR NURSING
Bibliographies on nursing. . . . Vol. III. Psychology and mental health; sociology and anthropology. New York, The League, 1957.

NATIONAL LEAGUE FOR NURSING
Bibliographies on nursing. Vol. VI. Medical nursing; nursing in diseases of the eye, ear, nose and throat; tropical disease nursing; tuberculosis nursing. New York, The League, 1957.

NATIONAL LEAGUE FOR NURSING
Bibliographies on nursing. Vol. X. Psychiatric nursing. New York, The League, 1957.

NATIONAL LEAGUE FOR NURSING
Bibliographies on nursing. Vol. XI. Public health nursing. New York, The League, 1957.

NATIONAL LEAGUE FOR NURSING
Bibliographies on nursing. Vol. XII. Occupational health nursing. New York, The League, 1957.

NATIONAL LEAGUE FOR NURSING
Bibliographies on nursing. Vol. XIV. Practical nursing. New York, The League, 1957.

NATIONAL LEAGUE OF NURSING EDUCATION
Source materials in nursing education, No. 1. [New York], National League of Nursing Education, 1952.
[Source materials in nursing education, No. 2, was prepared by the National League for Nursing, q.v.]

NATIONAL LEAGUE FOR NURSING
Source materials in nursing education, No. 2. [New York], National League for Nursing, 1954.
[Source materials in nursing education, No. 1, was prepared by the National League of Nursing Education, q.v.]

Collegiate Schools

BRAUN, ANNE E., and LARKIN, CONSTANCE M.
A maternal and child health program in the collegiate basic curriculum. *Nursing Outlook*, Dec. 1960, p. 677-80.

BRIDGMAN, MARGARET
Collegiate education for nursing. New York, Russell Sage Foundation, 1953.

CATHOLIC UNIVERSITY OF AMERICA
[Proceedings of the] workshop on administration of college programs in nursing, June 12 to 24, 1944. Washington, The University, 1944.

HENRIKSEN, HEIDE L.
Curriculum study of the occupational health aspects of nursing; an adventure in co-operation. A report of an educational project in six collegiate schools of nursing in Minnesota. Minneapolis, Minnesota League for Nursing, 1959.

NATIONAL LEAGUE FOR NURSING
Self-evaluation guide for collegiate schools of nursing. New York, The League, 1954.

NATIONAL LEAGUE OF NURSING EDUCATION
Descriptions of eight collegiate basic programs in nursing. New York, National League of Nursing Education, 1952.

NATIONAL LEAGUE OF NURSING EDUCATION
Guide for the organisation of collegiate schools of nursing. Rev. edn. New York, The League, 1946.

NATIONAL LEAGUE OF NURSING EDUCATION
Problems of collegiate schools of nursing offering basic professional programs. New York, The League, 1945.

NATIONAL NURSING COUNCIL FOR WAR SERVICE
and
ASSOCIATION OF COLLEGIATE SCHOOLS OF NURSING
Guide for the organisation of collegiate schools of nursing. New York, The Council, 1942.

STEPHENSON, ELSIE
A collegiate program in nursing in Scotland. *Nursing Outlook*, Aug. 1959, p. 457-9.
[Edinburgh University, Nursing Studies Unit.]

Community Colleges

FREEMAN, RUTH
Junior community college programmes in nursing. *Nursing Outlook*, Dec. 1956, p. 689-91.

MONTAG, MILDRED L.
Community college education for nursing: an experiment in technical education for nursing; report of the Co-operative Research Project in Junior Community College Education for Nursing, by Mildred L. Montag, with Part II by Lassar G. Gotkin. New York, McGraw-Hill, 1959.

Counselling

GORDON, H. PHOEBE, and others
Counseling in schools of nursing: a study of the principles and techniques of personnel services for students, by H. Phoebe Gordon, Kathrine J. Densford and E. G. Williamson. New York, McGraw-Hill, 1947.

JORDAN, CLIFFORD H., and KENNEDY, JANE
Counseling that enriches. *American Journal of Nursing*, Feb. 1960, p. 231-3.

KABACK, GOLDIE RUTH
Guidance and counseling perspectives for hospital schools of nursing. New York, National League for Nursing, 1958.

LEWIS, G. K.
Counseling? or criticizing? *American Journal of Nursing*, Oct. 1958, p. 1408-9.

MCCRACKEN, MABEL CARROLL
Biblio-counseling as a guidance technique in schools of nursing. Washington, Catholic University of America Press, 1950.

ST. MARY'S SCHOOL OF NURSING, MILWAUKEE, WISCONSIN, GUIDANCE COMMITTEE
The development of a guidance program in St. Mary's School of Nursing, Milwaukee, Wisconsin, by the Guidance Committee. . . . New York, National League for Nursing, 1956.

SPALDING, EUGENIA KENNEDY
The student nurse in this post-war period and her guidance. Ennisburg, Maryland, Institute for Directors of Nurses, St. Joseph's Central House, 1946.

TRIGGS, FRANCES ORALIND
Personnel work in schools of nursing. Philadelphia, Saunders, 1945.

WOOD, M. M.
The nurse as a part-time counselor. *Military Medicine*, Feb. 1960, p. 120-5.

Curricula

BENNE, KENNETH D., and MUNTYAN, BOZIDAR, editors
Human relations in curriculum change: selected readings with especial emphasis on group development. New York, Dryden Press, 1951.

BLACK, KATHLEEN
Human relations content in the basic curriculum. *Nursing Research*, June 1956, p. 4-17.

BROWN, AMY FRANCES
Curriculum development. Philadelphia, Saunders, 1960.

CANADIAN NURSES' ASSOCIATION
A proposed curriculum for schools of nursing in Canada. (A tentative report of the Curriculum Committee of the Nursing Education Section.) Montreal, The Association, 1936.

CARDEW, EMILY C., editor
Study guide for clinical nursing: a co-ordinated survey integrated with essentials of the basic sciences. Philadelphia, Lippincott, 1953.

CARTER, G. B.
Nursing education. Some considerations on the basic nursing curriculum. Canadian Nurse, May 1956, p. 357-61.

COVILLE, W.
The psychological approach in medical and surgical nursing. Hospital Progress, Dec. 1958, p. 76-9.

COWAN, F. P., and LYON, H. F.
Public health nursing in the collegiate basic curriculum. Nursing Outlook, Dec. 1957, p. 706-7.

DELEURAN, H.
The basic curriculum for the first year. International Nursing Review, April 1958, p. 54-6.

DENNY, FRANCIS P.
The need of an institution for the education of nurses independent of the hospitals. British Journal of Nursing, Aug. 15, 1903, p. 125-7.

DITCHFIELD, A. L.
Occupational health in the nursing curriculum. Nursing Outlook, Nov. 1956, p. 622-4.

DOUGLAS, J.
Public health in the nursing curriculum. Nursing Times, April 29, 1955, p. 467-8.

DU GAS, BEVERLY W., and BLACKWOOD, BARBARA
Teaching community aspects of nursing; their inclusion in the basic curriculum. Canadian Nurse, Oct. 1959, p. 932-6.

ELLIOTT, FLORENCE E.
Setting the stage. Canadian Nurse, Oct. 1960, p. 930-3.

ELLIOTT, FLORENCE E.
Viewpoints on curriculum development, expressed at the 1957 curriculum conferences of the National League for Nursing. New York, The League, 1957.

FARQUHARSON, M. D.
The minimum curriculum of education and standard qualifying for the registration of trained nurses. British Journal of Nursing, Sept. 17, 1904, p. 229-30.

HAWKINS, N. G.
A measure of empirical validity. Nursing Research, Winter 1959, p. 13-17.

HEYSE, M. F.
We share curriculum planning. Nursing Outlook, Sept. 1957, p. 532-5.

HULL, E. J., and ISAACS, B.
An experiment with the curriculum. Nursing Times, Dec. 9, 1960, p. 1540-3.

LAUNCESTON GENERAL HOSPITAL, LAUNCESTON, TASMANIA
Curriculum of nursing education. Nursing Record, April 24, 1897, p. 343.

MCCORKLE, MAE D.
A curriculum study in social hygiene for nurses. New York, Columbia University, Teachers' College, 1934.

MCKECHNIE, M. W.
What has been accomplished in the direction of a uniform curriculum. Questionaire sent to American and Canadian training schools and their replies. Nursing Record, May 29, 1897, p. 437-9; June 5, 1897, p. 455-6; June 12, 1897, p. 476-8.

NATIONAL LEAGUE FOR NURSING. DEPARTMENT OF DIPLOMA AND ASSOCIATE DEGREE PROGRAMS
Developing a basic nursing curriculum: the process and the problems; developed at a Workshop on Associate Degree Programs in Nursing; sponsored by the Extension Division, University of California, June 23-July 11, 1958. New York, The League, 1958.

NATIONAL LEAGUE OF NURSING EDUCATION
Standard curriculum for schools of nursing: prepared by the Committee on Education of the National League of Nursing Education. Baltimore, Waverly Press, n.d.

NATIONAL LEAGUE OF NURSING EDUCATION. COMMITTEE ON CURRICULUM
A curriculum guide for schools of nursing. New York, The League, 1917.
2nd edn., 1927.
3rd edn., 1937.

NATIONAL LEAGUE OF NURSING EDUCATION. DEPARTMENT OF SERVICES TO SCHOOLS OF NURSING
Nursing organization curriculum conference: report of proceedings of conference, Dec. 3-5, 1949, at Henry Hudson Hotel, New York. New York, The League, 1950.

NATIONAL LEAGUE OF NURSING EDUCATION. DEPARTMENT OF SERVICES TO SCHOOLS OF NURSING
Joint nursing curriculum conference; report of proceedings of conference, Nov. 13-15, 1950, at Teachers' College, Columbia University. New York, The League, 1951.
[A continuation of the nursing organization curriculum conference held in 1949.]

NURSES' ASSOCIATION OF CHINA. EDUCATION COMMITTEE
Curriculum outlines for use in the training schools for nurses of the Nurses' Association of China. Shanghai, Kwang Hsueh Publishing House, 1925.

PITTMAN, HELLEN, and KLUTAS, EDNA MAY
Continued story in Texas. Nursing Outlook, Nov. 1960, p. 608-11.
[Occupational health nursing in curriculum.]

RABO, M.
Integrating public health in schools of nursing. Preparation for the integration of public health in Swedish schools of nursing. International Nursing Review, Jan. 1958, p. 23-7.

RUNDLE, M. S.
The curriculum of training schools and the University of America [Abridged]. British Journal of Nursing, April 27, 1912, p. 329-30.

SAND, OLE
Curriculum study in basic nursing education. New York, Putnam, 1955.

SCHMITT, MARY
A curricular study of psychological problems encountered by students in the basic professional program in nursing. Pittsburgh, University of Pittsburgh, 1948.

SEYFFER, CHARLOTTE
Management content in the basic nursing curriculum. American Journal of Nursing, Aug. 1959, p. 1125-9.

SHETLAND, MARGARET L.
A method for exploring bases of curriculum development: the study preceding the reorganization of the Public Health Nursing Curriculum in the State University of New York. New York, National League for Nursing, 1955.

SNIVELY, MARY AGNES
A uniform curriculum for training schools. Nursing Record, April 6, 1895, p. 214-5, and April 13, 1895, p. 235-6.

SOCIALIST MEDICAL ASSOCIATION
Suggested syllabus for a two-year basic training in nursing. Socialist Medical Association, 1949.

SPALDING, EUGENIA KENNEDY
Developing curricula for nursing education. Hospital Progress, Nov. 1956, p. 68-72.

STEWART, ISLA
A uniform curriculum of education for nurses. *Nursing Record*, Nov. 2, 1895, p. 311-13; Nov. 9, 1895, p. 330-2; Nov. 16, 1895, p. 349-51.

TREASURE, EDNA H., *editor*
Implementation of the nursing curriculum in the clinical fields (the proceedings of the Workshop in Implementation of the Nursing Curriculum in the Clinical Fields, conducted at the Catholic University of America, June 15 to June 26, 1956). Washington, Catholic University of America Press, 1957.

ZURRER, GERTRUDE
A study of the social content in the basic nursing curriculum. New York, Columbia University, Teachers' College, 1934.

Diploma Schools

ALOYSIA, SISTER
A day school for diploma students. *Nursing Outlook*, July 1960, p. 379.

KINGSBURY, V.
Comprehensive education in diploma programs. *Hospital Progress*, Oct. 1957, p. 64-6.

SLEEPER, RUTH
A reaffirmation of belief in the diploma school of nursing. *Nursing Outlook*, Nov. 1958, p. 616-8.

Inservice Education

ANDERSON, R.
Inservice training for the nursing service. *Medical Bulletin of the U.S. Army, Europe*, Feb. 1957, p. 30-4.

BENNETT, B. A.
T.W.I. methods and their possibilities for nursing. *Nursing Mirror*, June 8, 1956, p. 721-2.

BREDENBERG, V.
Inservice nursing service programs in Catholic hospitals. *Hospital Progress*, Feb. 1958, part II, p. 362 and 364.

BRIDGES, DAISY C.
The needs and methods of inservice training. *Royal Society for the Promotion of Health Journal*, Sept. 1956, p. 632-4.

DE PAUL, SISTER
Inservice education and training. *Hospital Progress*, Aug. 1957, p. 64-6.

DONOVAN, HELEN MURPHY
Inservice programs and their evaluation. *Nursing Outlook*, Nov. 1956, p. 633-5.

DONOVAN, HELEN MURPHY
Making inservice education attractive. *American Journal of Nursing*, Oct. 1959, p. 1442-3.

HEIDGERKEN, LORETTA
Inservice education and research. *Nursing Outlook*, Aug. 1959, p. 474-5.

HICKEY, N. M.
Training within industry applied to hospital problems; report of a recent course at Guy's Hospital, London. *Nursing Mirror*, July 22, 1955, p. v-vi.

HINER, B.
Inservice education for good service. *Nursing Outlook*, April 1957, p. 218-9.

LAUGHLIN, HUGH D.
Education programs in service-centered hospital schools. *Nursing Outlook*, May 1956, p. 269-71.

LONG, L. M.
Motivating personnel for inservice education. *Nursing Outlook*, June 1959, p. 333-5.

MACRAE, M. C.
Inservice education for general staff nurses. *Canadian Nurse*, Nov. 1957, p. 1013-6.

MARY AGNES, SISTER
Inservice program meetings. *Hospital Progress*, Dec. 1960, p. 64-5.

MARY ALBERT, SISTER
Inservice program. *Hospital Management*, May 1959, p. 113-4.

MILLER, MARY ANNICE
Inservice education for hospital personnel. New York, National League for Nursing, 1958.

REDMOND, MARY M.
Is inservice education the answer? *American Journal of Nursing*, Nov. 1956, p. 1430-4.

RUTAN, E. L.
A co-operative program of inservice education. *Nursing Outlook*, Sept. 1956, p. 522-4.

WARSTLER, MARTHA E.
An adventure with inservice education. *Nursing Outlook*, Oct. 1955, p. 558-60.

Integrated Courses

GOODYEAR, K.
Four-year scheme of integrated training in psychiatric and general nursing fields. *Nursing Mirror*, May 11, 1956, p. viii-ix.

MERRY, E. J.
Integrated nursing course at Hammersmith Hospital Postgraduate Medical School of London, Battersea College of Technology and Queen's Institute of District Nursing. *Nursing Times*, Feb. 15, 1957, p. 193-4.

O'CONNELL, P. E.
The development of integrated schemes of training for nursing and health visiting. *Royal Society for the Promotion of Health Journal*, Nov.-Dec. 1957, p. 865-71.

ROYAL COLLEGE OF NURSING and KING'S COLLEGE HOSPITAL
General nursing and health visiting: integrated training. *Nursing Times*, Feb. 27, 1959, p. 256-8.
[See also UNIVERSITY COURSES p. 50]

Pre-Nursing Courses

ASSOCIATION OF WOMEN SCIENCE TEACHERS
The pre-nursing course: syllabuses, equipment and books; together with further recommendations of the Association of Women Science Teachers. John Murray, [1943]. 2nd edn., 1947.

CUTHBERT, T. M.
An experiment in psychiatric pre-nurse training. *Lancet*, Feb. 13, 1954, p. 357-9.

GENERAL NURSING COUNCIL FOR ENGLAND AND WALES
Pre-nursing courses, their purpose, function and history. The General Nursing Council for England and Wales, 1950.

LOGAN, J. S.
The vexed question of nursing cadets. *Nursing Mirror*, April 10, 1959, p. 117-8, and April 17, 1959, p. 199-200.

McCOULL, G.
Cadet scheme at a mental deficiency hospital. *Nursing Times*, May 15, 1959, p. 573-5.

MARCHANT, E. P.
Pre-nurse training. *Nursing Times*, Jan. 2, 1959, p. 11-12.

YORK, EDUCATION COMMITTEE
Junior nursing course in York. *Hospital*, Sept. 1959, p. 786-7.

Student Status

ANDERSON, BERNICE E.
The question of student employment. *American Journal of Nursing*, Nov. 1959, p. 1575-9.

HENTSCH, YVONNE
The student nurse in the community. *Canadian Nurse*, Mar. 1957, p. 205-7.

REGAN, W. A.
Student nurse status: legal considerations. *Hospital Progress*, June 1957, p. 70-2.

Teaching

AGATE, M. A., *and* COOPER, C.
Dramatics in the classroom. *Nursing Times*, Dec. 2, 1960, p. 1508-9.

AIKENS, CHARLOTTE A.
Training school methods for institutional nurses. Philadelphia, Saunders, 1919.

AUFHAUSER, T. R.
Giving assignments meaning. *American Journal of Nursing*, April 1957, p. 479-80.

BRAGDON, JANE SHERBURN, *and* SHOLTIS, LILLIAN A.
Teaching medical and surgical nursing. Philadelphia, Lippincott, 1955.

BREGG, E. A.
How can we help students learn? *American Journal of Nursing*, Aug. 1958, p. 1120-2.

BRETHORST, ALICE B.
Methods of teaching in schools of nursing. Philadelphia, Saunders, 1949.

BRIESS, L.
Diagram jig-saw puzzle: a learning aid for student nurses. *Nursing Mirror*, Nov. 25, 1955, p. viii-ix.

BROOKS, S. M.
The textbook; big or little? *Nursing Outlook*, July 1959, p. 406-7.

BROWN, AMY FRANCES
Clinical instruction. Philadelphia, Saunders, 1949.

BROWN, AMY FRANCES
Organization of clinical learning experiences. *Nursing Outlook*, Feb. 1957, p. 95-7.

BROWN, BILLYE J.
Evaluating the text book. *Nursing Outlook*, Oct. 1959, p. 601-3.

CARDEW, EMILY C.
Patient-centered teaching. Philadelphia, Lippincott, 1958.

CATHOLIC UNIVERSITY OF AMERICA
Dynamics of clinical instruction in nursing education (the proceedings of the Workshop on the Dynamics of Clinical Instruction . . . June 11 to June 22, 1954); edited by Mary Grace Gabig and Barbara T. Lanigan. Washington, Catholic University of America Press, 1956.

CATHOLIC UNIVERSITY OF AMERICA
Symposium on clinical experience in medical and surgical nursing in the Providence Division of the School of Nursing Education. . . . Washington, Catholic University of America Press, 1940.

CHARLES, E.
Co-ordinating ward and classroom teaching in a mental hospital. *Nursing Mirror*, Dec. 30, 1955, p. v-vi.

CLAY, M. J. H.
Teaching of students at varying intelligence levels. *Nursing Mirror*, Sept. 20, 1957, p. 1793-4.

COSTON, H. M.
Patient-centered teaching. *Nursing Outlook*, Dec. 1958, p. 697-9.

COULTER, PEARL PARVIN
The teaching-learning process in nursing education. *Nursing Outlook*, Oct. 1960, p. 575-8.

COURTNEY, M. E.
The effectiveness of the classroom laboratory in the teaching of nursing arts. *Nursing Research*, Summer 1959, p. 148-54.

DOMAN, GLENN J., WARNOCK, ROSEMARY BOYLE, *and* DELACATO, CARL H.
Making classroom teaching glow. *Nursing Outlook*, Mar. 1960, p. 156-7.

ELLIOTT, FLORENCE E.
The selection of learning experiences. *Canadian Nurse*, Dec. 1960, p. 1094-5.

FADDIS, M. O.
Nursing education today. On clinical teaching: how, within a generation, teaching has become centered on patients rather than procedures. *American Journal of Nursing*, Oct. 1960, p. 1461-4.

FEENEY, E.
The changing role of the nurse as a teacher. *Military Medicine*, Nov. 1957, p. 304-7.

FOLEY, M. M.
Patient centered nursing education. *Hospital Progress*, Aug. 1958, p. 92-3.

FRIEND, C. P.
The X-ray department as a teaching tool. *Virginia Medical Monthly*, Aug 1960, p. 461-2.

GABRIEL, SISTER JOHN
Practical methods of study: a textbook for student nurses. New York, Macmillan, 1930.

GABRIEL, SISTER JOHN
Principles of teaching in schools of nursing. New York, Macmillan, 1928.

GABRIEL, SISTER JOHN
Teachers' work organization book for schools of nursing. Philadelphia, Saunders, 1931.

GEDDES, J. D. C.
The potential clinical instructor. *Nursing Times*, June 24, 1960, p. 781-2 and 787.

HALL, B. H.
Creating a climate for learning. *Nursing Outlook*, July 1959, p. 421-2.

HARMER, BERTHA
Methods and principles of teaching the principles and practice of nursing. New York, Macmillan, 1926.

HEIDGERKEN, LORETTA E.
The nursing student evaluates her teachers. Philadelphia, Lippincott, 1952.

HEIDGERKEN, LORETTA E.
Teaching in schools of nursing, principles and methods. Philadelphia, Lippincott, 1946. 2nd end., 1953.

HOLLAND, D. L.
Teaching social aspects of disease. 4. The integration of preventive medicine in the basic training. *Nursing Times*, May 9, 1953, p. 458-60.

INGLES, THELMA
An experience in learning. *Nursing Research*, Oct. 1957, p. 77-8.

INGLES, THELMA
Understanding instructors. *Nursing Outlook*, Dec. 1956, p. 692-3.

INGMIRE, ALICE E., *and* HART, BERNICE HUDSON
Student centred teaching in nursing. New York National League for Nursing, 1959.

JACKSON, ALICE M., *and* ARMSTRONG, KATHERINE F.
Teaching in schools of nursing. Faber, 1934. 2nd edn., 1952.

JENSEN, DEBORAH MACLURG, *and others*
Principles and practice of ward teaching. Henry Kimpton, 1942.
2nd edn., Principles and practice of clinical instruction in nursing, 1946.
3rd edn., Clinical instruction and its integration in the curriculum, 1952.

KNEPLER, H. W.
Communication in nursing education. Teaching English to nursing students. *Nursing Outlook*, Nov. 1955, p. 613-4.

LEICESTER ROYAL INFIRMARY
The Leicester Experiment. An account of the experiment (at Leicester Royal Infirmary) of appointing four clinical instructors in addition to the tutors. *Nursing Times*, Oct. 23, 1959, p. 1034.

LENNON, SISTER MARY ISADORE
Teaching in the outpatient department. New York, Putnam, 1954.

McCUNE, HELEN L., *and* MEYER, RUTH T.
The bulletin board: an effective teaching aid. *Nursing Outlook*, Sept. 1959, p. 532-3.

McINTYRE, P. H.
Ward teaching packets. *American Journal of Nursing*, April 1959, p. 524-6.

McNAUGHT, E.
Clinical instruction. *Nursing Times*, June 7, 1957, p. 644-5.

MARY, SISTER
Teaching religion in professional schools of nursing. *Hospital Progress*, Nov. 1958, p. 88-92.

METHUEN, DOLORES, *and* STRAYER, CONSTANCE H.
Teaching dynamics of human behavior; the clinical potential. *Nursing Outlook*, Jan. 1960, p. 47-50.

MOHAN, T., *Jr.*
Integrated methods of teaching. *Hospital Progress*, Sept. 1959, p. 112-6.

MORRISON, RUTH M.
Providing for depth of learning. *Canadian Nurse*, Aug. 1960, p. 730-4.

MULLER, T., *and* SCHOLDER, A. P.
Teaching with closed circuit television. *Nursing Outlook*, Dec. 1957, p. 698-700.

NITE, GLADYS
Learning every day: nursing service provides the ideal setting in which nurses can improve their clinical competence. *American Journal of Nursing*, Dec. 1960, p. 1761-4.

NORRIS, C. M.
A structure for learning. *Nursing Outlook*, July 1958, p. 379-81.

OUSELEY, M. H.
The teaching of nursing skills and procedures. *Nursing Times*, Sept. 13, 1957, p. 1027-8.

PATMORE, E.
Problems of nurse teaching and training. *Nursing Mirror*, Mar. 15, 1957, p. 1753.

PEPLAU, HILDEGARD E.
What is experimental teaching? *American Journal of Nursing*, July 1957, p. 884-6.

PFEFFERKORN, BLANCHE, *and* ROTTMAN, MARIAN
Clinical education in nursing. New York, Macmillan, 1932.

PLOGSTED, H.
Using nursing records to teach. *Nursing Outlook*, Jan. 1959, p. 43-5.

REID, A. E.
Nurses as teachers of science. *Canadian Nurse*, Mar. 1956, p. 187-91.

ROHWEDER, ANNE W., *and* HART, BETTY C.
How attitudes are taught and caught. *American Journal of Nursing*, June 1960, p. 806-9.

ROHWEDER, ANNE W., *and* OLSEN, B. M.
A new approach to teaching nursing arts. *Nursing Outlook*, Aug. 1958, p. 462-5.

ROYAL COLLEGE OF NURSING. EDUCATION DEPARTMENT
The use of visual aids in schools of nursing. The College, [195?].

SMITH, DOROTHY M., HINES, MADELINE, *and* TOURTILLOT, ELEANOR
Instruction in history of nursing. *Nursing Outlook*, Nov. 1960, p. 631-5.

SPANEY, EMMA, *and* JENNINGS, LOUISE A.
The art of studying; a guide for student nurses. Philadelphia, Lippincott, 1958.

SPIESEKE, A. W.
How should the textbook be used? *Nursing Outlook*, May 1958, p. 276-7.

STAUBLE, W. J.
Teaching group sessions for nurses. *Nursing Mirror*, Dec. 27, 1957, p. 933-4.

TAYLOR, ANNA M.
Ward teaching: methods of clinical instruction. Philadelphia, Lippincott, 1941.

THOMAS, J. L.
The spirit of a teaching program.
I. *Hospital Progress*, Mar. 1960, p. 108-12.
II. *Hospital Progress*, April 1960, p. 114-20.

WIGGINS, VIRGINIA L.
The teaching team. *American Journal of Nursing*, June 1956, p. 764-6.

WILLIAMS, R. C.
Communication in clinical instruction. *Hospital Progress*, Dec. 1956, p. 54-6.

WILSON, LOLA
The centralized teaching program for nursing students in Saskatchewan: the story of the first three years, prepared under the direction of the Steering Committee for the Board of Administration for the centralized teaching program for nursing students in Saskatchewan. Regina, Saskatchewan Registered Nurses' Association, 1957.

WILSON, R.
Challenge to the nurse tutor—importance to nursing of modern educational ideal. *Nursing Mirror*, Jan. 27, 1956, p. 1129.

University Courses

BEARD, RICHARD OLDING
The university education of the nurse. New York, National League of Nursing Education, 1919.

BLACK, A.
The development of integrated schemes of training for nursing and health visiting. *Royal Society for the Promotion of Health Journal*, Nov.-Dec. 1957, p. 871-4.

BOYD, LOUIE CROFT
The universities and the education of the nurse. Albuquerque, New Mexico, University of New Mexico, 1916. *Bulletin of the University of New Mexico*, vol. 1, no. 10, Sept. 1916.

CAFFERTY, K. W.
An associate degree program in nursing. *Journal of the American Dietetic Association*, May 1960, p. 473-4.

HASSENPLUG, LULU WOLF
Nursing education in universities. *Nursing Outlook*, Feb. 1960, p. 92-5.
2. Programs for graduate nurses. *Nursing Outlook*, Mar. 1960, p. 154-5.

KIRKCONNELL, N. E., *and* McCAIN, R. F.
The development of the degree program in nursing at the University of Michigan. *University of Michigan Medical Bulletin*, Sept. 1956, p. 390-7.

McDOWELL, EDITH M.
The profession and the university. *Canadian Nurse*, Feb. 1960, p. 129-31.

MANCHESTER REGIONAL HOSPITAL BOARD *and*
UNIVERSITY OF MANCHESTER
Course for a "community nurse". *Nursing Mirror*, April 10, 1959, p. 119 and 118.

MANCHESTER REGIONAL HOSPITAL BOARD *and*
UNIVERSITY OF MANCHESTER
Integrated scheme of training for state registration and health visiting. *Hospital and Social Service Journal*, Jan. 23, 1959, p. 82.

MANCHESTER UNIVERSITY/CRUMPSALL HOSPITAL
The Manchester scheme from four angles. *Nursing Times*, July 22, 1960, p. 906-8.

NEWMAN, C.
University education for nurses. *Nursing Times*, Aug. 29, 1958, p. 1002-3.

NEWTON, MILDRED E.
The relation of the educational unit in nursing to other departments of the university. *Nursing Outlook*, May 1958, p. 264-6.

O'CONNELL, P. E.
Integrated course of nurse/health visitor training prepared by Southampton University and the Nightingale School, St. Thomas' Hospital. *Nursing Times*, Sept. 21, 1956, p. 922-5.
[*See also* INTEGRATED COURSES p. 48]

LIBRARIES

ALTSCHUL, A.
Libraries in schools of nursing. In a mental hospital. *Nursing Times*, April 22, 1955, p. 433-4.

AMERICAN LIBRARY ASSOCIATION *and others.*
JOINT COMMITTEE ON STANDARDS FOR HOSPITAL LIBRARIES
Hospital libraries; objectives and standards, by committees of the American Library Association, the Medical Library Association and the Special Libraries Association, Chicago. A.L.A., Hospital Libraries Division, 1953.

BEATTY, W. K.
The Medical Centre Library: a symposium; the new Medical Centre Library. *Bulletin of the Medical Library Association*, Oct. 1958, p. 514-8.

BROOKLYN HOSPITAL, ORTHOPAEDIC DISPENSARY AND
TRAINING SCHOOL FOR NURSES.
List of donations to Training School includes many books for the nurses' library. Also contains rules for admission to the school and syllabus of training. The Dispensary, 1894.

BROWN, AMY FRANCES
The importance of hospital and nursing school libraries to the nursing profession. *Bulletin of the Medical Library Association*, July 1959, p. 258-63.

COLBURN, E. W.
Ward libraries. *American Journal of Nursing*, Mar. 1951, p. 193.

FORD, B. M.
Books alive. *Nursing Outlook*, Jan. 1957, p. 27-8.

FRANCIS XAVIER, SISTER
The library function in nursing education. *Hospital Progress*, July 1958, p. 66-7.

GAINES, M. JOSEPHINE
Preserving the structures of the past. *Nursing Outlook*, Feb. 1958, p. 103-4.

GORDON, BR.
Libraries, scholarship and the student in nursing. *Hospital Progress*, June 1959, p. 129 and 131-2.

GROVE, L.
A world to discover. The library is a richly rewarding "world" for nursing students if they are taught how to use its wealth of resources effectively. *Nursing Outlook*, April 1960, p. 220-1.

JANE, M. A.
A developmental reading course for nursing students. *Nursing Outlook*, Sept. 1960, p. 493-5.

LAGE, L. C., MILLER, L. B., *and* WASHBURN, D.
Dental, nursing and pharmaceutical libraries, 1947-1957. *Bulletin of the Medical Library Association*, July 1957, p. 371-7.

MACLEOD, A. ISOBEL
A profession and its journal. *Canadian Nurse*, Feb. 1958, p. 101-2.

MANOCH, H., *and* CORCORAN, J.
A library-centred program assists student-nurse development. *Hospital Progress*, Nov. 1959, p. 86, 156, 158.

MOLLETT, NINA
The nurse's library. *Nursing Record*, Jan. 19, 1893, p. 42-4.

MORRISSEY, M.
Relation of librarian to nursing school staff. *Bulletin of the Medical Library Association*, Oct. 1956, p. 452-4.

NATIONAL LEAGUE FOR NURSING
Basic book list. New York, The League, 1937.

NATIONAL LEAGUE FOR NURSING
Guide for the development of libraries in schools of nursing. New York, The League, 1952.

NATIONAL LEAGUE OF NURSING EDUCATION
Books suggested for libraries in schools of nursing. New York, The League, 1944.

NATIONAL LEAGUE OF NURSING EDUCATION
A library handbook for nursing schools. New York, The League, 1936.

NATIONAL LEAGUE OF NURSING EDUCATION
Manual for the nursing school library. New York, The League, 1947.

NURSING RECORD
Suggested list of books for a library for nursing staff in hospital. *Nursing Record*, Sept. 27, 1888, p. 350-1.

PORTER, ELIZABETH K.
The prospect before you. *American Journal of Nursing*, Jan. 1959, p. 56-9.
[This article considers education as a continuous process and stresses the need for extensive and thoughtful reading.]

RAISIG, L. M.
Keeping up with professional literature. *American Journal of Nursing*, April 1959, p. 544-5.
[Abstracting and indexing.]

ROYAL COLLEGE OF NURSING
Nursing libraries in hospitals and libraries in schools of nursing. R.C.N., [195?].

ROYAL COLLEGE OF NURSING. SISTER TUTOR SECTION
Libraries in 19 schools of nursing. *Nursing Times*, June 3, 1960, p. 689.

SOMERSET NURSES' SOCIAL UNION
The nurses' lending library. *Nursing Times*, April 27, 1907, p. 359-61.

TERESA, LOUISA, SISTER, *and* BRANDON, ALFRED N.
The integrated library: in a hospital school; in a college. *Nursing Outlook*, Nov. 1956, p. 619-22.

THOMPSON, A. M. C.
Nursing libraries in hospitals and libraries in schools of nursing. *Nursing Journal of India*, May 1960, p. 135-7.

WORTHY, E. J.
Libraries in schools of nursing: in a paediatric hospital. *Nursing Times*, April 15, 1955, p. 409-10.

POST-BASIC EDUCATION

ALLEN, D. E.
Opinions and plans of a group of graduate nurses in relation to graduate nurse education. *Nursing Research*, Feb. 1957, p. 121-9.

BIXLER, GENEVIEVE K., *and* SIMMONS, LEO W.
The regional project in graduate education and research in nursing: a report. Atlanta, Georgia, Southern Regional Education Board, 1960.

BRACKETT, M. E.
Where and how should head nurses be prepared?*Nursing Outlook*, Nov. 1957, p. 644-7.

BRIDGE, B. C.
A central training college for nurses. *Nursing Times*, Mar. 2, 1907, p. 182.

CAMPBELL, MARGARET
Why statistics? *Canadian Nurse*, Aug. 1960, p. 726-8.

CAWS, A. G.
The training of nurse tutors in mental hospitals. *Nursing Mirror*, Sept. 28, 1956, p. v-vii.

CHARLETON, J. W.
Clinical instructors' course. *Nursing Times*, Sept. 25, 1959, p. 898-900.

CHITTICK, RAE
University courses for graduate nurses. *Canadian Nurse*, Mar. 1955, p. 202-4.

COLUMBIA UNIVERSITY. TEACHERS' COLLEGE.
DIVISION OF NURSING EDUCATION
Problems of graduate nurse education: report of a work conference. [New York], Columbia University, 1952.

CUNNINGHAM, E. V.
Education for leadership in nursing: 1899-1959. *Nursing Outlook*, May 1959, p. 268-72.

EDINBURGH UNIVERSITY
Nursing studies unit—University of Edinburgh. *Nursing Times*, Feb. 1, 1957, p. 125.

EDINBURGH UNIVERSITY
Nurse teaching unit. *Nursing Times*, July 29, 1955, p. 825, Dec. 2, 1955, p. 1355.

ELKINS, W. H., *and* McMANUS, R. L.
Doctoral education in nursing. *Nursing Outlook*, Oct. 1960, and p. 542-6.

ELLIOTT, F. E.
The dietitian on the nursing faculty. *Journal of the American Dietetic Association*, Oct. 1959, p. 1052-4.

ERICKSON, MARY EDWARD
The inservice hospital sister needs continuing education. *Hospital Progress*, Aug. 1959, p. 82-3 and 113.

FAWKES, BARBARA N.
A day for study. *American Journal of Nursing*, Dec. 1956, p. 1546-7.
[In-service training for ward sisters in Great Britain.]

FIDLER, N. D.
Post-basic nursing education. *International Nursing Review*, Jan. 1958, p. 6-10.

FRANCES PAYNE BOLTON SCHOOL OF NURSING
Curriculum study of the graduate nurse programs. Cleveland, Ohio, Western Reserve University, 1954.

FREEMAN, RUTH B.
A plan for the continuing education of nurses. New York, National League for Nursing, 1956.

FRODSHAM, W., *and* O'ROARKE, E. M.
Seconding the sister to the teaching department. *Nursing Mirror*, Mar. 20, p. ii-iv.

GIPS, C. D.
An evaluation of graduates of an associate degree program. *Nursing Outlook*, Dec. 1959, p. 701-2.

GREAT BRITAIN. MINISTRY OF HEALTH *and others*
Report of the committee set up to consider the function, status and training of nurse tutors. H.M.S.O., 1954.

GUY'S HOSPITAL NURSES' LEAGUE
A scheme for post-graduate lectures to nurses started by Guy's Hospital Nurses' League. *British Journal of Nursing*, Sept. 26, 1903, p. 242.

HASSENPLUG, LULU WOLF
How can we prepare our teachers better. *Nursing World*, April 1960, p. 18-9 and 34.

HASSENPLUG, LULU WOLF
Nursing education in universities. *Nursing Outlook*, Feb. 1960, p. 92-5, and Mar. 1960, p. 154-5.

HEIDGERKEN, LORETTA
Preparing teachers of nursing. *Nursing Outlook*, Dec. 1955, p. 635-8.

INTERNATIONAL COUNCIL OF NURSES. EDUCATION COMMITTEE
Developing graduate nurse education; a guide for educational planners, [prepared during the years 1937-1947]. I.C.N., 1951.

INTERNATIONAL COUNCIL OF NURSES.
FLORENCE NIGHTINGALE INTERNATIONAL FOUNDATION
An international list of advanced programmes in nursing education (1951-1952) prepared by the Florence Nightingale International Foundation. I.C.N., 1954.

INTERNATIONAL COUNCIL OF NURSES.
FLORENCE NIGHTINGALE INTERNATIONAL FOUNDATION
Supplement to an international list of advanced programmes in nursing education (1957). I.C.N., 1958.

INTERNATIONAL COUNCIL OF NURSES.
FLORENCE NIGHTINGALE INTERNATIONAL FOUNDATION
Post-basic nursing education; principles of administration as applied to advanced programmes in nursing education. A report prepared under the auspices of the Florence Nightingale International Foundation, by Yvonne Schroeder, assisted by the staff of the Florence Nightingale International Foundation. International Council of Nurses, 1957. 2 vols.

INTERNATIONAL COUNCIL OF NURSES.
FLORENCE NIGHTINGALE INTERNATIONAL FOUNDATION
The report of a study of the facilities for advanced nursing education in London, both professional and academic, and the future educational policy of the Florence Nightingale International Foundation, May 1936. I.C.N., 1936.

KELBER, MAGDA
Principles and practice of adult education.
1. Basic facts about the learning process.
2-7. Important forms of presentation.
8. How to run a training conference.
Nursing Mirror, Feb. 1, 1957, p. 1269-70; Feb. 8, 1957, p. 1349-50; Feb. 15, 1957, p. 1431-2; Feb. 22, 1957, p. 1507-8; Mar. 1, 1957, p. vi-vii; Mar. 8, 1957, p. v-vi; Mar. 15, 1957, p. v-vi; Mar. 22, 1957, p. iii and 1830.

KELLEHER, R. P.
General nursing programs for graduate nurses. *Hospital Progress*, Aug. 1960, p. 68-71.

LAMBERTSEN, ELEANOR CATHERINE
Education for nursing leadership. Philadelphia, Lippincott, 1958.

LAMBERTSEN, ELEANOR CATHERINE
Professional education for leadership in nursing practice. New York, Columbia University, Teachers' College, 1957.

LERSNER, O. VON
The Heidelberg University School of Nursing. *International Nursing Review*, Oct. 1955, p. 27-32.

LEVINE, E.
How many nurses now have college degrees. *Nursing Outlook*, Dec. 1958, p. 688-9.

McDOWELL, E. M.
The profession and the university. *Canadian Nurse*, Feb. 1960, p. 129-31.

McGLOTHLIN, WILLIAM J.
Towards a regional program of graduate education and research in nursing. New York, National League for Nursing, 1953.

MACKENZIE, NORAH
The value of educational psychology to sister tutors: a series of lectures given in the special course for sister tutors at the Royal College of Nursing. *Nursing Times*, 1946.

McMILLAN, M. HELENA
Post-graduate instruction for nurses. *Nursing Record*, Jan. 18, 1902, p. 46-7.

MacQUEEN, E. U. *and* I. A. G.
The status of nurse tutors. *Nursing Times*, Dec. 7, 1956, p. 1256-7.

MANSFIELD, L.
Clinical nursing course for graduate nurses. *Nursing Outlook*, Sept. 1958, p. 518-20.

MARTIN, J.
Post-basic preparation of nurses: the preparation of teachers. *Nursing Times*, June 28, 1957, p. 725-7.

MARY EMIL, SISTER
The place of the nursing sister in the Sister Formation Movement. *Hospital Progress*, Sept. 1956, p. 57-60.

MEIR, E. M.
Nurses with degrees. *Nursing Times*, May 30, 1958, p. 629.

MILES, H. B.
University education for nurse teachers; an account of the University of Hull Sister Tutor's Diploma. *Nursing Mirror*, Mar. 11, 1955, p. x-xii.

MINNESOTA UNIVERSITY. SCHOOL OF NURSING
A study of the graduates of the University of Minnesota School of Nursing, by the Faculty of the School of Nursing. University of Minnesota, 1953?

MUDGE, J.
The tutor sister and her place in the teaching team. *Australian Nurses' Journal*, April 1960, p. 90-3 and 103.

MURRAY, J. G.
The functions of a sister tutor. *U.N.A. Nursing Journal*, Jan. 1959, p. 8-15.

MUSSELMAN, GRACE
A continuation program in nursing education. *Nursing Outlook*, Aug. 1960, p. 428-30.

MUSSON, E. M.
Post-graduate training for nurses. *British Journal of Nursing*, July 12, 1913, p. 23-5.

NATIONAL LEAGUE FOR NURSING.
DEPARTMENT OF BACCALAUREATE AND HIGHER DEGREE PROGRAMS
Characteristics of graduate education in nursing. New York, National League for Nursing, [1959].

NATIONAL LEAGUE FOR NURSING.
DIVISION OF NURSING EDUCATION
Report of work conference on graduate nurse education: a conference of schools offering programs leading to a degree for graduate nurses. [New York], National League for Nursing, 1952.

NATIONAL LEAGUE OF NURSING EDUCATION
Faculty positions in schools of nursing and how to prepare for them. New York, The League, 1946.

NATIONAL LEAGUE OF NURSING EDUCATION.
EDUCATION COMMITTEE
The nursing school faculty: duties, qualifications and preparation. New York, The League, 1933.

NURSING OUTLOOK
Educational programs for graduate nurses. *Nursing Outlook*, Nov. 1955, p. 601-7.

NURSING TIMES
University of London Diploma in Nursing. *Nursing Times*, Jan. 7, 1955, p. 7-8.

NUTINI, S.
Advanced nursing education in Italy. *Nursing Times*, May 17, 1957, p. 547-8.

ORME, S. E.
The matron's course: an introduction to hospital and private nursing. Scientific Press, 1897.

PALMER, M. E.
A learning exercise for senior nursing students: learning the method of investigating a problem is as important as its solution. *Nursing World*, April 1960, p. 10-11 and 32.

PATTERSON, T. K.
Flexible scholarships to improve nursing care. *Nursing Outlook*, Mar. 1957, p. 170-1.

POTTER, R. M.
Faculty work load in the clinical fields in nursing degree programs. *Nursing Research*, Summer 1959, p. 160-8.

POWERS, RUTH A.
A refresher program in a community hospital. *American Journal of Nursing*, June 1960, p. 821-3.

ROYAL COLLEGE OF NURSING
Memorandum on the sister tutor, her function, scope, responsibilities and conditions of service. Royal College of Nursing, 1953.

ROYAL COLLEGE OF NURSING. EDUCATION DEPARTMENT
The tutor's preparation in the Education Department, R.C.N. *Nursing Times*, Jan. 20, 1956, p. 60-2 and 75.

SEARLE, C.
B.A. and B.Sc. nursing degrees. Four and a half years' course at University of Pretoria. *South African Nursing Journal*, April 1956, p. 20-6.

SEYFFER, C.
Revision of a university nursing curriculum. *W.H.O. Chronicle*, Feb. 1960, p. 63-6.
[An account of the Higher Institute of Nursing at the Faculty of Medicine, University of Alexandria, Egypt.]

SMET, H.
Preparation of nurses for their administrative role. *Nursing Times*, June 28, 1957, p. 728-9.

SMITH, RUTH L., *and* STOUT, EDNA
Using community resources for refresher courses. *Nursing Outlook*, Jan. 1960, p. 22-3.

SOUTHERN REGIONAL EDUCATION BOARD
Continuity in nursing education for better patient care. Atlanta, Georgia, The Board, 1956.

SOUTHERN REGIONAL EDUCATION BOARD
Regional programs in professional and graduate education: principles and procedures. Atlanta, Georgia, The Board, 1952.

SOUTHERN REGIONAL EDUCATION BOARD.
REGIONAL COMMITTEE ON GRADUATE EDUCATION AND RESEARCH IN NURSING
Graduate education and research in nursing. Atlanta, Georgia, The Board, 1957.

SOUZA, L. E., MATHEWS, B., *and* REUELL, C. H.
Future nurse administrators learn by doing. *American Journal of Nursing*, Jan. 1956, p. 76-8.

STEPHENSON, E.
Nursing Studies Unit of Edinburgh University. *Nursing Mirror*, July 26, 1957, p. vi-vii.

SYKEPIEIERSKENES SAMARBEID I NORDEN
Survey of advanced education in the Northern Countries, Autumn, 1952. [Stockholm?], Svensk Sjukskoverskeforenings Forlag, 1956.
[Association of Nurses of the Northern Countries of Europe.]

VANDERBILT UNIVERSITY. SCHOOL OF NURSING
A study of the professional activities of the Faculty of the School of Nursing of Vanderbilt University, 1952-1953. Nashville, Tennessee, Vanderbilt University, 1955.

WALLACE, G. S.
Back to the bedside. *Nursing Outlook*, Oct. 1956, p. 555-8.

WILLIAMS, M. M.
Faculty development. *Nursing Outlook*, June 1957, p. 350-1.

WILSON, R.
The preparation of the nurse-tutor. *Nursing Mirror*, Jan. 27, 1956, p. 1129.

WORLD HEALTH ORGANIZATION
Post-basic nursing education programmes for foreign students: report of a Conference, Geneva, 5-14 October, 1959. Geneva, W.H.O., 1960.
[Technical Report Series, No. 199.]

WORLD HEALTH ORGANIZATION.
REGIONAL OFFICE FOR EUROPE
Post-basic nursing education: report of a Conference . . . Peebles, 19-26 June, 1956. Geneva, W.H.O., 1956.

TRAINING SCHOOLS

General Works

ALLINE, ANNA L.
Registration of nurse training schools in the State of New York, U.S.A. *British Journal of Nursing*, Sept. 25, 1909, p. 253-5.

BURGESS, MAY AYRES
A five-year programme for the Committee on the Grading of Nursing Schools. New York, The Committee, 1926.

CAIRNS, E.
An adequate budget. *Hospital Progress*, June 1960, p. 122-4.

CANFIELD, S. A. MARTHA
The inception, organization and management of training schools for nurses. Washington, U.S. Govt. Printing Office, 1882.

COMMITTEE ON THE GRADING OF NURSING SCHOOLS
Nurses, production, education, distribution and pay. New York, The Committee, 1930.

COMMITTEE ON THE GRADING OF NURSING SCHOOLS
Nursing schools today and tomorrow: final report. New York, The Committee, 1934.

DARCHE, LOUISE
Proper organization of training schools in America.
In
HAMPTON, ISABEL A., *and others*
Nursing of the sick, 1893.

DOCK, L. L.
The relation of training schools to hospitals.
In
HAMPTON, ISABEL A., *and others*
Nursing of the sick, 1893.

EATON, JOHN
Training schools for nurses. Washington, U.S. Govt. Printing Office, 1879.
[An address delivered before the Washington Training School.]

FOLEY, M. M.
Catholic schools of nursing. *Hospital Progress*, Feb. 1960, part 2, p. 159-69.

FOLEY, M. M.
What does the student pay? The report of a study of certain elements of cost in Catholic hospital schools of nursing. *Hospital Progress*, Nov. 1957, p. 88-92.

GENERAL NURSING COUNCIL FOR ENGLAND AND WALES
Notes on the planning, building and equipping of hospitals drawn up by the Council as an indication of the standards to be aimed at in hospitals approved as training schools for nurses. G.N.C., 1959.

GILHOOLEY, MARY A. N., *and* ELLIOTT, FLORENCE E.
The status of organizations in schools of nursing. *American Journal of Nursing*, May 1958, p. 703-5.

GIVEN, LEILA I., *and* FAVREAU, CLAIRE
A guide for supervision of State Approved Schools of Nursing. New York, American Nurses' Association, 1948.

GOODRICH, ANNIE W.
The introduction of salaried instruction in the training schools. *British Journal of Nursing*, June 17, 1905, p. 473-4.

HAMILTON, T. S.
What is ahead for the hospital school of nursing? Healthy now, it needs joint leadership to keep it strong. *Hospitals*, Aug. 16, 1960, p. 36 *passim*.

HURD, HENRY M.
Shall training schools for nurses be endowed? *British Journal of Nursing*, Sept. 22, 1906, p. 225-7, and Sept. 29, 1906, p. 245-7.

HURST, IRENE
Nursing schools and service in American Hospitals. (i) and (ii). *Hospital and Social Service Journal*, Nov. 4, 1960, p. 1205-6, and Nov. 11, 1960, p. 1235-6.

INTERNATIONAL COUNCIL OF NURSES.
FLORENCE NIGHTINGALE INTERNATIONAL FOUNDATION
How to survey a school of nursing: a suggested method, illustrated with samples of five post-basic schools. International Council of Nurses, 1954.

KING EDWARD'S HOSPITAL FUND FOR LONDON
Suggestions for the use of hospitals considering the establishment of central preliminary training schools for nurses. King Edward's Hospital Fund for London, [194?].

LEAHY, K. M.
Selecting the dean of a nursing school. *Nursing Outlook*, Dec. 1958, p. 705.

LEFEBVRE, DENISE
Behind the scenes on accreditation. *Canadian Nurse*, Oct. 1960, p. 893-8.
[Report of the special committee on the pilot project of evaluating schools of nursing in Canada.]

LESPARRE, M.
Accrediting a school of nursing. *Hospitals*, April 1955, p. 72-9.

McFADDEN, G. M., MILLER, H. A., CHAPMAN, M. P., *and* RICH, F. R.
How do nurses spend their time in schools? *American Journal of Public Health and the Nation's Health*, Aug. 1957, p. 937-43.

MACMAHON, R. P.
Schools of nursing on the Continent. *Hospital and Social Service Journal*, June 19, 1959, p. 635-6.

McMANUS, R. LOUISE
Study guide on evaluation. New York, National League Nursing Education, 1944.

McQUARRIE, FRANCIS
To evaluate schools of nursing. *Canadian Hospital*, April 1957, p. 42-3.

MAGUIRE, SISTER MARY ALMA
Contractual relationships existing between schools of nursing and participating agencies. Washington, Catholic University of America Press, 1949.

MANSFIELD, E. O.
Economics affecting the growth of hospital schools of nursing. *Hospital Management*, July 1957, p. 43 *passim*.

MUSSALLEM, HELEN K.
Evaluating schools of nursing. *Canadian Hospital*, Aug. 1959, p. 44-5.

MUSSALLEM, HELEN K.
A pilot project for evaluation of schools of nursing. *Canadian Journal of Public Health*, Aug. 1958, p. 348-50.

MUSSALLEM, HELEN K.
Spotlight on nursing education: the report of the pilot project for the evaluation of schools of nursing in Canada. Ottawa, Canadian Nurses' Association, 1960.

NAHM, HELEN
An evaluation of selected schools of nursing with respect to certain educational objectives. Palo Alto, Stanford University Press, 1948.

NATIONAL COMMITTEE FOR THE IMPROVEMENT OF NURSING SERVICES.
SUB-COMMITTEE ON SCHOOL DATA ANALYSIS
Nursing schools at the mid-century: a report prepared ... by Margaret West and Christy Hawkins. New York, The Committee, 1950.

NATIONAL LEAGUE FOR NURSING.
DIVISION OF NURSING EDUCATION
Accrediting your school of nursing. New York, The League, 1956.

NATIONAL LEAGUE FOR NURSING.
DIVISION OF NURSING EDUCATION
Report on the program of temporary accreditation of the National Nursing Accrediting Service. Part 1, study of basic programs offered by schools of nursing. [New York], The League, 1952.

NATIONAL LEAGUE OF NURSING EDUCATION
Committee of the six national nursing organizations on unification of accrediting activities—manual of accrediting educational programmes in nursing. New York, The League, 1949.

NATIONAL LEAGUE OF NURSING EDUCATION
Essentials of a good school of nursing. New York, The League, 1945.

NATIONAL LEAGUE OF NURSING EDUCATION
Fundamentals of administration for schools of nursing. New York, The League, 1940.

NATIONAL LEAGUE OF NURSING EDUCATION
Guidance programs for schools of nursing. New York, The League, 1946.

NATIONAL LEAGUE OF NURSING EDUCATION
State accredited schools of nursing. New York, The League, 1946.

NATIONAL LEAGUE OF NURSING EDUCATION.
COMMITTEE ON CURRICULUM
Essentials of a good school of nursing. New York, The League, 1942.

NATIONAL LEAGUE OF NURSING EDUCATION.
COMMITTEE ON VOCATIONAL GUIDANCE
Program for schools of nursing. New York, The League, 1946.

NATIONAL LEAGUE OF NURSING EDUCATION.
COMMITTEE TO STUDY ADMINISTRATION IN SCHOOLS OF NURSING
Fundamentals of administration for schools of nursing: report of the committee.... New York, The League, 1940.

NATIONAL NURSING COUNCIL
A thousand think together: a report of three regional conferences ... 1947, held in connection with the study of schools of nursing.... New York, The Council, 1948.

NATIONAL ORGANIZATION OF HOSPITAL SCHOOLS OF NURSING
A study of the educational programs of hospital schools of nursing, by Kenneth R. Williams, Fred Couey, James E. Greene. Atlanta, Georgia, National Organization of Hospital Schools of Nursing, 1954.

NURSING RECORD
Directory of training schools in London and the provinces. *Nursing Record*, Oct. 6, 1894, p. 217-38.

NURSING RECORD
Hospitals as training schools. *Nursing Record*, Jan. 19, 1893, p. 34-6.

NUTTING, MARY ADELAIDE
A sound economic basis for schools of nursing, and other addresses. New York, Putnam, 1926.

OLSON, J. F., and YORK, M. E.
Co-operation: keystone for success in planning a school of nursing. *American Journal of Nursing*, June 1959, p. 862-3.

RICHARDS, LINDA
The superintendent of the training school. *Nursing Record*, Aug. 13, 1898, p. 126-8.

RIDDLE, MARY M.
Relations of training schools to hospital administration. *Nursing Record*, Nov. 2, 1901, p. 353-6.

ROSE, D. E., and SCHWIER, M. E.
Administrator and nurse debate accreditation. *Modern Hospital*, Mar. 1959, p. 100-3.

ROYAL COLLEGE OF NURSING
Memorandum on the establishment of education committees in schools of nursing. The College, 1954. 2nd edn., 1959.

ROYAL COLLEGE OF NURSING and
BRITISH HOSPITALS ASSOCIATION
Preliminary training schools for student nurses: memorandum prepared jointly by the Royal College of Nursing and the British Hospitals Association on the advice of their liaison committee. [The College and The Association, 1944.]

SCHUMACHER, M. E.
The adviser to schools of nursing. *Canadian Nurse*, April 1959, p. 332, 334 and 336.

SCHWIER, MILDRED E.
Ten thousand nurse faculty members in basic professional schools of nursing, prepared by M. E. Schwier and others. New York, National League for Nursing, 1953.

Sisterhoods. Reprinted from *Pall Mall Gazette*. Schools for nurses, reprinted from *Saturday Review*, with notes by a physician. Benmore, 1866.

SLEEPER, RUTH P.
What is ahead for the hospital school of nursing? Its survival depends on new methods and facilities. *Hospitals*, Aug. 16, 1960, p. 37-9.

SMITH, DOROTHY M., and EGLOFF, FRANK R. L.
Something new in nursing arts. *Nursing Outlook*, Feb. 1957, p. 92-5.

SMITH, LOUISE C.
An approach to evaluating the achievement of one objective of an educational programme in nursing. *Nursing Research*, Feb. 1957, p. 115-20.

STEWART, ISABEL MAITLAND, and others
Educational programme of the school of nursing. Geneva, International Council of Nurses, 1934.

SUPERINTENDENTS OF TRAINING SCHOOLS
Discussion on the three years' course, and the working of the eight-hour system [in America]. *Nursing World*, Nov. 3, 1900, p. 355-6, and Nov. 10, 1900, p. 380-1.

TATE, BARBARA L.
Credit for military training in schools of nursing. *Nursing Outlook*, June 1960, p. 323-5.

THOMPSON, WILLIAM GILMAN
Training schools for nurses, with notes on twenty-two schools. New York, Putnam, 1883.

VODEV, E. D.
Financing the school of nursing. *Hospital Management*, Sept. 1957, p. 104 *passim*.

WILLIAMS, DOROTHY ROGERS
Administration of schools of nursing, edited by Isabel M. Stewart. New York, Macmillan, 1950.

WORCESTER, ALFRED
The advantages of separate organizations for training schools and hospitals. Boston, Heath, 1906.
[Repr. *Boston Med. and Surg. Journal*, vol. CLV, Aug. 23, 1906, p. 195-9.]

WORCESTER, ALFRED
The first American training school.
In
WORCESTER, ALFRED
Nurses and nursing. 1927, chap. VII.

Individual Training Schools

AHLA, M.
College of Nursing, Helsinki, Finland. *International Nursing Review*, Jan. 1957, p. 7-11.

BELLEVUE HOSPITAL NURSING SCHOOLS
A candle in her hand: a story of the nursing schools of Bellevue Hospital, by Dorothy Giles. New York, Putnam, 1949.

BELLEVUE HOSPITAL, NEW YORK
Bellevue: a short history of Bellevue Hospital and of the training schools, by the Pension Fund Committee of the Alumnae Association of Bellevue. New York, Alumnae Association of Bellevue, 1915.

BELLEVUE HOSPITAL TRAINING SCHOOL FOR NURSES
A new profession for women, by Franklin H. North. *The Century Illustrated Monthly Magazine*, Nov. 1882 to April 1883.
[This article deals with the Bellevue Hospital Training School for Nurses.]

BOSTON CHILDREN'S HOSPITAL SCHOOL OF NURSING
Fifty years: a history of the School of Nursing, the Children's Hospital, Boston, by Stella Goostray. Boston, Mass., the Alumnae Association of the Children's Hospital School of Nursing, 1940.

CAMBRIDGE SCHOOL OF NURSING, MASS.
The Cambridge School of Nursing, Massachusetts, U.S.A., by C. J. Wood. *Nursing Times*, Aug. 12, 1905, p. 265-6.

CAMBRIDGE SCHOOL OF NURSING, MASS.
Addresses, relative to the Cambridge School of Nursing, read before the Cambridge Medical Improvement Society, the Colonial Club of Cambridge and the students of Radcliffe College, by Alfred Worcester. Waltham, Mass., Press of E. L. Barry, 1905.

CHARING CROSS HOSPITAL
Charing Cross Hospital as a training school for nurses. *Nursing Times*, Dec. 30, 1905, p. 596-8.

CHURCH HOME AND HOSPITAL, BALTIMORE
Ensign on a hill: the story of the Church Home and Hospital and its School of Nursing, 1854-1954, by Judith Robinson. Baltimore, The Hospital, 1954.

COLONIAL HOSPITAL, PORT-OF-SPAIN, TRINIDAD
A century of service, by I. D. Waterman. *Caribbean Medical Journal*, 1958, p. 36-41.

COLUMBIA UNIVERSITY TEACHERS' COLLEGE
Teachers' College, Department of Nursing Education. Nursing education: twenty-five years of nursing education at Teachers' College, 1899-1925. New York, Teachers' College, 1926. (*T.C. Bull.*, 17th series, no. 3, Feb. 1926.)

CONNECTICUT TRAINING SCHOOL
The past, present and future of the Yale University School of Medicine and affiliated institutions including the New Haven Dispensary and the Connecticut Training School for Nurses. New Haven, The University, 1922.

CORNELL UNIVERSITY—NEW YORK HOSPITAL SCHOOL OF NURSING
Cornell University—New York Hospital School of Nursing, 1877-1952, by Helene Jamieson Jordan. [New York, Society of the New York Hospital?], 1952.

DUBLIN METROPOLITAN TECHNICAL SCHOOL FOR NURSES
Rules and regulations. *Nursing Record*, July 20, 1895, p. 8.

EVANSTON SCHOOL OF NURSING, ILLINOIS
Evanston School of Nursing 1898-1948, by C. L. Smith. Chicago, 1948?

FARRAND TRAINING SCHOOL FOR NURSES, DETROIT, MICHIGAN
The Farrand Training School for Nurses. *British Journal of Nursing*, Oct. 3, 1903, p. 267-9.

FARRAND TRAINING SCHOOL FOR NURSES
The history of the Farrand Training School for Nurses, by Agnes G. Deans and Anne L. Austin. Detroit, Mich., Alumnae Association of the Farrand Training School for Nurses, 1936.

GUY'S HOSPITAL
Preliminary nursing school at Guy's Hospital, by Margaret Breay. *British Journal of Nursing*, Feb. 26, 1910, p. 167-8.

HAMILTON GENERAL HOSPITAL SCHOOL OF NURSING
The Hamilton General Hospital School of Nursing, 1890-1955, by Marjorie Freeman Campbell. Toronto, Ryerson Press, 1956.

IBADAN. UNIVERSITY COLLEGE SCHOOL OF NURSING
1. Developing the school, by L. M. Bell.
2. Introducing district nursing into the basic training, by D. Goodwin. *Nursing Times*, Feb. 10, 1956, p. 139-42 and 147.

ILLINOIS TRAINING SCHOOL FOR NURSES
A history of the Illinois Training School for Nurses, 1880-1929, by Grace Fay Schryver. Chicago, The School, 1930.

JOHNS HOPKINS HOSPITAL SCHOOL OF NURSING
The Johns Hopkins Hospital School of Nursing, 1889-1949, by Ethel Johns and Blanche Pfefferkorn. Baltimore, Johns Hopkins Press, 1954.

KAISERSWERTH INSTITUTE
The institute of Kaiserswerth-on-the-Rhine; for the practical training of deaconesses under the direction of the Rev. Pastor Fliedner, embracing the support and care of hospital infant and industrial schools and a female penitentiary, by Florence Nightingale. London, Ragged Colonial Training School, 1851.

LA SOURCE, LAUSANNE
La Source, 1859-1959, Lausanne. *Nursing Times*, May 29, 1959, p. 635-9.

LA SOURCE SCHOOL OF NURSING, LAUSANNE
La Source Normal Evangelical School for Independent Nurses for the Sick at Lausanne, Switzerland, by Dr. Charles Krafft.
In
HAMPTON, ISABEL A., *and others*
Nursing of the sick, 1893.

LIVERPOOL NURSES' TRAINING SCHOOL
Organisation of nursing: an account of the Liverpool Nurses' Training School: its foundation, progress and operation in hospital, district and private nursing; by a member of the committee of the Home and Training School, with an introduction and notes by Florence Nightingale. Liverpool, Holder, 1865.

MACK TRAINING SCHOOL, ST. CATHERINE'S HOSPITAL, ONTARIO
St. Catherine's General Hospital—the Mack Training School for Nurses. Seventy-fifth anniversary—1874-1949. St. Catherine's General Hospital, St. Catherine's, Ontario, *St. Catherine's Standard*, n.d.

MASSACHUSETTS GENERAL HOSPITAL SCHOOL OF NURSING
History of the Massachusetts General Hospital School of Nursing, by Sara E. Parsons. Boston, Whitcomb & Barrows, 1922.

MINNESOTA UNIVERSITY. SCHOOL OF NURSING
A study of the graduates of the University of Minnesota School of Nursing by the Faculty of the School of Nursing. Minneapolis, University of Minnesota Press, 1953.

MINNESOTA UNIVERSITY. SCHOOL OF NURSING
Education for nursing; a history of the University of Minnesota School, by James Gray. Minneapolis, Univ. of Minnesota Press, [1960].

MISSOURI UNIVERSITY
The school of nursing at the University of Missouri, by R. Potter and J. Hoffmann. *Missouri Medicine*, April 1960, p. 469-72.

MONTREAL GENERAL HOSPITAL
History of the school for nurses of the Montreal General Hospital, by Hugh Ernest MacDermot. Montreal Alumnae Association, 1940.

NEWTON HOSPITAL, MASSACHUSETTS
Addresses delivered at the dedication of the training school for nurses, Feb. 14, 1894. Newton, The Hospital, 1894.

NEW BRUNSWICK UNIVERSITY
University of New Brunswick school of nursing, by Katherine E. MacLaggan. *Canadian Nurse*, May 1960, p. 424-6.

NEW YORK CITY TRAINING SCHOOL FOR NURSES
Curriculum. *Nursing Record*, Oct. 19, 1895, p. 268-9; Oct. 26, 1895, p. 288-9; Nov. 9, 1895, p. 329.

NEW YORK CITY TRAINING SCHOOL FOR NURSES
Preparatory teaching for nurses in the New York City Training School for Nurses, by Mary Gilmour. *British Journal of Nursing*, Mar. 7, 1903, p. 188-9.

NEW YORK HOSPITAL SCHOOL OF NURSING
New York Hospital School of Nursing, 1877-1927, by Lydia Anderson and others. New York, The Alumnae Association, n.d.

NEW YORK POSTGRADUATE MEDICAL SCHOOL AND HOSPITAL
History of nursing at the New York Postgraduate Medical School and Hospital, by Lena Dufton. New York, The Alumnae Association, 1944.

NIGHTINGALE TRAINING SCHOOL
Centenary of nurses' training, by Lucy R. Seymer. *Nursing Mirror*, May 13, 1960, p. vii-x and 606.

NIGHTINGALE TRAINING SCHOOL
1860-1960: centenary of the Nightingale Training School. *Nightingale Fellowship Journal*, no. LXIII, July 1960.

NIGHTINGALE TRAINING SCHOOL
Florence Nightingale's nurses: the Nightingale Training School 1860-1960, by Lucy Seymer. Pitman, 1960.

NIGHTINGALE TRAINING SCHOOL
Growth of the Nightingale School, by M. E. Gould. *Nursing Times*, May 13, 1960, p. 590-2.

NIGHTINGALE TRAINING SCHOOL
The Nightingale Training School, St. Thomas' Hospital, 1860-1960. Privately printed for the Nightingale Training School for Nurses, 1960.

NIGHTINGALE TRAINING SCHOOL
One hundred years ago, by Lucy R. Seymer. *American Journal of Nursing*, May 1960, p. 658-61.

NIGHTINGALE TRAINING SCHOOL
The wider influence of the Nightingale Training School, by O. Baggallay. *Nursing Times*, May 13, 1960, p. 604-7.

NIGHTINGALE TRAINING SCHOOL, ST. THOMAS'S HOSPITAL, *and* GUY'S HOSPITAL TRAINING SCHOOL
The origin and early development of two English training schools for nurses: the Nightingale Training School, St. Thomas's Hospital, the Guy's Hospital Training School, by Virginia M. Dunbar. Florence Nightingale International Foundation, 1936. [Typescript.]

ORANGE TRAINING SCHOOL FOR NURSES, ORANGE, NEW JERSEY
Some account of the Orange Training School for Nurses Orange, New Jersey, The School, 1899.

PASANEN, U.
A Finnish nursing school. *Nursing Outlook*, Oct. 1959. p. 594-5.

PRESBYTERIAN HOSPITAL SCHOOL OF NURSING, NEW YORK
History of the School of Nursing of the Presbyterian Hospital, New York, 1892-1942, by Eleanor Lee New York, Putnam, 1942.

RED CRESCENT SCHOOL OF NURSING, ISTANBUL
A short history of the Red Crescent School of Nursing, by Asuman Turer. Istanbul, The School, 1949. [Typescript.]

RHODE ISLAND HOSPITAL
Historical sketch of the Rhode Island Hospital Training School for Nurses. Nurses' Alumnae Association, 1932?

RICHARDS, LINDA
Mission training schools and nursing.
In
HAMPTON, ISABEL A., *and others*
Nursing of the sick, 1893.

ROOSEVELT HOSPITAL, NEW YORK, SCHOOL OF NURSING
Fifty years of service: history of the School of Nursing of the Roosevelt Hospital, New York City, 1906-1946, by Evelyn G. Fraser. [New York, Alumnae of the Roosevelt Hospital School of Nursing, 1946.]

ST. JOSEPH HOSPITAL SCHOOL OF NURSING
History of St. Joseph Hospital School of Nursing, Kansas City, Missouri, by Sister Mary Giles Phillips. Kansas, The Hospital, 1929.

ST. LOUIS CITY HOSPITAL TRAINING SCHOOL FOR NURSES
History of the St. Louis Training School for Nurses, which later became the St. Louis City Hospital Training School for Nurses, by Elizabeth Green. St. Louis, Missouri, The School, 1941.

ST. LUKE'S HOSPITAL SCHOOL OF NURSING
The history of St. Luke's Hospital School of Nursing, by Marie G. Merrill. Oak Park, Illinois, Hub Printing Service, 1946.

ST. LUKE'S HOSPITAL TRAINING SCHOOL FOR NURSES, NEW YORK
History of the St. Luke's Hospital Training School for Nurses: fiftieth anniversary, May 28th, 1888-May 28th, 1938, by Manelna Keller. New York, The Hospital, 1938.

ST. MARY'S HOSPITAL, LONDON
A hundred years of nursing at St. Mary's Hospital, Paddington, by Zachary Cope. Heinemann, 1955.

SHADYSIDE HOSPITAL SCHOOL OF NURSING
Through the years with the nurses at Shadyside Hospital—a history of the Pittsburgh Training Schools for Nurses, now the Shadyside Hospital School of Nursing, by Miriam Charlotte Miller. Pittsburgh, Pa., 1946.

SIMPSON, H. M.
A visit to the College of Nursing in Delhi. *Nursing Times*, May 27, 1960, p. 657-8.

SUTCLIFFE, IRENE
History of American training schools.
In
HAMPTON, ISABEL A., *and others*
Nursing of the sick, 1893.

TORONTO. NIGHTINGALE SCHOOL OF NURSING
The Nightingale School of Nursing, Toronto, by B. Duncanson. *Canadian Nurse*, Sept. 1960, p. 802-4.

VANCOUVER GENERAL HOSPITAL—SCHOOL OF NURSING
Our School of Nursing, 1899-1949, by Anne S. Cavers. Vancouver, The School, 1949.

WALTHAM TRAINING HOME AND SCHOOL FOR NURSES. MASS.
The Waltham Training School. *Nursing Record*, Mar. 15, 1902, p. 209-13.

WESTMINSTER TRAINING SCHOOL
The Westminster Training School, by Sarah A. Tooley. *Nursing Times*, June 16, 1906, p. 494-7.

WINNIPEG GENERAL HOSPITAL SCHOOL OF NURSING
The Winnipeg General Hospital School of Nursing, 1887-1953, by Ethel Johns. Winnipeg, The Alumnae Association of the Winnipeg General Hospital School of Nursing, 195?.

NURSING RESEARCH

ABDELLAH, FAYE G.
Methods of identifying covert aspects of nursing problems; a key to improved clinical teaching. *Nursing Research*, June 1957, p. 4-23.

ADAMS, APOLLONIA O.
Current status of nursing research. *Hospitals*, Jan. 11, 1960, p. 57-8.

ADAMS, APOLLONIA O.
Research—the "R" in nursing. *Journal of the American Medical Association*, May 7, 1960, p. 49-52.

AMERICAN NURSES' ASSOCIATION.
RESEARCH AND STATISTICS UNIT
Clearing house for studies in nursing, 1950-1953, and Supplement 1954-1955. New York, American Nurses' Association, 1955.
Supplement 1955-1956, 1956.
Supplement 1957-1958, entitled "Studies in nursing", 1959.

AMERICAN NURSES' FOUNDATION
The first three years [1955-58]. New York, The Foundation, 1958.

AMERICAN NURSES' FOUNDATION
Research—pathway to future progress in nursing care. *Nursing Research*, Winter 1960, p. 4-7.

ANDERSON, L. C.
The nurse and research. *Military Medicine*, Nov. 1957, p. 308-11.

ARNSTEIN, M. G.
Improving nursing service. *Canadian Nurse*, Nov. 1956, p. 869-74.

ARNSTEIN, M. G.
Training nurses for research work. *International Nursing Review*, Oct. 1959, p. 38-42.

AUSTIN, ANNE L.
The historical method in nursing. *Nursing Research*, Feb. 1958, p. 4-10.

BAILEY, J. T.
The critical incident technique in identifying behavioural criteria of professional nursing effectiveness. *Nursing Research*, Oct. 1956, p. 52-64.

BENZ, E. G.
A nursing staff studies its services. *American Journal of Nursing*, Oct. 1958, p. 1389-91.

BERTOZZI, E., and SAGE, V.
A study of the older nurse in Rhode Island. *Nursing Research*, Feb. 1958, p. 11-22.

BLAKE, E. L.
Walking records on the ward. *Nursing Mirror*, Feb. 5, 1960, p. vii.

BOYLE, RENA E.
The International Seminar in Delhi. *Nursing Research*, Fall 1960, p. 196-7.

BREDENBERG, VIOLA CONSTANCE
Nursing service research: experimental studies with the nursing service team. Philadelphia, Lippincott, 1951.

BRODMAN, E.
Abstracting tools in the sciences. *Nursing Research*, Fall 1959, p. 198-201.

BROWN, AMY FRANCES
Research in nursing. Philadelphia, Saunders, 1958.

BUNGE, HELEN L.
The Institute of Research and Service in Nursing Education, Teachers' College, Columbia University. *Nursing Research*, Oct. 1958, p. 113-5.

BUNGE, HELEN L.
Is research the answer. *Nursing World*, July 1958, p. 18-20.

BUNGE, HELEN L.
The meaning and importance of research in nursing. *Canadian Nurse*, Dec. 1955, p. 945-8.

BUNGE, HELEN L.
Research in nursing: is there a need. *International Nursing Review*, Oct. 1959, p. 33-7.

BUNGE, HELEN L.
Research is every professional nurse's business. *American Journal of Nursing*, June 1958, p. 816-9.

BUNGE, HELEN L.
Research in nursing in the United States: some reflections on its development. *Teachers' College Record*, April 1957, p. 371-6.

CANADIAN NURSES' ASSOCIATION
Studies relating to nursing in Canada. Montreal, C.N.A., 1959.

CARTER, G. B.
A study of the course for nurse tutors organized by the Royal College of Nursing (Scottish Branch) leading to the certificate awarded by the University of Edinburgh to nurse tutors. 1956.
[Boots Research Fellowship in Nursing at the University of Edinburgh.]

CATHOLIC UNIVERSITY OF AMERICA
The improvement of nursing through research (the proceedings of the Workshop on the Improvement of Nursing through Research . . . June 14 to 24, 1958), edited by Loretta E. Heidgerken. Washington, Catholic University of America, 1958.

CHITTICK, RAE, and ALLEN, MOYNA
Let us find some answers and tell others. *Canadian Nurse*, Jan. 1957, p. 40-1.

COX, B. R.
Student nurse in a research team. *Nursing Mirror*, April 8, 1960, p. 147-8.

CROSSEY, B., and others
Nurses in the psychiatric research team. *Nursing Times*, July 26, 1957, p. 835-8.

DAGSLAND, H.
Learning to undertake research: a personal view of the problems involved. *International Nursing Review*, Oct. 1959, p. 43-5.

DECARY, M.
Nursing research. *Canadian Hospital*, Jan. 1957, p. 48 *passim*.

DECARY, M., and OUIMET, J.
Research into better patient care. *Canadian Nurse*, Dec. 1958, p. 1115-8.

ERON, LEONARD D.
The effect of nursing attitudes. *Nursing Research*, Jun. 1955, p. 24-7.

FIDLER, N. D.
The need for research in nursing. *Canadian Nurse*, Mar. 1959, p. 224-6.

FISHER, W.
Nursing research in a local health department. *Nursing Outlook*, Nov. 1958, p. 643-5.

FLITTER, H.
How to develop a questionnaire. *Nursing Outlook*, Oct. 1960, p. 566-9.

FRY, V.
A conference on research in nursing. *Nursing Research*, June 1958, p. 52-6.

GODBOUT, ROSE A., *and* HURWITZ, IRVING
The role of the infirmary in a therapeutic camp for boys. *Nursing Research*, Winter 1960, p. 23-31.

GORDON, RICHARD E.
Electroencephalographic and social psychological indicators of nursing student performance. *Nursing Research*, Winter 1960, p. 46-8.

GREENBLATT, MILTON
The nurse in research. *Nursing Research*, Feb. 1957, p. 36-40.

HALL, G. M., *and* STREET, M. M.
Survey of a hospital nursing service. *International Nursing Review*, Oct. 1959, p. 46-54.

HARDIN, CLARA A.
Expansion of research to focus on nursing problems. *American Journal of Nursing*, Nov. 1960, p. 1629-30.

HARDIN, CLARA A.
Using the studies of nursing functions. *American Journal of Nursing*, May 1957, p. 622-3.

HEIDGERKEN, LORETTA E.
Inservice education and research. *Nursing Outlook*, Aug. 1959, p. 474-5.

HENDERSON, VIRGINIA
An overview of nursing research. *Nursing Research*, Oct. 1957, p. 61-71.

HILBERT, HEIDE
A trial plan for abstracting reports of studies in nursing. A project report. *Nursing Research*, Summer 1960, p. 172-5.

HOCHBAUM, G. M.
The nurse in research. *Nursing Outlook*, April 1960, p. 192-5.

INTERNATIONAL COUNCIL OF NURSES
Learning to investigate nursing problems: report of an international seminar on research in nursing. I.C.N., 1960.

JENSEN, ALFRED C.
Determining critical requirements for nurses. *Nursing Research*, Winter 1960, p. 8-11.

JONES, J. A.
Methods research in nursing. *Nursing Outlook*, May 1957, p. 294-5.

KLINGELHOFER, ANN
A.N.A. approaches to research. *American Journal of Nursing*, Jan. 1960, p. 56-7.

LEE, P. F.
Research in nursing. *Journal of the West Australian Nurses*, Nov. 1959, p. 3-10.

LENTZ, EDITH M., *and* MICHAELS, ROBERT G.
Comparative ratings of medical and surgical nurses. *Nursing Research*, Fall 1960, p. 198-202.

LENTZ, EDITH M., *and* MICHAELS, ROBERT G.
Comparisons between medical and surgical nurses. *Nursing Research*, Fall 1959, p. 192-7.

LEONE, LUCILE PETRY
Necessary ingredients for solution of problems in nursing. *Military Medicine*, April 1960, p. 275-80.

MACDONALD, WILLIAM J., *and others*
A symposium on research in nursing, April 18, 1958. Washington, Catholic University of America, 1958.

MENDOZA, R.
Development of the research attitude among basic nursing students. *International Nursing Review*, Oct. 1959, p. 58-62.

MEYER, GENEVIEVE R.
The attitude of student nurses toward patient contact and their images of and preferences for four nursing specialities. *Nursing Research*, Oct. 1958, p. 126-30.

MEYER, GENEVIEVE R.
Conflict and harmony in nursing values. *Nursing Outlook*, July 1959, p. 398-9.

MEYER, GENEVIEVE R.
Some preliminary results from a questionnaire survey of registered nurses in the Los Angeles Metropolitan Area. [Los Angeles, University of California, 195?]

MORGAN, M. P.
Nursing education; research in basic nursing in Canada. *Canadian Nurse*, Dec. 1955, p. 962-6.

NATIONAL LEAGUE FOR NURSING
Its role in nursing research. *Nursing Research*, Fall 1960, p. 190-5.

NAVRAN, LESLIE, *and* STAUFFACHER, JAMES C.
A comparative analysis of the personality structure of psychiatric and non-psychiatric nurses. *Nursing Research*, June 1958, p. 64-7.

NAVRAN, LESLIE, *and* STAUFFACHER, JAMES C.
The personality structure of psychiatric nurses. *Nursing Research*, Feb. 1957, p. 109-14.

NELSON, KATHRYN J., *and* GRAF, CATHERINE N.
Introduction to the elements of research. *Nursing Outlook*, Sept. 1955, p. 500-2.

NURSING RESEARCH
The ingredients of research. *Nursing Research*, Oct. 1955, p. 51.

OUSELEY, M. H.
The case for a nursing research council. *Nursing Mirror*, Dec. 4, 1959, p. xi-xii.

POULOS, E. S., *and* MCCABE, G. S.
The nurse in the role of the research observer. *Nursing Research*, Summer 1960, p. 137-40.

Research—pathway to future progress in nursing care. *Nursing Research*, Winter 1960, p. 4-7.

SAFREN, M. A., *and* CHAPANIS, A.
A critical incident study of hospital medication errors. *Hospitals*, May 1, 1960, p. 32-4.
Hospitals, May 16, 1960, p. 53.

SANFORD, TILLMORE H.
The behavioural sciences and research in nursing. *Nursing Research*, Oct. 1957, p. 52-6.

SCHLOTFELDT, R. M.
Reflections on nursing research. *American Journal of Nursing*, April 1960, p. 492-4.

SHELDON, E. B., *and others*
An experimental program in nursing research. *Nursing Research*, Summer 1959, p. 169-71.

SIMON, J. R., *and* OLSON, M. E.
Assessing job attitudes of nursing service personnel. *Nursing Outlook*, Aug. 1960, p. 424-7.

SIMPSON, H. M.
Studying a salary structure: some initial problems. *International Nursing Review*, Oct. 1959, p. 55-8.

UNITED STATES PUBLIC HEALTH SERVICE.
DIVISION OF NURSING RESOURCES
Design for statewide nursing surveys: a basis for action; a manual prepared . . . under the direction of Margaret G. Arnstein. Washington, Govt. Printing Office, 1956.

UNITED STATES PUBLIC HEALTH SERVICE.
DIVISION OF NURSING RESOURCES
How to study nursing activities in a patient unit: a manual prepared . . . under the direction of Margaret G. Arnstein. Washington, Govt. Printing Office, 1954.

UNITED STATES PUBLIC HEALTH SERVICE.
DIVISION OF NURSING RESOURCES
How to study supervisor activities in a hospital nursing service; a manual prepared by Elinor D. Stanford . . . and other members of the staff of the Division of Nursing Resources. Washington, U.S. Govt. Printing Office, 1957.

UPRICHARD, M.
The nature of research. *Canadian Nurse*, April 1959, p. 318-20.

VREELAND, E. M.
The nursing research grant and fellowship program of the public health service. *American Journal of Nursing*, Dec. 1958, p. 1700-2.

WATT, JAMES
The biological sciences and research in nursing. *Nursing Research*, Oct. 1957, p. 57-60.

WEBSTER, R. C.
The nurse's role in clinical research. *Nursing Outlook*, Dec. 1960, p. 681-3.

WHITING, J. F., *and others*
Some practical aspects of nursing research. *American Journal of Nursing*, Feb. 1960, p. 199-203.

NURSING ETHICS
GENERAL WORKS

AIKENS, CHARLOTTE A.
Studies in ethics for nurses. Philadelphia, Saunders, 1916.
2nd edn., 1923.
3rd edn., 1930.
4th edn., 1937.
5th edn., 1943.

AMERICAN NURSES' ASSOCIATION
The code for professional nurses. *American Journal of Nursing*, Sept. 1960, p. 1287.

AMERICAN NURSES' ASSOCIATION
Making ideals tangible. *American Journal of Nursing*, May 1960, p. 672-6.

AMERICAN NURSES' ASSOCIATION
Revision proposed in code for professional nurses. *American Journal of Nursing*, Jan. 1960, p. 77-81.

BECK, MARY BERENICE, SISTER
The nurse, handmaid of the Divine Physician: a handbook of the religious care of the patient. Philadelphia, Lippincott, 1945.
2nd edn., 1952, called "Handmaid of the Divine Physician", pub. by Bruce, Milwaukee.

BECK, MARY BERENICE, SISTER
What's in our Code? *American Journal of Nursing*, Nov. 1956, p. 1406-7.
[A.N.A. Code for professional nurses.]

BLAIR, J.
Opening address to nurses: with notes to nurses and rules for nurses under training added. Melbourne, 1880.

BOYD, HARRY, *and* FREY, THOMAS E.
The press and the hospital. *Nursing Outlook*, Feb. 1958, p. 80-3.

BROGAN, JAMES M.
Ethical principles for the character of a nurse. Milwaukee, Bruce, 1924.

CATHERINE DE JESUS CHRIST
At the bedside of the sick: precepts and counsels for hospital nurses; translated by E. F. Peeler. Burns Oates & Washbourne, 1938.

A collection of prayers for use in hospitals. Nottingham, Derry, 1951.

CRAVEN, M. E.
The work of the Ethics of Nursing Committee. *International Nursing Review*, Oct. 1958, p. 33-9.

CREIGHTON, H.
Nursing ethics and the law. *American Association of Industrial Nurses' Journal*, Mar. 1960, p. 8-15.

DICKS, RUSSELL L.
Who is my patient? A religious manual for nurses. New York, Macmillan, 1947.

DRAKE, E. M.
The nurse and citizenship. *Canadian Nurse*, July 1957, p. 629-31.

EDGELL, BEATRICE
Ethical problems: an introduction to ethics for hospital nurses and social workers. Methuen, 1929.

FINK, LEO. GREGORY, *editor*
Graduate nurses symposium of ethical inspiration. 3rd edn. New York, Paulist Press, 1938.

FOX, E. MARGARET
Nursing ethics. *Nursing Times*, May 4, 1912, p. 475-8.

GABRIEL, SISTER JOHN
Professional problems: a textbook for nurses. Philadelphia, Saunders, 1932.

GARESCHÉ, EDWARD FRANCIS
Corners of mercy, friendly talks to nurses. Milwaukee, Bruce, 1925.

GARESCHÉ, EDWARD FRANCIS
Ethics and the art of conduct for nurses. Philadelphia, Saunders, 1929.
2nd edn., 1944.

GLADWIN, MARY ELIZABETH
Ethics: talks to nurses. Philadelphia, Saunders, 1930.
2nd edn., 1937, entitled "Ethics, a textbook for nurses".

GLIDDON, PAUL, *and* POWELL, MURIEL B.
Called to serve. Hodder & Stoughton, 1952.

GOODRICH, ANNIE WARBURTON
The social and ethical significance of nursing: a series of addresses. New York, Macmillan, 1932.

GRETTER, E. L.
Ethics of nursing. *Nursing Record*, July 13, 1901, p. 28-30.

HARDING, A.
Hospital church sister. *Nursing Times*, Nov. 7, 1958, p. 1328.

HARDING, GERTRUDE
The higher aspect of nursing. Philadelphia, Saunders, 1919.

HARRISON, GENE
Ethics in nursing. Kimpton, 1932.

HAYES, EDWARD J., *and others*
Moral handbook of nursing: a compendium of principles, spiritual aids, and concise answers regarding Catholic personnel, patients and problems; by the Reverend Edward J. Hayes, the Reverend Paul J. Hayes and Dorothy Ellen Kelly. New York, Macmillan, 1956.

HOLLAND, SYDNEY
Two talks to the nurses of the London Hospital, December 1897. [Whitehead, n.d.]

HYDE, R. W., *and* COGGAN, N. E.
When nurses have guilt feelings. *American Journal of Nursing*, Feb. 1958, p. 233-6.

INTERNATIONAL COUNCIL OF NURSES
Nursing ethics: an international code. *Nursing Times*, Mar. 11, 1955, p. 258.

JOHNS HOPKINS HOSPITAL, BALTIMORE, ALUMNAE ASSOCIATION OF NURSES
Code of ethics. *Nursing Record*, Oct. 3, 1896, p. 268-70.

JOHNSON, BRIAN D.
The Catholic nurse. Burns Oates & Washbourne, 1950.

KING, EDWARD, BISHOP OF LINCOLN
Counsels to nurses by Edward King. Being his addresses and letters to the Guild of St. Barnabas for Nurses. Ed. . . . E. F. Russell. Mowbray, 1911.

KIRKPATRICK, THOMAS PERCY CLAUDE
Nursing ethics: a lecture. Dublin, University Press, 1917.

LANCASTER, A.
The International Code of Nursing Ethics. *International Nursing Review*, Feb. 1960, p. 13-17.

LETOURNEAU, CHARLES
The nurse's duty to the hospital. *Hospital Management*, July 1958, p. 46 and 64-6.

MCALLISTER, JOSEPH B.
Catholicism and some moral problems in obstetric nursing. Washington, National Council of Catholic Nurses, 1953.

MCALLISTER, JOSEPH B.
Ethics: with special application to the nursing profession. Philadelphia, Saunders, 1947.
2nd edn., 1955, entitled "Ethics: with special application to the medical and nursing professions".

MCALLISTER, JOSEPH B.
Vocation of the Christian nurse. St. Cloud, Minnesota, St. Cloud Hospital School of Nursing, 1948.

MCISSAC, ISABEL
Ethics in nursing. *Nursing Record*, May 25, 1901, p. 412-3.

MARTIN, D. V.
Divine healing: religion, healing and the nurse. *Nursing Times*, Aug. 21, 1959, p. 761-3.

MERCIER, CHARLES ARTHUR
The ideal nurse: an address to nurses delivered to the nursing staff of the Retreat at York, 1909. London Mental Culture Enterprise, 1909.

MEYER, GENEVIEVE ROGGE
Tenderness and technique: nursing values in transition. Los Angeles, Institute of Industrial Relations, University of California, [c. 1960].

MITCHELL, SILAS WEIR
. . . Address delivered . . . to the graduating class of the New York Hospital Training School for Nurses, February 28th, 1908. New York, Society of the New York Hospital, 1908.

MOLLETT, M.
Nursing ethics. *Nursing Record*, June 4, 1902, p. 469-471.

MORRELL, M. A.
Our work for Christ among his suffering people: a book for hospital nurses. Rivingtons, 1877.

MURPHY, R. J.
The Catholic nurse, her spirit and her duties. Milwaukee, Bruce, 1923.

NIGHTINGALE, FLORENCE
Address from Florence Nightingale to the probationer-nurses in the "Nightingale Fund" School at the St. Thomas's Hospital and the nurses who trained there, July 23, 1874. Spottiswoode, 1874.
[London, printed for private circulation, 1872.]

NURSING MIRROR
Should the nurse tell. *Nursing Mirror*, June 22, 1956, p. 863-4.

NURSING TIMES
Divine healing: a series of articles devoted to the spiritual aspects of health and healing, which appeared in the *Nursing Times* in 1959. Macmillan, [1960].

OLD INTERNATIONALS' ASSOCIATION
Human relationships in international nursing affairs: the *Nursing Times* report of addresses given at the summer school held by the Old Internationals' Association (Florence Nightingale International Foundation) in July 1952. . . . *Nursing Times*, 1952.

PARSONS, SARA E.
Nursing problems and obligations. Boston, Whitcomb & Barrows, 1916.

PEARCE, DOREEN
A little book of devotion for nurses. Mowbray, 1948.

ROBB, ISABEL HAMPTON
Nursing ethics: for hospital and private use. Cleveland, Ohio, Savage, 1903.

ROBB, ISABEL HAMPTON
The quality of thoroughness in nurses' work. *British Journal of Nursing*, Jan. 2, 1904, p. 7-10, and Jan. 9, 1904, p. 26-7.

ROBB, ISABEL HAMPTON
Talks on ethics in nursing. *Nursing Record*, Nov. 19, 1898, p. 409-11.

SOUTH AFRICA
Apartheid: a background picture from the African Bureau. *Nursing Times*, April 18, 1958, p. 449-50.

SOUTHARD, SAMUEL
Religion and nursing. Nashville, Tennessee, Broadman, 1959.

STANDARD, SAMUEL, and NATHAN, HELMUTH, editors
Should the patient know the truth? A response of physicians, nurses, clergymen and lawyers. New York, Springer, 1955.

SULLIVAN, C.
Spiritual principles in the life of a sister. *Hospital Progress*, June 1958, p. 67-8.

TALLEY, CHARLOTTE
Ethics: a textbook for nurses. New York, Putnam, 1925.

THURMAN, H.
The responsibility of the professional person to society. *Nursing Outlook*, June 1957, p. 334-5.

TUFTS, MARY H.
Hospital discipline and ethics. *Nursing Times*, Oct. 20, 1917, p. 1231-2; Nov. 24, 1917, p. 1338-9; Dec. 1, 1917, p. 1422-5.

VAUGHAN, SISTER ROSE HELENE
The actual incidence of moral problems in nursing. A preliminary study in empirical ethics. New York, Catholic University of America, 1935.

WAY, H.
Ethics for nurses.
1. A sense of duty. *Nursing Times*, April 1, 1960, p. 402-3.
2. Duty to ourselves. *Nursing Times*, April 8, 1960, p. 438-9.
3. The nurse's virtues. *Nursing Times*, April 15, 1960, p. 477-8.
4. Duty to others. *Nursing Times*, April 22, 1960, p. 519-20.
5. Authority and discipline. *Nursing Times*, April 29, 1960, p. 545-6.

WESTBERG, GRANGER
Nurse, pastor and patient: a hospital chaplain talks with nurses. Rock Island, Ill., Augustana Press, 1955.

WILSON, MICHAEL
The Christian nurse. Edinburgh House Press, 1960.

WOLFF, ILSE S.
Should the patient know the truth? *American Journal of Nursing*, May 1955, p. 546-9.

WOOD, CATHERINE J.
Ethics in the profession.
1. Ethics in training. *Nursing Times*, Jan. 23, 1909, p. 67-8.
2. Ethics in hospital. *Nursing Times*, Jan. 30, 1909, p. 87.
3. Ethics in teaching. *Nursing Times*, Feb. 6, 1909, p. 106-7.
4. Ethics in practice. *Nursing Times*, Feb. 13, 1909, p. 126.

WORCESTER, ALFRED
Nursing as a distinct form of Christian service. Cleveland, Ohio, n.p., 1924.
[An address at the service held under the auspices of St. Barnabas Guild in Trinity Cathedral, Cleveland, Ohio, May 12, 1924. Reprinted from the *News Letter*, June 1924.]

PATIENT-STAFF RELATIONSHIPS

ABDELLAH, FAYE G., *and* LEVINE, EUGENE
Effect of nurse staffing on satisfactions with nursing care. Chicago, American Hospital Association, 1958.

BERNARD, JESSIE, *and* JENSEN, DEBORAH MACLURG
Sociology. St. Louis, Mosby, 1939.
2nd edn., 1943.
3rd edn., 1947.
4th edn., 1954.
5th edn., 1958.

BIRD, BRIAN
Talking with patients. Philadelphia, Lippincott, 1955.

BLACKLOCK, CATHERINE
Nurse-patient relationships. *Canadian Nurse*, Feb. 1960, p. 148-54.

BOGARDUS, EMORY S., *and* BRETHORST, ALICE B.
Sociology applied to nursing. Philadelphia, Saunders, 1941.
2nd edn., 1945.
3rd edn., 1952.

BOYLE, RENA E.
A study of student nurse perception of patient attitudes. Washington, Govt. Printing Office, 1960.

BOYLE, RENA E.
Who says its important? *American Journal of Nursing*, Oct. 1960, p. 1450-3.

BROWN, FRANCES J.
Sociology, with application to nursing and health education. Englewood Cliffs, N.J., Prentice-Hall, 1957.

BURTON, GENEVIEVE
Personal, impersonal and interpersonal relations, a guide for nurses. New York, Springer, 1958.

CENTRAL COUNCIL FOR HEALTH EDUCATION
Coming into hospital. The Council, 1957.

CENTRAL HEALTH SERVICES COUNCIL
The reception and welfare of in-patients in hospitals. H.M.S.O., 1953.

CLARK-KENNEDY, A. E.
Patients as people: being more clinical stories for students, nurses and practitioners. Faber, 1957.

DODGE, JOAN S.
Nurse-doctor relations and attitudes toward the patient. *Nursing Research*, Winter 1960, p. 32-8.

ELDRED, S. H.
Improving nurse-patient communication. *American Journal of Nursing*, Nov. 1960, p. 1600-2.

FIDLER, FLORENCE G.
The patient looks at the hospital. Hale, 1936.

FREEMAN, RUTH B.
Nurses, patients and progress. *Nursing Outlook*, Jan. 1959, p. 161-8.

FREEMAN, RUTH B.
The patient and the nurse. *Hospital Management*, Feb. 1960, p. 94-6.

GABRIEL, SISTER JOHN
Through the patient's eyes: hospitals, doctors, nurses. Philadelphia, Lippincott, 1935.

GEORGE, G. R., *and* GIBSON, R. W.
Patient-staff relationships change with environment. *Mental Hospitals*, Nov. 1959, p. 18-19.

GOULD, —
The personal factor in nursing: patient, doctor, nurse. *Nursing Times*, Mar. 5, 1910, p. 186-9.

HAYES, WAYLAND J., *and* GAZAWAY, RENA
Human relations in nursing. Philadelphia, Saunders, 1955. 2nd edn., 1959.

HEIL, LOUIS M., *and* CAVAGLIERI, NORMA
An investigation of student-nurse achievement in nurse-patient relations and problem-solving in emotional aspects of cancer nursing. [Bethesda, Md., National Cancer Institutes, 1956.]

HOLMES, MARGUERITE J.
What's wrong with getting involved? *Nursing Outlook*, May 1960, p. 250-1.

HOUTS, D. C.
The patient has something to say. *Hospitals*, Dec. 16, 1958, p. 38-40.

HOWELL, SARA K.
Are you my nurse? *American Journal of Nursing*, Oct. 1960, p. 1456-7.

INGLES, THELMA
Do patients feel lost in a general hospital. *American Journal of Nursing*, May 1960, p. 648-51.

JACOBSON, F. N.
The voice of the patients: an early report. *Mental Hygiene*, Oct. 1956, p. 551-4.

JOURARD, SIDNEY M.
The bedside manner: a psychologist comments on the reasons why nurses develop modes of behaviour that interfere with giving successful nursing care, and suggests some ways of improving nurse-patient relationships. *American Journal of Nursing*, Jan. 1960, p. 63-6.

JOURARD, SIDNEY M.
How well do you know your patients? *American Journal of Nursing*, Nov. 1959, p. 1568-71.

KATHLEEN MARY, SISTER
The apostate to the living. *Hospital Progress*, Aug. 1958, p. 161-4.

KERRIGAN, SISTER M. RUTH
Analysis of conversations between selected students and their assigned patients. *Nursing Research*, June 1957, p. 43-5.

KING EDWARD'S HOSPITAL FUND FOR LONDON
Patient's waking hours in London voluntary hospitals, being a report by a subcommittee of the Distribution Committee. George Barber (for the Fund), 1931.

KNOWLES, L. N.
How can we reassure patients. *American Journal of Nursing*, June 1959, p. 834-5.

KOONTZ, A. R.
What has happened to nursing? *Maryland State Medical Journal*, July 1958, p. 365-8.

KRANOCK, A., *and others*
A method for the study of social interaction on the hospital ward. *Nursing Research*, Summer 1959, p. 172-6.

KULP, DANIEL HARRISON
Introductory sociology for students of nursing. New York, Macmillan, 1936.

LEE, VIOLET T.
When the nurse and patient are together. *American Journal of Nursing*, Dec. 1960, p. 1786-8.

LENNON, SISTER MARY ISIDORE
Sociology and social problems in nursing. Kimpton, 1951.
2nd edn., 1955.
3rd edn., 1959.

LESSER, MARION S., *and* KEANE, VERA R.
Nurse-patient relationships in a hospital maternity service. St. Louis, Mosby, 1956.

LISTON, M. F.
Communications and their value in health nursing. *Military Medicine*, Nov. 1958, p. 366-70.

LOCKERBY, FLORENCE K.
Communication: inhibitor or catalyst? *Hospital Management*, May 1957, p. 132-3.

MANZER, HELEN G.
Practical sociology and social problems. Philadelphia, Lippincott, 1942.

MATTHEWS, OLIVE
Hospital improvements, how to improve the daily life of the patient in the ward. Twickenham, Riverside Press, printers, 1950.

MORIMOTO, FRANCOISE R.
A technique for measuring interactions of patients and personnel in mental hospitals. *Nursing Research*, Oct. 1955, p. 74-8.

NEWSHOLME, H. P.
Nurse and patient. The Guild of Health, [1934].

NURSING MIRROR
A new attitude towards the patient. *Nursing Mirror*, Nov. 13, 1959, p. 548.

PAINE, L. H. W.
Putting the patient in perspective. *Hospital*, Dec. 1959, p. 981-4.

PARKER, S.
Disorganization on a psychiatric ward: the natural history of a crisis. *Psychiatry*, Feb. 1959, p. 65-79.

PEARCE, EVELYN CLARE
Nurse and patient: an ethical consideration of human relations. Faber, 1953.

PEPLAU, HILDEGARD E.
Interpersonal relations in nursing: a conceptual frame of reference for psychodynamic nursing. New York, Putnam, 1952.

PEPLAU, HILDEGARD E.
Talking with patients. *American Journal of Nursing*, July 1960, p. 964-6.

PREHER, SISTER LEO MARIE, *and*
CALVEY, SISTER M. EUCHARISTA
Sociology with social problems applied to nursing. Philadelphia, Saunders, 1949.

REINHARDT, JAMES M.
Society and the nursing profession: an introductory sociology; with contributions by Paul Meadows. Philadelphia, Saunders, 1953.

RENDER, HELENA WILLIS
Nurse-patient relationships in psychiatry. New York, McGraw-Hill, 1947.
2nd edn., 1959, by H. W. Render and M. Olga Weiss.

ROBERTS, D. I.
A psychiatrist helps them to understand their patients. *American Journal of Nursing*, Oct. 1956, p. 1302-5.

SABSHIN, MELVIN
Nurse-doctor-patient relationships in psychiatry. *American Journal of Nursing*, Feb. 1957, p. 188-92.

SAMSON, H. P.
The patient as a person. *International Nursing Review*, Jan. 1958, p. 49-52.

SCOTTISH HEALTH SERVICES COUNCIL
The reception and welfare of in-patients: report by the Standing Advisory Committee on Hospital and Specialist Services. Edinburgh, H.M.S.O., 1951.

SELLEW, GLADYS, *and* FURFEY, PAUL HANLEY
Sociology and social problems in nursing service. Philadelphia, Saunders, 1941.
2nd edn., 1946.
3rd edn., 1951.
4th edn., 1957, called "Sociology and its use in nursing service".

SHEAR, H. J.
Nurses' positive-negative attitudes towards patients. *Delaware State Medical Journal*, Mar. 1959, p. 74-6.

SMITH, DOROTHY M.
A nurse and a patient. *Nursing Outlook*, Feb. 1960, p. 68-72.

STARR, D. S.
Interpersonal relationships: a classroom subject. *Canadian Nurse*, Feb. 1960, p. 145-8.

TRUDEAU, JULIA
The nurse and the new patients. *Canadian Nurse*, Jan. 1960, p. 37-9.

VAN KAMM, ADRIAN L.
The nurse in the patient's world. *American Journal of Nursing*, Dec. 1959, p. 1708-10.

WEBB, J.
The nurse and the reception of out-patients. *Nursing Mirror*, Mar. 22, 1957, p. i-ii.

WHITING, J. FRANK
Needs, values, perceptions and the nurse-patient relationship. *Journal of Clinical Psychology*, April 1959, p. 146-50.

WHITING, J. FRANK, *and others*
The nurse-patient relationship and the healing process; a progress report to the American Nurses' Foundation, Inc., June 1955 to December 1957. Pittsburgh, American Nurses' Foundation, [c. 1958].

WHITING, J. FRANK
Patients' needs, nurses' needs, and the healing process. *American Journal of Nursing*, May 1959, p. 661-5.

WILLIE, C. V.
Patient and nurse; members of a group. *Nursing Outlook*, Oct. 1957, p. 585-7.

ZBORAY, D. E.
The hospital patient opinion poll. *Medical Technicians' Bulletin*, Jan.-Feb. 1957, p. 34-8.

PROFESSIONAL AND STAFF RELATIONSHIPS

ALABAMA UNIVERSITY. COMMITTEE ON HUMAN RELATIONS
Institutional nurses: roles, relationships and attitudes in three Alabama hospitals: a study conducted ... for the Alabama State Nurses' Association under sponsorship of the American Nurses' Association; [by] Thomas R. Ford and Diane D. Stephenson. Montgomery, University of Alabama Press, 1954.

BLUMBERG, ARTHUR, *and* BUSCHE, MARGARET J.
An inservice program in human relations. *Nursing Outlook*, Dec. 1957, p. 703-5.

BOWERS, L.
The relationship of the registered nurse and the practical nurse from the point of view of the practical nurse. *Hospital Management*, Jan. 1960, p. 88-91.

BURLING, TEMPLE, *and others*
The give and take in hospitals: a study of human organiza-tion in hospitals, by Temple Burling, Edith M. Lentz, Robert N. Wilson; a study conducted by the New York State School of Industrial and Labour Relations . . . with the support and co-operation of the American Hospital Association. New York, Putnam, 1956.

CHRIST, EDWIN A.
Interpersonal relationship between nurses. *Practical Nursing*, Jan. 1956, p. 10-12.

COBB, BEATRIX, *and* PATTERSON, MARY G.
Inservice training in interpersonal relationships: an experi-mental approach. *American Journal of Nursing*, May 1957, p. 614-6.

DANIEL, M. P.
The almoner and the ward sister. *The Almoner*, June 1957, p. 89-93.

DIETZ, LENA DIXON
Professional adjustments 1. Philadelphia, F. A. Davis, 1940.
2nd edn., 1943.
3rd edn., 1948.
4th edn., 1957.

DIETZ, LENA DIXON
Professional adjustments 2. Philadelphia, F. A. Davis, 1940.
2nd edn., 1946.
3rd edn., 1950.
4th edn., 1954.
5th edn., 1959.

DIETZ, LENA DIXON
Professional problems of nurses. Philadelphia, Davis, 1939.

DENSFORD, KATHERINE J., *and* EVERETT, MILLARD S.
Ethics for modern nurses: professional adjustments 1. Philadelphia, Saunders, 1946.

FLORES, F.
The nurse: handmaiden or partner? *Boston Medical Quarterly*, June 1957, p. 33-43.

HANSEN, HELEN F.
Professional relationships of the nurse. Philadelphia, Saunders, 1942.
2nd edn., 1947.

HARRISON, GENE
Professional adjustments II. Kimpton, 1942.

JOHN GABRIEL, SISTER
Professional problems: a textbook for nurses. Philadelphia, Saunders, 1932.

KEMPF, FLORENCE C.
The person as a nurse (professional adjustments). New York, Macmillan, 1950.
2nd ed., 1957.

LANCET
Doctor, nurse and hospital. *Lancet*, May 21, 1955, p. 1062-3.

LENNON, SISTER MARY ISIDORE
Professional adjustments. Kimpton, 1946.

LIVERPOOL UNIVERSITY, DEPARTMENT OF SOCIAL SCIENCE
Employment relations in a group of hospitals, by Joan Woodward. Institute of Hospital Administrators, 1950.

MCFARLAND, JOSEPH
Physician and nurse—an idealization: an address to nurses. Philadelphia, 1909.

MARTIN, S. E.
The personal touch in nursing staff communications. *Hospitals*, Jan. 16, 1959, p. 60-4.

MOLLETT, M.
The relations of nursing and medicine. *British Journal of Nursing*, May 14, 1910, p. 389-91.

Nurse and doctor. *Lancet*, Jan. 26, 1957, p. 199-200.

POPE, FRANK M.
The relation of the nursing to the medical profession, being the concluding portion of a course of lectures to the probationers of the School of Nursing of the Leicester Infirmary. *Nursing Record*, April 11, 1889, p. 235-6.

PURDY, K. E.
Interpersonal relations in the hospital. *United States Armed Forces Medical Journal*, Sept. 1956, p. 1337-43.

SEVESTRE, ROBERT
The relations of nursing and medicine. *British Journal of Nursing*, May 21, 1910, p. 409-11.

SPALDING, EUGENIA KENNEDY
Professional adjustments in nursing for senior students. Philadelphia, Lippincott, 1939.
2nd edn., 1941.
3rd edn., 1946.
4th edn., 1950, called "Professional nursing trends and adjustments".
5th edn., 1954, called "Professional nursing trends and relationships".
6th edn., 1959.

STURGES, OCTAVIUS
Nurses and doctors: an address to the British Nurses' Association. *Nursing Record*, Mar. 28, 1889, p. 197-9, and April 4, 1889, p. 213-5.

ZUCKER, E. M. M.
The nurse and the almoner. *Nursing Mirror*, June 14, 1957, p. ii-iv and vi.

WORK OF THE NURSE

GENERAL WORKS

ABDELLAH, FAYE G.
How we look at ourselves. *Nursing Outlook*, May 1959, p. 273-5.

AMERICAN NURSES' ASSOCIATION
Nurses invest in patient care; a preliminary report [on a five-year program of studies of nursing functions conducted by the American Nurses' Association]. New York, The Association, 1956.

AMERICAN NURSES' ASSOCIATION AND NATIONAL LEAGUE OF NURSING EDUCATION JOINT COMMITTEE
The general staff nurse: information concerning the status of the general staff nurse in the hospital, based on current literature and data received from superintendents of nursing. . . . New York, 1941.

ANDRELL, M., CARPENTER, H., *and* MARIN, A.
The role of the nurse in the total health program. *Inter-national Nursing Review*, Oct. 1957, p. 19-40.

B.C.H.
Thoughts for nurses: their life and work difficulties and encouragements by one who has worked among them, published under the direction of the Tract Committee, London. Society for Promoting Christian Knowledge, 1900.

BAKER, S. M.
Nursing in homes, private hospitals and sanitariums.
In
HAMPTON, ISABEL A., *and others*
Nursing of the sick, 1893.

BRIDGES, DAISY C.
Nursing in the World Health Organization. *Nursing Mirror*, July 30, 1949, p. 278.

CHANT, ORMISTON
Nursing scrubbers. *Nursing Record*, Jan. 12, 1893, p. 29.

COPE, ZACHARY
Florence Nightingale and district nursing.
Florence Nightingale and nurses' duties.
District Nursing, Nov. 1958, p. 179-80, and Dec. 1958, p. 213-4.

DAN MASON NURSING RESEARCH COMMITTEE
The work of recently qualified nurses: report of an inquiry into the work undertaken by state-registered nurses within two and a half years of qualifying. The Committee, 1956.

DAN MASON NURSING RESEARCH COMMITTEE
The work, responsibilities and status of the staff nurse. The Committee, 1960.

FENWICK, ETHEL GORDON
A practical standard of nursing. *Nursing Record*, July 16, 1898, p. 45-8, and July 23, 1898, p. 64-6.

FLYNN, C. W.
The P.R. role of nurses. *Hospital Progress*, Jan. 1960, p. 76.

FOX, E. MARGARET
The nurse in voluntary hospitals.
See
NURSING TIMES
The nurse and the nation: a survey of her position in the State today. *Nursing Times*, Nov. 5, 1910, p. 904-31.

FOX, E. MARGARET
The responsibilities of the probationer. *Nursing Times*, June 19, 1909, p. 502-3.

GERDS, GRETCHEN
Public and professional interests meet. *American Journal of Nursing*, Feb. 1960, p. 210-4.

HABENSTEIN, ROBERT W., and CHRIST, EDWIN A.
Professionalizer, traditionalizer and utilizer; an interpretive study of the work of the general duty nurse in non-Metropolitan Central Missouri general hospitals. A study conducted under the auspices of the Institute for Research in the Social Sciences, for the Missouri State Nurses' Association, under sponsorship of the American Nurses' Association. Columbia, Mo., University of Missouri, 1955.

HARDY, C. H.
Introductory lectures on the duties of nurses, delivered at the Alfred Hospital, Melbourne, 1881.

HAWARD, WARRINGTON
On the division of labour—nursing. *Nursing Record*, May 1, 1890, p. 209-13.

HILL, ELIZABETH
Nursing in the World Health Organization. *American Journal of Nursing*, April 1958, p. 528-30.

HONE, ROSAMOND
What are the needs for nursing care of the individual, the family and the community? *Nursing Times*, April 1, 1955, p. 344-7.

JOHNS, ETHEL, and PFEFFERKORN, BLANCHE
Activity analysis of nursing. New York, Committee on the Grading of Nursing Schools, 1934.

KANSAS STATE NURSES' ASSOCIATION.
NURSING FUNCTIONS COMMITTEE
A study of the activities of registered professional nurses in small Kansas hospitals, prepared . . . by the Government Research Center, University of Kansas. . . . Topeka, Kansas, Kansas State Nurses' Association, [1953].

LEAHY, K. M.
Nursing and the W.H.O. *Public Health Nursing*, April 1952, p. 185-6.

LEONE, LUCILLE PETRY
Wanted: good nursing. *Nursing Outlook*, Oct. 1957, p. 576-8.

LUDLAM, REUBEN
The nurse: her natural history, duties and responsibilities as an aid to the physician; being a lecture introductory to the course delivered in Hahnmann Medical College for the session 1866-67. Chicago, C. S. Halsey, 1866.

McIVER, P.
Nursing in world health programs. *Journal-Lancet*, June 1958, p. 245-7.

NATIONAL LEAGUE OF NURSING EDUCATION
A study on the use of the graduate nurse for bedside nursing in the hospital. New York, The League, 1933.

NATIONAL LEAGUE OF NURSING EDUCATION.
DEPARTMENT OF STUDIES
A study of nursing service in one children's hospital and 21 general hospitals. New York, The League, 1948.

NURSING TIMES
The nurse and the nation: a survey of her position in the State today.
  1. Fox, E. Margaret. The nurse in voluntary hospitals.
  2. Barton, Eleanor C. The Poor Law nurse.
  3. Drakard, M. The nurse in fever hospitals.
  4. Head, Phoebe. The nurse in mental hospitals.
  5. Browne, Sidney. The military nurse at home and abroad.
  6. Browne, Sidney. The Army Reserve and Territorial nurse; the naval nurse; Lady Minto's Indian nurses.
  7. The private nurse.
  8. Boge, Else. The nurse on district.
  9. Hay, M. E. Dalrymple. The Colonial Association nurse.
  10. A Medical Officer. The school nurse.
  11. Monkhouse, Mary. The nurse as health visitor and sanitary inspector.
  12. Crabbe, Violet Eyre. The nurse in schools for mothers.
  13. Windsor, A. E. The Mission nurse.
  14. Windsor, A. E., The nurse in the fight against tuberculosis.
  15. Haydon, M. Olive. The midwife and maternity nurse.
Nursing Times, Nov. 5, 1910, p. 904-31.

O'NEILL, H. C., and BARNETT, EDITH A.
Our nurses and the work they have to do. Ward Lock, 1888.

PICTURE FACTS ASSOCIATES
Nurses at work. New York, Harper, 1939.

POORMAN, ANN
The hospital consultant nurse. *Nursing Outlook*, July 1955, p. 382-5.

REILLY, CATHERINE E.
Night nursing. Philadelphia, Davis, 1940.

RICE, FLORENCE FRANCES
Hospital and nurses—compiled and written by F. F. Rice. Read before the Worcester Women's Club, Dec. 23, 1891. Boston, Darwell & Upham, 1892.

ROBERTS, KATHERINE
Five months in a London hospital. Letchworth, Garden City Press, 1911.

SOUTH-EAST METROPOLITAN AREA NURSE-TRAINING COMMITTEE
The work of student nurses and pupil assistant nurses, being a report submitted . . . to the General Nursing Council for England and Wales. . . . South-East Metropolitan Area Nurse-Training Committee, 1957. [Chairman: H. A. Goddard.]

TREGARTHEN, MARY
On nurses and their work. *Nursing Record*, Nov. 13, 1890, p. 232-4.

VERHONICK, P. J., and ROWLAND, M. A.
Problem solving approach to a nursing situation. *Military Medicine*, Oct. 1960, p. 685-8.

WALKER, V. H.
Nursing functions and activities. *American Journal of Nursing*, Jan. 1957, p. 79-80.

ADMINISTRATION

General Works

AMERICAN HOSPITAL ASSOCIATION AND NATIONAL LEAGUE OF NURSING EDUCATION
Administrative cost analysis for nursing service and nursing education: a study to develop methods for finding out the costs of nursing service and nursing education; by Blanche Pfefferkorn and Charles A. Rovetta. Chicago, American Hospital Association, New York, National League of Nursing Education, 1940.

ANDERSON, L. C., and MIDDLETON, A. B.
The supervisory process in administration. *Military Medicine*, Nov. 1956, p. 292-5.

ASSOCIATION OF HOSPITAL MATRONS
The office of matron: guidance for matrons and hospital authorities. The Association, 1944.

ATTEBERRY, M.
Addicted to administration. *Nursing Outlook*, Aug. 1957, p. 464-5.

BAILEY, SISTER M. EDITH
A study of the patterns of administrative organization in a selected number of schools of nursing in institutions of higher learning offering clinical experience in two or more hospitals or other agencies. Washington, The Catholic University of America, 1948.

BARRETT, JEAN
Ward management and teaching. New York, Appleton-Century-Crofts, 1949.
2nd edn., 1954.

BEATTY, M. M.
Training for leadership. *Nursing Outlook*, Sept. 1956, p. 504-6.

BERG, M. J.
Head nurse leadership role. *Military Medicine*, Jan. 1960, p. 52-7.

BLAKE, F. G.
The supervisor's task. *Nursing Outlook*, Nov. 1956, p. 641-3.

BRECH, E. F. L.
Principles of administration. Elements of administration and some applications to nursing. *Nursing Mirror*, June 28, 1957, p. xi-xii.

BREDENBERG, V.
Ward management in practice and theory. *Hospital Progress*, April 1957, p. 77-8.

CANADIAN NURSES' ASSOCIATION
Manual for head nurses in hospitals. Ottawa, Canadian Nurses' Association, 1960.

COCKAYNE, E.
Policy-making. *Nursing Times*, Jan. 4, 1957, p. 4-5.

COLETTI, A. C.
The head nurse is a manager . . . of both human and non-human resources. *Hospital Progress*, Mar. 1960, p. 100-1.

COPE, Z.
The changing functions of hospital matrons. *Nursing Times*, Oct. 21, 1955, p. 1182-4.

DONOVAN, HELEN MURPHY
What is supervision? *Nursing Outlook*, June 1957, p. 371-4.

FERGUSON, M.
The ward book. *Canadian Nurse*, Oct. 1957, p. 917-9.

FEY, LEOLA HIRSCH
The process of change: a case study of one institution. New York, N.L.N., 1960.

FINER, HERMAN
Administration and the nursing services. New York, Macmillan, 1952.

FLORENCE, M.
Nursing administration's role in the problem of hospital infection. *Nursing Outlook*, Nov. 1959, p. 644-7.

FORMAN, D. H.
Learning leadership in workshops. *American Journal of Nursing*, Feb. 1958, p. 205-7.

FOX, E. MARGARET
The responsibility of a senior nurse towards other nurses. *Nursing Times*, Jan. 16, 1908, p. 46-9.

FRANCOISE DE CHANTAL, SISTER
The director of nurses. *Canadian Hospital*, April 1957, p. 56-7.

FREEMAN, RUTH B.
Leadership in nursing. *Nursing World*, April 1958, p. 8-11.

FREEMAN, RUTH B.
Meeting nursing needs through citizen participation. *Nursing Outlook*, Jan. 1957, p. 43-4.

GERMAIN, L. D.
The nurse administrator in education and service. *Nursing Outlook*, Dec. 1958, p. 678-9.

GIPE, FLORENCE MEDA, and SELLEW, GLADYS
Ward administration and clinical teaching. St. Louis, Mosby, 1949.

GIRARD, ALICE
Wanted: leaders. *Canadian Nurse*, Jan. 1960, p. 17-18.

GLADSTEIN, SOLOMON, and others
A floor-manager-pattern for the nursing unit: an experiment conducted at Sinai Hospital of Baltimore . . . by Solomon Gladstein, Genevieve Prasatek and Morris N. Throne. Baltimore, Sinai Hospital, 1959.

JENKINS, P.
Nursing administration. *Australian Nurses' Journal*, Jan. 1960, p. 13-16.

JENSEN, DEBORAH MacLURG
Ward administration. Kimpton, 1952.

JENSEN, FAUNTELLA T.
The chief nurse in the small hospital. New York, Springer, [1960].

KANDEL, PHOEBE MILLER
Hospital economics for nurses. New York, Harper, 1930.

LANDALE, E. J. R.
A few hints to sisters. *Nursing Record*, July 4, 1896, p. 5-6.

LEES, FLORENCE S.
Handbook for hospital sisters; edited by Henry W. Acland. Ibister, 1874.

LEONE, LUCILE PETRY
Accent on leadership. *American Journal of Nursing*, Oct. 1958, p. 1419-21.

LIVERPOOL UNIVERSITY. DEPARTMENT OF SOCIAL SCIENCE
Employment relations in a group of hospitals, a report of a survey . . . carried out by Joan Woodward. Institute of Hospital Administrators, 1950.

LOGSDON, A.
The head nurse. *American Journal of Nursing*, June 1959, p. 825-7.

LUCKES, EVA C. E.
Hospital sisters and their duties. Churchill, 1886.
2nd edn., 1888.
3rd edn., 1893.
4th edn., 1912.

MARY LOUISE, SISTER
Head nursing is middle management. *Hospital Progress*, Nov. 1959, p. 71-3.

66

MARY MARGARELLA, SISTER
Communication: the catalyst. *Hospital Progress*, May 1960, p. 53-4.

The matron: her duties and responsibilities, including principles of economy in institutions. *Scientific Press*, 1907.

NATIONAL LEAGUE FOR NURSING
Preparation of nursing leaders. *Nursing Outlook*, Sept. 1956, p. 517-21.

NATIONAL LEAGUE FOR NURSING.
DEPARTMENT OF HOSPITAL NURSING
The head nurse at work. New York, National League for Nursing, 1953.

NEWTON, MILDRED E.
Developing leadership potential. *Nursing Outlook*, July 1957, p. 400-3.

NORTON, FELICIE
The duties of sisters in small hospitals. Bailliere, Tindall & Cox, 1920.

PHILLIPS, L. F. MARCH
English matrons and their profession: with some considerations as to their various offices, their national importance and the education they require. Gordon Sampson, Low, 1873.

RADZIALOWSKI, R.
Administrative planning. *Hospital Progress*, Aug. 1959, p. 74-7.

RANDALL, MARGARET
Ward administration. Philadelphia, Saunders, 1950.

RICHWAGEN, LESTER E., *and* DAY, PHILLIP E.
Wanted: managers in nursing. *Hospitals*, Aug. 16, 1958, p. 28-31.

RIDDLE, MARY M.
How to attain greater uniformity in ward work. *Nursing Record*, May 14, 1898, p. 397-8; May 21, 1898, p. 414-5; May 28, 1898, p. 434-5.

RUNELL, E. S.
The balance of power in hospital management. *Nursing Record*, July 9, 1891, p. 29-31.

RUNELL, E. S.
Distribution of responsibility in small hospitals. *Nursing Record*, Dec. 3, 1891, p. 290-1.

RYLE, A. E., *and* SNOKE, A. W.
Communications and relations between hospital administration and nursing administration. *Nursing Outlook*, May 1957, p. 282-3.

SCALES, MARGARET
Handbook for ward sisters. Bailliere, Tindall & Cox, 1952. 2nd edn., 1958.

SELLEW, GLADYS
A textbook of ward administration. Philadelphia, Saunders, 1930.

STANFORD, E. D.
Management responsibilities of the head nurse. *Hospital Management*, July 1957, p. 97-8, and Aug. 1957, p. 100-1.

STEARNS, L.
Changing concepts in nursing supervision. *American Journal of Nursing*, Jan. 1959, p. 63-5.

STEWART, ISLA
The training of the nurse in the wards and the position and duties of the matron. *British Journal of Nursing*, July 27, 1907, p. 62-5.

TIESSELINCK, J.
The director of nursing. *Hospital Management*, July 1958, p. 40-1.

UNITED STATES DEPARTMENT OF NATIONAL HEALTH AND WELFARE, RESEARCH DIVISION
A study of the functions and activities of head nurses in a general hospital. Washington, Govt. Printing Office, 1954.

UNITED STATES PUBLIC HEALTH SERVICE
The head nurse looks at her job: a manual prepared by Ruth I. Gillan, Helen G. Tibbitts and Dorothy Sutherland, under the direction of Margaret Arnstein. Washington, Govt. Printing Office, 1952.

UNITED STATES PUBLIC HEALTH SERVICE
A study of head nurse activities in a general hospital, 1950, by Apollonia Frances Olson and Helen G. Tibbitts. Washington, U.S. Govt. Printing Office, 1951.

VESTAL, A.
How many supervisors? *Hospital Progress*, May 1960, p. 174-6.

WAYLAND, MARY MARVIN
The hospital head nurse: her function and her preparation; edited by Isabel M. Stewart. New York, Macmillan, 1938. 2nd edn., 1944, by M. M. Wayland, R. Louise Metcalfe McManus, Margine O. Faddis.

WEED, W. W.
Reducing talk in the nurses' station. *Hospital Management*, April 1959, p. 96-9.

WELLENKAMP, J.
All groups benefit by group nursing plan. *Modern Hospital*, April 1959, p. 67-70.

Why good nurses make bad bosses. *Modern Hospital*, Sept. 1956, p. 79-81.

Job Analysis

ARKANSAS STATE NURSES' ASSOCIATION
Source book for the function of the general-duty nurse in ten Arkansas hospitals, [by] Donald D. Stewart [and] Christine E. Needham. Fayetteville, Arkansas, University of Arkansas, College of Arts and Sciences, Dept. of Sociology, 1955.

BECKETT, J. D. H.
Work study to help nurses' duty rotas. *Nursing Mirror*, Dec. 19, 1958, p. 885.

BERNSTEIN, EDNA, *and others*
How long is the nurse at the patient's bedside. *American Journal of Nursing*, Sept. 1954, p. 1115-6.

BERNSTEIN, EDNA, *and others*
. . . A study of direct nursing care consumed by patients with varying degrees of illness. Submitted . . . for the course "Problems in nursing education" in the School of Education, New York University, 1952. New York, University Bookstore, 1953.

BOSHOWERS, H.
The evaluation of personnel. *Canadian Nurse*, June 1959, p. 532-6.

CALIFORNIA STATE NURSES' ASSOCIATION
Nursing practice in California hospitals: a report based on a study of actual practice in forty California hospitals. . . . Sponsored by the California State Nurses' Association; conducted by Louis J. Kroeger and associates. [California, The Association, 1953.]

CANADIAN NURSES' ASSOCIATION
Job analysis and job evaluation. Ottawa, The Association, 1948.
Rev. edn., 1957.

CANADIAN NURSES' ASSOCIATION
Orientation: a guide to better nursing. Ottawa, The Association, 1956.

CANADIAN NURSES' ASSOCIATION
A study of the functions and activities of head nurses in a general hospital. . . . Planned and conducted by the Research Division, Dept. of National Health and Welfare, at the request of the Canadian Nurses' Association, and with the co-operation of the Ottawa Civic Hospital. Ottawa, [The Association?], 1954.

CHRIST, EDWIN A.
Nurses at work: a study of tasks-attitude concensus, work disparagement, and work tension . . . conducted under the auspices of the Institute of Research in the Social Sciences [University of Missouri]. Columbia, University of Missouri, 1956.

COLUMBIA UNIVERSITY TEACHERS' COLLEGE.
DIVISION OF NURSING EDUCATION
Nursing team organization and functioning . . . result of a study . . . [by] Eleanor C. Lambertsen. New York, Columbia University, Bureau of Publications, 1953.

DODGE, J. S.
The nurse and her patient. *Hospitals*, June 1, 1959, p. 30-4.

FALCK, H. S.
Job satisfaction in the professions. *Canadian Nurse*, Feb. 1957, p. 130-8.

FREY, M.
A look at job descriptions. *American Journal of Nursing*, Dec. 1960, p. 1782-3.

GRIVEST, M. T.
A personnel inventory of supervisors, head nurses, and staff nurses in selected hospitals: educational implications. *Nursing Research*, June 1958, p. 77-87.

JOSIE, G. H.
Job analysis of nursing personnel. *Medical Services Journal, Canada*, July-Aug. 1960, p. 573-82.

KAKOSH, M. E.
A method for studying the utilization of nursing service personnel in veterans' administration hospitals. *Nursing Research*, Oct. 1957, p. 79-81.

KEITH, HAZEL
A time and activity analysis of the functions of a director and assistant director of nursing service. *Nursing Research*, June 1958, p. 57-63.

KITCHIN, J. B.
Nursing and work study. *Nursing Times*, Sept. 13, 1957, p. 1022-3.

KLUMP, O. M.
The application of work measurement and performance budgeting to nursing. *Nursing Outlook*, Oct. 1959, p. 573-6.

KURTZ, G.
Nurse guide: a new approach to staff orientation. *American Journal of Nursing*, Nov. 1958, p. 1564-5.

MARYO, J. S., and LASKY, J. J.
A work satisfaction survey among nurses. *American Journal of Nursing*, April 1959, p. 501-3.

MEYER, B.
Development of a method for determining estimates of professional nurse needs. *Nursing Research*, June 1957, p. 24-8.

MORLAN, V.
Job analysis; what and why. *American Journal of Nursing*, Oct. 1956, p. 1285-7.

NEW YORK UNIVERSITY. DEPARTMENT OF NURSE EDUCATION
A study of nursing functions in twelve hospitals in the State of New York: a study to determine the functions of the professional and the practical nurse; submitted . . . by eighteen nurses as part of their advanced study. . . . New York, The University, 1952.

NORRIS, S.
A faculty looks at its orientation program. *American Journal of Nursing*, Jan. 1958, p. 80-1.

NUFFIELD PROVINCIAL HOSPITALS TRUST
The work of nurses in hospital wards: report of a job analysis. The Trust, 1953.

ROYAL COLLEGE OF NURSING
Comment on the Nuffield Provincial Hospitals Trust Job Analysis of the work of nurses in hospital wards. Royal College of Nursing, 1953.

SCOTTISH HEALTH SERVICES COUNCIL.
STANDING NURSING AND MIDWIFERY ADVISORY COMMITTEE
The work of nurses in hospital wards; report by the Standing Nursing and Midwifery Advisory Committee on "job analysis of the work of nurses in hospital wards", prepared by the Nuffield Provincial Hospitals Trust. Edinburgh, H.M.S.O., 1955.

O'BOYLE, MYRTLE
A study of practices in orientating staff nurses: a survey of personal experiences of fifty-five nurses in becoming oriented in new positions. . . . New York, National League for Nursing, 1956.

PICKENS, M. ELIZABETH, and TAYBACK, MATHEW
A job satisfaction survey. *Nursing Outlook*, Mar. 1957, p. 157-9.

PRATT, D. L.
A supervisor analyses her job. *Hospital Progress*, Feb. 1960, p. 58-9.

REID, MARGARET
Evaluating the services of the nurse: a handbook for staff nurses and supervisors. New York, Metropolitan Life Insurance Company, 1948.

REVANS, R. W.
Training work-study staff in hospitals. *Nursing Times*, Oct. 3, 1958, p. 1144-5, and Oct. 10, 1958, p. 1177-8.

TRACY, MARGARET A.
Time study of nursing procedures used in the care of a variety of surgical cases. New Haven, Yale University School of Nursing, 1928.

UNITED STATES. DEPARTMENT OF HEALTH, EDUCATION AND WELFARE
How to study nursing activities in a patient unit, by Margaret Amstein. Washington, Govt. Printing Office, 1954.

WEBER, H. J.
Aspects of job satisfaction through orientation and in-service programmes. *Hospital Progress*, Dec. 1956, p. 62-4.

What nurses like and dislike about their jobs. *Modern Hospital*, Dec. 1957, p. 53-8.

WORLD HEALTH ORGANIZATION.
REGIONAL OFFICE FOR SOUTH-EAST ASIA
Seminar on categories and functions of nursing personnel, organized by the Regional Office for South-East Asia of the W.H.O., Delhi, India, 6-25 August, 1956. New Delhi, W.H.O. Regional Office for South-East Asia, 1957.

Nursing Service Organization

ADAMS, APOLLONIA O.
How to study the nursing service of an out-patient department. Washington, Govt. Printing Office, 1957.

AMERICAN HOSPITALS ASSOCIATION and
NATIONAL LEAGUE OF NURSING EDUCATION
Hospital nursing service manual; prepared . . . with the assistance of Stella Goostray. New York, The League, 1950.

AMERICAN HOSPITAL ASSOCIATION, DIVISION OF NURSING, and NATIONAL LEAGUE OF NURSING EDUCATION
Manual of the essentials of good hospital nursing service. Chicago, The Association, 1942. 2nd edn., 1945.

ARMIGER, B.
Nursing service. Supervisory development. Part 2. Personnel management. *Hospital Progress*, Oct. 1960, p. 94-101.

ARNSTEIN, MARGARET G.
Improving nursing service. *Canadian Nurse*, Nov. 1956, p. 869-74.

BARNOWE, T. J.
The human relations involved in administering nursing service in a large modern hospital. *Nursing Research*, Oct. 1957, p. 72-4.

BENZ, E. G.
A nursing staff studies its service. *American Journal of Nursing*, Oct. 1958, p. 1389-91.

BOSTON UNIVERSITY. SCHOOL OF NURSING
Case studies in nursing service administration: collected and compiled by faculty and graduate students in nursing service administration. Boston University Press, 1956.

BREDENBURG, VIOLA CONSTANCE
A functional analysis of the nursing service team. . . . Washington, Catholic University of America Press, 1949.

BREDENBURG, VIOLA CONSTANCE
Hospital nursing service organization. *Hospital Progress*, Dec. 1957, p. 71 and 145.

BREDENBURG, VIOLA CONSTANCE
Supervisory training in nursing service. *Hospital Progress*, Nov. 1957, p. 80-1.

BUSH, C. K.
Nursing service criteria. *Mental Hospitals*, Mar. 1960, p. 13.

CATHOLIC UNIVERSITY OF AMERICA
The organization of hospital nursing services (the proceedings of the Workshop on the Organization of Hospital Nursing Services, conducted . . . from June 12 to June 22, 1951), edited by Charlotte Seyffer. Washington, Catholic University of America Press, 1952.

EDDLESON, R. B.
Organizing the nursing service for a new hospital. *American Journal of Nursing*, Feb. 1955, p. 198-202.

GODDARD, H. A.
Principles of administration applied to nursing service. Geneva, W.H.O., 1958.

GORDON, P.
Evaluation: a tool in nursing service. *American Journal of Nursing*, Mar. 1960, p. 364-6.

HANLON, M. R.
Nursing service: functions of the supervisor. *Hospital Progress*, Nov. 1960, p. 74-6.

HESLIN, L.
Nursing service: the personnel function in supervision. *Hospital Progress*, Jan. 1960, p. 66-7.

INTERDEPARTMENTAL COMMITTEE ON THE NURSING SERVICES
Interim report. H.M.S.O., 1939.
[Set up by the Ministry of Health and the Board of Education. Chairman: The Earl of Athlone.]

ROYAL COLLEGE OF NURSING
Memorandum relating to conditions in the nursing profession for submission to the Interdepartmental Committee on the Nursing Services. The College, 1938.

JONES, G. C., *and* WALDRUM, A. F.
Present-day concepts in nursing service administration in hospitals for the mentally ill. *American Journal of Psychiatry*, Oct. 1960, p. 329-35.

MARGARET VINCENT, SISTER
The functions of a nursing service department. *Hospital Progress*, April 1958, p. 90-2.

MARY MAURITA, SISTER
An administrator looks at nursing service. *Hospital Progress*, Sept. 1958, p. 90-2, and Oct. 1958, p. 65-7.

MENZIES, ISABEL E. P.
A case study in the functioning of social systems as a defence against anxiety: a report on a study of the nursing service of a general hospital. *Human Relations*, vol. 13, no. 2, 1960.

MONAHAN, SYLVIA
Budgetary practices in nursing service. *Nursing Outlook*, April 1957, p. 213-5.

MONGRAIN, L., SISTER
Nursing service in the hospital: its responsibility to the educational program. *Canadian Nurse*, Feb. 1955, p. 106-9.

MULLANE, MARY KELLY
Education for nursing service administration; an experience in program development by fourteen universities. Michigan, W. K. Kellogg Foundation, 1959.

OSGOOD, G. A.
Study of clinic nursing service. *Nursing Research*, Feb. 1958, p. 33-7.

REISSMAN, LEONARD, *and* ROHRER, JOHN H., *editors*
Change and dilemma in the nursing profession; studies of nursing services in a large general hospital. New York, Putnam, 1957.

ROYAL COLLEGE OF NURSING
The problem of providing a continuous nursing service especially in relation to night duty. R.C.N., 1958.

SCHWIER, M. E.
Creative nursing. *Canadian Nurse*, Nov. 1956, p. 875-80.

SCOTLAND. DEPARTMENT OF HEALTH
Report of the Scottish Departmental Committee on Nursing. H.M.S.O., 1938.
[Chairman: Lord Alness.]

WASHINGTON STATE NURSES' ASSOCIATION.
JOINT COMMITTEE ON NURSING SERVICES
Report of nursing functions study; an analysis of the nursing activities of a medical service in two urban hospitals. . . . Study carried out under the auspices of the American Nurses' Association. Washington, The Association, 1953.

WREN, G. R.
How we compute our nursing service expenses. *Hospitals*, June 1, 1957, p. 37-8.

Staffing

ABDELLAH, FAYE G., *and* LEVINE, EUGENE
Effect of nurse staffing on satisfaction with nursing care. . . . Chicago, American Hospital Association, 1958.

GEISTER, JANET M.
The trouble is not lack of nurses, it's lack of sense in using them. *Modern Hospital*, Aug. 1957, p. 63-5.

JENKINS, B.
Nurses' permanent rotation schedule. *Canadian Nurse*, Oct. 1957, p. 907-10.

KING EDWARD'S HOSPITAL FUND FOR LONDON
Nursing staff: considerations on standards of staffing. George Barber, for the Fund, 1945.

LEVINE, EUGENE
Turnover among nursing personnel in general hospitals *Hospitals*, Sept. 1, 1957, p. 50-3.

MANCHESTER REGIONAL HOSPITAL BOARD
Nurse staffing standards. *Hospital and Social Service Journal*, Dec. 13, 1957, p. 1304.

MANCHESTER REGIONAL HOSPITAL BOARD
Report of the Working Party on Standards of Nursing Staff for Hospitals. [Manchester, The Board, 1957.]

NEW, PETER KONG-MING, *and others*
Nursing service and patient care: a staffing experiment, by Peter Kong-Ming New, Gladys Nite and Josephine M. Callahan. Kansas City, Community Studies, 1959.

NEW, PETER KONG-MING, *and* NITE, GLADYS
Staffing and interaction. *Nursing Outlook*, July 1960, p. 396-400.

PERRODIN, CECILIA M.
Supervision of nursing service personnel. New York, Macmillan, 1954.

POTTER, R. M.
Faculty work load in the clinical fields in nursing degree programs. *Nursing Research*, Summer 1959, p. 160-8.

REIMANN, CHRISTIANE
Some observations on the ratio of nurses to patients. *Nosokomeion*, Supplementary Number, 1931, p. 91-168.

RITCHIE, J. A.
Fluctuating the nursing staff according to patient load. *Canadian Hospital*, May 1960, p. 62 *passim*.

SCHAFFER, MARGARET K.
Staffing the general hospital, 25-100 beds. Chicago, American Hospital Association, 1949.

SCHOELLER, V. D.
Work simplification applied to nursing. *American Journal of Nursing*, Aug. 1957, p. 1034-6.

SIMON, I. RICHARD, *and* OLSON, MARIAN E.
Assessing job attitudes of nursing service personnel. *Nursing Outlook*, Aug. 1960, p. 424-7.

SKELLERN, EILEEN
Report of an investigation carried out "to study, report and make recommendations on the practical application toward administration of modern methods in the instruction and handling of staff and student nurse". *Royal College of Nursing*, 1953.

UNITED STATES. DIVISION OF NURSING RESOURCES AND DIVISION OF PUBLIC HEALTH METHODS
Health manpower source book. [Section] 2: Nursing personnel. Prepared by Helen G. Tibbitts and Eugene Levine. Washington, U.S. Govt. Printing Office, [1953].

UNITED STATES. DIVISION OF PUBLIC HEALTH METHODS
Health manpower source book. [Section] 9: Physicians, dentists, and professional nurses. [Washington], U.S. Govt. Printing Office, [1959].

UNITED STATES. FEDERAL SECURITY AGENCY
Measuring nursing resources; prepared by Lois E. Gordner. Washington, The Agency, 1949.

UNITED STATES PUBLIC HEALTH SERVICE.
DIVISION OF NURSING RESOURCES
Nursing resources: a progress report on the program of the Division of Nursing Resources, prepared by Apollonia O. Adams. Washington, Govt. Printing Office, [1958].

"The way we've always done it" isn't the way to solve the problem of staffing the floors. *Modern Hospital*, Sept. 1957, p. 72-6.

WORLD HEALTH ORGANIZATION
Guide for national studies of nursing resources, by Margaret G. Arnstein. Geneva, W.H.O., 1953.

AUXILIARIES

AMERICAN HOSPITAL ASSOCIATION
Pattern and principles for hospital auxiliaries. Chicago, The Association, 1957.

AMERICAN HOSPITAL ASSOCIATION
The training of auxiliary workers for nursing service. Chicago, The Association, 1952.

American Nurses' Association and non-professional workers in nursing. *American Journal of Nursing*, Jan. 1955, p. 44-5.

AMERICAN NURSES' ASSOCIATION *and others*
Nursing aides and other auxiliary workers in nursing services, prepared by the Joint Committee on Practical Nurses and Auxiliary Workers in Nursing Services of the American Nurses' Association, and others. New York, The Association 1950.

BERKE, MARK
Where volunteers fit into the programme. *Modern Hospital*, Feb. 1957, p. 80-2.

BERKE, MARK
Why do volunteers volunteer? *Hospitals*, Aug. 16, 1958, p. 32-6.

BOLLIGER, W.
A brief survey of unskilled female nursing staff (nurse assistants) in three sanatoria for tuberculosis in Victoria. *Medical Journal of Australia*, Oct. 6, 1956, p. 520-1.

BOTTS, W. H.
Getting the volunteer program off to a good start. *Hospitals*, Mar. 1, 1959, p. 43-4.

BOYER, V. S.
Paid teen-age aides pay nursing dividends. *Hospitals*, Sept. 16, 1959, p. 34-6.

CHARLOTTE, SISTER
A nursing aide inservice program. *Hospital Progress*, May 1959, p. 118-20.

DOWDING, M. K.
The nurse-assistant. *Nursing Record*, Mar. 10, 1894, p. 162-3.

ELLSWORTH, ROBERT, BRYANT, ARTHUR, *and* BUTLER, GRACE
Psychiatric aide inservice training: an experimental approach. *Nursing Research*, Winter 1960, p. 12-16.

GUREL, LEE, *and* MORGAN, MOIRELINE M.
A project in psychiatric aide evaluation:
The process. *Nursing Outlook*, Oct. 1958, p. 590-2.
The outcome. *Nursing Outlook*, Nov. 1958, p. 619-21.

HASSENPLUG, LULU WOLF, *and* BRESNAHAN, D.
Part-time work for basic university nursing students. *Nursing Outlook*, Nov. 1959, p. 630-3.

HOBAN, L.
Why not a school for non-professional personnel? *Hospital Progress*, Jan. 1960, p. 68-9.

IWAMOTO, SURU
Operating room technicians. *Canadian Nurse*, Aug. 1960, p. 710.

JENSEN, F. T.
Experience is the best teacher for nurses' aides. *Modern Hospital*, Feb. 1959, p. 83-5.

KOZMA, W. A.
Even the best volunteers need good training. *Modern Hospital*, Feb. 1958, p. 77-8.

LEE, ANNE NATALIE
How to train nursing aides and orderlies. *Hospitals*, Nov. 16, 1958, p. 39-40.

LEE, ANNE NATALIE
The training of non-professional personnel. *Nursing Outlook*, April 1958, p. 222-5.

LEWIS, G. K.
Report on the seminar project for teachers of psychiatric aides. *American Journal of Psychiatry*, Sept. 1960, p. 224-7.

McGOLRICK, BETTY
Nursing aide instructor's guide. Washington, Govt. Printing Office, 1954.

MACLEOD, CHRISTINA
Manitoba Women's Hospital Auxiliaries Association. *Canadian Nurse*, Feb. 1960, p. 138-41.

MILLS, K. A., *and* STEFFEY, P.
The organization and utilization of volunteer groups. *Military Medicine*, Nov. 1958, p. 352-5.

MONTAG, MILDRED L.
The education of nursing technicians. New York, Putnam, 1951.

MYERS, R. S.
Lay technicians could assume many more nursing functions. *Modern Hospital*, June 1960, p. 132.

PINANSKI, V. R.
New trends in training volunteers. *Modern Hospital*, Jan. 1957, p. 56-8.

ROBERTSON, ESTHER
The untrained nurse, by a graduate of Bellevue Hospital, New York. Boston, Angel Guardian Press, 1903.

ROSEMONT, V. L.
In-service training of nursing auxiliaries. *Nursing Mirror*, July 8, 1960, p. vi-vii.

SCOTT, JOSEPHINE
Illustrated practical nursing procedures for hospital assistants. Heinemann, 1955.
[Written for African nursing orderlies.]

SHAW, H. F.
Volunteers take a look at themselves. *Mental Hospitals*, June 1960, p. 40-2.

UNITED HOSPITAL FUND OF NEW YORK
A guide to the organization of women's auxiliaries in hospitals. New York, United Hospitals Fund, 1955.

WILSON, A. T. M.
Hospital nursing auxiliaries: notes on a background survey and job analysis. Tavistock Publications, [1951].

WOLCOTT, H.
Aide training works for the general welfare. *Modern Hospital*, April 1960, p. 115-7.

COLONIAL NURSING

HAY, M. E. DALRYMPLE
The Colonial Association nurse.
See
NURSING TIMES
The nurse and the nation: a survey of her position in the State today. *Nursing Times*, Nov. 5, 1910, p. 904-31.

ENROLLED NURSE

AMERICAN NURSES' ASSOCIATION *and others*
Practical nurses and auxiliary workers for the care of the sick, prepared by the Joint Committee on Auxiliary Nursing Service of the American Nurses' Association, and others. New York, The Association, 1947.

AMERICAN NURSES' ASSOCIATION *and others*
Practical nurses in nursing services, prepared by the Joint Committee on Practical Nurses and Auxiliary Workers in Nursing Services of the American Nurses' Association, and others. New York, The Association, 1951.

BURTON, D. E.
Part-time assistant nurse training scheme at Devizes Hospital, Devizes. *Nursing Mirror*, June 24, 1955, p. iii-v.

GOLD, RAYMOND L., *and* FORD, THOMAS R.
A survey of licensed practical nurses in Alabama. Alabama University Press, 1957.

GREAT BRITAIN CENTRAL HEALTH SERVICES COUNCIL.
STANDING NURSING ADVISORY COMMITTEE ON THE POSITION OF THE ENROLLED ASSISTANT NURSE WITHIN THE NATIONAL HEALTH SERVICE
Report. H.M.S.O., 1954.

HARRINGTON, G. M.
What it costs to train a practical nurse. *Hospitals*, Aug. 16, 1958, p. 50-4.

W. K. KELLOG FOUNDATION
An experience in practical nurse education. Battle Creek, Michigan, The Foundation, [1957?].

KELLY, C. W.
Today's practical nurse; how she is filling the nursing gap. *Hospitals*, Aug. 16, 1959, p. 47-50.

LEONE, LUCILE PETRY
Trends and problems in practical nurse training. *American Journal of Nursing*, Jan. 1956, p. 51-3.

McGIRR, P. O. M.
The place of the state-enrolled assistant nurse in industry. *Journal for Industrial Nurses*, Autumn 1958, p. 133-5.

NATIONAL ASSOCIATION FOR PRACTICAL NURSE EDUCATION
Clinical teaching guide for practical nurse education. New York, The Association, 1953.

NATIONAL ASSOCIATION FOR PRACTICAL NURSE EDUCATION
The practical nurse in a general hospital. New York, The Association, 1947.

NATIONAL ASSOCIATION OF STATE ENROLLED ASSISTANT NURSES
The position of the state-enrolled assistant nurse in the National Health Service: memorandum submitted to the Ministry of Health. The Association, 1953.

NURSING OUTLOOK
Practical nurse education. *Nursing Outlook*, July 1955, p. 366-9.

NURSING TIMES
The assistant nurse in the health service. *Nursing Times*, Dec. 12, 1953, p. 1259-60.

OREM, DOROTHEA E.
Guides for developing curricula for the education of practical nurses. Washington, Govt. Printing Office, 1959.

PRICE, EDNA D.
The hospital looks at the practical nurse. *Practical Nursing*, Sept. 1958, p. 9-10.

ROSS, C. F.
Practical nurse education. *Nursing World*, Mar. 1956, p. 18-21.

ROYAL COLLEGE OF NURSING
Problems of the assistant nurse in U.K. and in U.S.A. *Nursing Mirror*, June 21, 1957, p. 851-2.

SCOTTISH HEALTH SERVICES COUNCIL.
STANDING NURSING AND MIDWIFERY ADVISORY COMMITTEE
The state-enrolled assistant nurse in the National Health Service. Edinburgh, H.M.S.O., 1955.

SHERROD, H. H.
The role of the licensed practical nurse in the hospital. *Journal of the Tennessee Medical Association*, Jan. 1960, p. 31-2.

SMITH, GENEVIEVE WAPLES
The patient teaches class. *Nursing Outlook*, Jan. 1960, p. 28-9.

STEVENSON, NEVA M.
Perspective on developments in practical nursing. *Nursing Outlook*, January 1960, p. 34-7.

TORROP, HILDA M.
Today's practical nurse; concepts behind her education. *Hospitals*, Aug. 16, 1959, p. 46-7.

UNITED STATES. DIVISION OF VOCATIONAL EDUCATION
Practical nurse training comes of age, by Louise Moore. Washington, Govt. Printing Office, 1954.

UNITED STATES
DIVISION OF VOCATIONAL EDUCATION
Report on the training of practical nurses in the United States. *Industry and Labour*, Nov. 1958, p. 339.

UNITED STATES. OFFICE OF EDUCATION
Practical nursing: an analysis of the practical nurse occupation, with suggestions for the organization of training programs. Washington, Govt. Printing Office, 1947.

UNITED STATES. OFFICE OF EDUCATION
Practical nursing curriculum, suggestions for developing a program of instruction based upon the analysis of the practical nurse occupation. Washington, Govt. Printing Office, 1950.

UNITED STATES. OFFICE OF EDUCATION
Source materials for practical nurse education, prepared by the Practical Nurse Education Section, Division of Vocational Education. Washington, Govt. Printing Office, 1958.

WAIN, O. M.
The assistant nurse: her training and her value. *Nursing Times*, June 24, 1960, p. 779-80.

WAIN, O. M.
Training for the roll. *Nursing Times*, Aug. 5, 1960, p. 957-9.

MISSION NURSING

THE FLIEDNER INSTITUTE, KAISERSWERTH, GERMANY
The work of deaconesses in Germany.
In
HAMPTON, ISABEL A., *and others*
Nursing of the sick, 1893.

GIBBONS, CARDINAL
Work done by religious communities devoted to the relief of the sick.
In
HAMPTON, ISABEL A., *and others*
Nursing of the sick, 1893.

JOHNSON, MABEL
Missionary nurse. *Canadian Nurse*, Jan. 1960, p. 69-71.

WINDSOR, A. E.
The mission nurse.
See
NURSING TIMES
The nurse and the nation: a survey of her position in the State today. *Nursing Times*, Nov. 5, 1910, p. 904-31.

POOR-LAW NURSING

BARTON, ELEANOR C.
The poor law nurse.
See
NURSING TIMES
The nurse and the nation: a survey of her position in the State today. *Nursing Times*, Nov. 5, 1910, p. 904-31.

PRISON NURSING

ST. JOHN MAXWELL
Nursing in prisons. *British Journal of Nursing*, Aug. 1, 1914, p. 95-7.

PRIVATE NURSING

AMERICAN NURSES' ASSOCIATION
Functions, standards and qualifications for the practice of private duty nursing. New York, The Association, 1956.

AMERICAN NURSES' ASSOCIATION.
RESEARCH AND STATISTICS UNIT
Meet the professional private duty nurse. New York, The Association, n.d.

BREAY, MARGARET
How can private nurses keep in touch with modern methods? *Nursing Record*, Mar. 20, 1897, p. 232-4.

COUEY, ELIZABETH D., *and* STEPHENSON, DIANE D.
The field of private duty nursing; a study of the functions of the private duty nurse in the hospital environment, conducted by Couey and Couey, Educational Consultants, for the Georgia State Nurses' Association, under a grant, from the American Nurses' Association. Montgomery, Alabama, Cadden Advertizing Agency, 1955.

DE WITT, KATHARINE
Private duty nursing. Philadelphia, Lippincott, 1913.

FINER, HERMAN
Evaluating the private duty nurse's performance. *American Journal of Nursing*, Dec. 1956, p. 1564-6.

FOGGO-THOMPSON, HELEN
Private nursing: paper read before the British Nurses' Association. *Nursing Record*, Mar. 13, 1890, p. 126-7, and Mar. 20, 1890, p. 136-9.

GILBERTSON, H. C.
Private nursing in Great Britain. *Australian Nurses' Journal*, July 1959, p. 178-9.

HABEL, MARY LOUISE, *and* MILTON, HAZEL DORIS
The graduate nurse in the home. Philadelphia, Lippincott, 1939.

HOLMES, JESSIE
The private duty nurse: some reminiscences of eight years' private nursing. T. Fisher Unwin, 1899.

HUGHES, LORA WOOD
No time for tears. Boston, Houghton Mifflin, 1946.

KENT, BEATRICE
The nurse in private practice: the nurses' point of view. *British Journal of Nursing*, Jan. 1, 1910, p. 3-4, and Jan. 8, 1910, p. 23-4.

MOSES, E. B.
The care in private duty. *American Journal of Nursing*, Dec. 1960, p. 1784-5.

PENNSYLVANIA STATE NURSES' ASSOCIATION
Survey of professional nurses' registry practices in Pennsylvania. Pennsylvania, The Association, 1954.

PUMROY, SHIRLEY S., *and* SUTTELL, BARBARA J.
The private duty nurse: her role in the hospital environment of Washington, D.C. Sponsored by the American Nurses' Foundation. Pittsburgh, American Institute for Research, 1956.

RICHARDSON, W. L.
An address on the duties and conduct of nurses in private nursing. Boston, 1887.
[London, 1887, with some notes on preventing the spread of infectious disease.]

SALVADOR, ALPHEN
The nurse in private practice: the qualities of the nurse. *British Journal of Nursing*, Jan. 15, 1910, p. 45-6.

SPOHN, ROBERTA R.
A study of private duty nurses. New York, American Nurses' Association, 1954.

STONEY, EMILY A. M.
Practical points in nursing for nurses in private practice, with an appendix containing rules for feeding the sick; recipes for invalid foods and beverages; weights and measures; dose list; and a full glossary of medical terms and nursing treatment. Philadelphia, Saunders, 1896. 2nd edn., 1902.

WENDEN, MARIANNE
Private nursing. Faber, 1936.

WOOD, C. J.
Private nursing. *Nursing Record*, April 12, 1888, p. 14-17.

STEWARDESSES

YANTA, GERALDINE M.
Stewardess-nurse. *American Journal of Nursing*, Dec. 1958, p. 1699.

TECHNIQUES OF NURSING

GENERAL WORKS

ADAMS, RALPH
Prevention of infections in hospitals. *American Journal of Nursing*, Mar. 1958, p. 344-8.

AMERICAN HOSPITAL ASSOCIATION
Handbook for nursing aides in hospitals. Chicago, The Association, 1954.

AMERICAN HOSPITAL ASSOCIATION
Nursing aide instructor's guide. Chicago, The Association, 1952.

AMERICAN HOSPITAL ASSOCIATION *and*
NATIONAL LEAGUE OF NURSING EDUCATION
Hospital nursing service manual; prepared . . . with the assistance of Stella Goostray, New York, National League of Nursing Education, 1950.

ASHDOWN, A. MILLICENT
A complete system of nursing. Dent, 1917.
2nd edn., 1919.
3rd edn., 1921.
4th edn., 1922.
5th edn., 1924.
6th edn., 1925.
7th edn., 1927.
8th edn., 1928.
9th edn., 1929.
10th edn., 1931.
11th edn., 1932.
12th edn., 1939.
13th edn., 1943.

ASHDOWN, A. MILLICENT
A complete system of nursing for male nurses. Dent, 1934.

ASHDOWN, A. MILLICENT
The elementary practice of nursing. Dent, 1940.

BAGOT, RUTH A.
Nursing. Bailliere, Tindall & Cox, 1937.
2nd edn., revised by Elizabeth C. Wilson and Ethel Dodsworth, 1951.
[Bailliere's Medical Manuals for Africans.]

BARCLAY, M. K.
101 suggestions for ward instructions (specially adapted for use in military hospitals). Beck, 1933.

BARWELL, R.
The care of the sick: a discourse of practical lectures delivered at the Working Women's College. 2nd edn. London, 1857.

BATEMAN, F. J. A.
Prevention of bedsores with silicone barrier cream. *Nursing Mirror*, Nov. 16, 1956, p. 483-2.

BECKETT, JOHN S., *and* BERMAN, PHOEBUS
Sterilization and disinfection, with special emphasis on autoclave sterilization: a handbook for nurses. North Hollywood, Aseptic Thermo Indicator Co., Publishing Division, 1953.

BELILIOS, ARTHUR D., *and* DUNCAN-JOHNSTONE, DOROTHEA
A handbook of elementary nursing. Bailliere, Tindall & Cox, 1952.

BELLEVUE HOSPITAL TRAINING SCHOOL
A manual of nursing prepared for the Training School attached to Bellevue Hospital. New York, Putnam, 1878.

BENNETT, B. A.
Modern medicine and nursing care. *Hospital and Social Service Journal*, Nov. 19, 1954, p. 1199-1200.

BIEN, RUTH
Practical nursing procedures. Albany, Delmar, 1954.

BILLROTH, CHRISTIAN ALBERT THEODOR
The care of the sick at home and in the hospital: a handbook for families and for nurses. Translated by J. B. Ending. New York, Scribner & Welford, 1891.

BIRD, E. P.
Manual of nursing procedures. Philadelphia, Saunders, 1926.

BLAIR, L. B.
How we added practical training to professional training. *Hospitals*, Aug. 1, 1957, p. 38-41.

BRIDGE, HELEN LILLIAN
A manual of practical nursing—prepared by the Washington University Training School for Nurses at the Barnes and St. Louis Children's Hospital. St. Louis, Mosby, 1916.

BRIDGES, D. C.
Nursing the whole patient. *Nursing Mirror*, Oct. 19, 1956, p. iii-iv.

BRITTEN, JESSIE D.
Practical notes on nursing procedures. Edinburgh, Livingstone, 1957.
2nd edn., 1959.
3rd edn., 1960.

BROWN, AMY FRANCES
Medical and surgical nursing—II. Philadelphia, Saunders, 1959.

BROWN, AMY FRANCES
Medical nursing. Philadelphia, Saunders, 1945.
2nd edn., 1952.
3rd edn., 1957.

BROWN, CHARLOTTE AMBROSE
Principles of nursing. Philadelphia, Lea & Febiger, 1919.

BROWNELL, KATHRYN OSMOND
A textbook of practical nursing. Philadelphia, Saunders, 1939.
2nd edn., 1944.
3rd edn., 1949.
4th edn., 1954, by K. O. Brownell and Vivian M. Culver, entitled "The practical nurse".
5th edn., 1959.

BRUEN, E.
Practical lessons in nursing. Outlines for the management of diet, on the regulation of food to the requirements of health and the treatment of disease. Philadelphia, 1887.

BUCHANAN, M. EDITH
A study guide in nursing arts. Printed in the United States, 1953.
[Written for use in India.]

CABOT, R. C., *and* DICKS, R. L.
The art of ministering to the sick. New York, Macmillan, 1936.

CASELEY, D. J.
Trends in medical practice; their implications for nursing. *Nursing Outlook*, May 1957, p. 300-2.

CAUFIELD, WILLIAM BUCKINGHAM
The hygiene of the sick room. A book for nurses and others. Philadelphia, Blakiston, 1892.

C. H. C.
A reference book for trained nurses. Buffalo, New York, Lakeside Publ. Co., 1889.

CHETWYND, C. A.
Cross-infection in hospital wards and departments and its control. *Nursing Mirror*, July 15, 1955, p. 1065-6 and 1068.

CLEWES, E. S.
Barrier nursing and non-touch technique in domiciliary nursing. *Nursing Times*, Oct. 8, 1954, p. 1091-2.

COLTMAN, GALE
Textbook for male practical nurses. New York, Macmillan, 1941.

COOK, J. B.
Index of practical nursing. London, 1912.

CORRY, SARAH
Notes on nursing, by a nurse. New York, Appleton-Century, 1944.

CULLINGWORTH, CHARLES J.
The nurse's companion: a manual of general and monthly nursing. Churchill, 1876.
2nd edn., 1889.
3rd edn., 1890.

CURRAN, W. MARTIN
Sickness and accidents: modern methods of treatment. Information for nurses in home and hospital. Chicago, 1893.

DAKIN, FLORENCE
Simplified nursing. Philadelphia, Lippincott, 1925.
2nd edn., 1930.
3rd edn., 1931.
4th edn., 1941, by F. Dakin and E. M. Thompson
5th edn., 1951.
6th edn., 1956, assisted by M. LeBaron.
7th edn., 1960, by E. M. Thompson and M. LeBaron.

DALRYMPLE-SMITH, M.
Making a bed. *Nursing Times*, April 17, 1959, p. 472-4.

DARMADY, E. M., *and others*
Portsmouth Central Sterile Supply Service and the Wessex dressing technique. *Nursing Mirror*, Dec. 2, 1960, p. x-xiii.

DAVIES, MARY
The nurse's companion to the sick room. Virtue, 1889.

DAY, MARY AGNITA CLAIRE
Basic science in nursing arts. Kimpton, 1943.
2nd edn., 1947.

DAY, MARY AGNITA CLAIRE
Principles and techniques of nursing procedures as developed in St. Mary's Group of Hospitals of St. Louis University. Kimpton, 1943.

DEMING, DOROTHY
The practical nurse. New York, Commonwealth Fund, 1947.

DICKIE, HELEN M.
Pocket book on tray and trolley setting. Livingstone, 1959.

DOCK, LAVINIA L.
Short papers in nursing subjects. New York, Longeway, 1900.

DOHERTY, MURIEL KNOX, *and others*
Modern practical nursing procedures. Sydney, Dymocks Book Arcade, 1944.
2nd edn., 1946.
3rd edn., 1946.
4th edn., 1949.
5th edn., 1953.
6th edn., 1954.
7th edn., 1956.
8th edn., 1959, by M. K. Doherty, M. B. Sirl and O. I. Ring.

DOMVILLE, EDWARD J.
A manual for hospital nurses and others engaged in attending on the sick. Philadelphia, Blakiston, 1888.

DONAHOE, MARGARET FRANCES
A manual of nursing. New York, Appleton-Century, 1910.

DUDER, RICHARD, *and* GAILANI, DOROTHY M.
Frequency of nursing procedures performed at the bedside. *Nursing Research*, Winter 1960, p. 43-5.

DURRANT, M. M.
The nurse's responsibility concerning cross-infection. *Nursing Mirror*, Jan. 15, 1954, p. xi-xiii.

EDWARDS, WILLIAM
Here's your medicine: nursing for novices. Macmillan, 1960.

ELIASON, ELDRIDGE L.
Practical bandaging, including adhesive and plaster-of-paris dressings. Philadelphia, Lippincott, 1914.
2nd edn., 1921.
3rd edn., 1924.
4th edn., 1930.
5th edn., 1938.
6th edn., 1943.

ESAU, MARGARET C., *and others*
Practical nursing today: attitudes, knowledge, skills. New York, Putnam, 1957.

FADDIS, MARGENE O., *and* HAYMAN, JOSEPH M.
Care of the medical patient: a textbook for nurses. New York, McGraw-Hill, 1952.

FARNWORTH, MARY
Roller and triangular bandaging illustrated. Faber, 1939.

FISHER, ESTHER
The nurse's textbook: a manual of medical and surgical nursing. Faber, 1937.

FOX, E. MARGARET
First lines in nursing: being a handbook for junior probationers and all who contemplate entering the nursing profession. Scientific Press, 1914.
2nd edn., 1924.
3rd edn., 1930, called "First steps in nursing".

FREDERICK, HESTER K.
A textbook of nursing technique. New York, Macmillan, 1928.
2nd edn., 1938, called "A textbook of nursing practice".

FREEDMAN, MARILYN GOTTEHRER, *and* HANNAN, JUSTINE
Medical-surgical workbook for practical nurses. Philadelphia, Davis, 1960.

FREEMAN, EDNA
Teaching the administration of medications to practical nurse students. *Nursing Outlook*, May 1959, p. 305-6.

FUERST, ELINOR V., *and* WOLFF, LU VERNE
Teaching fundamentals of nursing: method, content and evaluation. Philadelphia, Lippincott, 1956.
2nd edn., 1958.
3rd edn., 1960.

GIBSON, M., *and* MANN, T. P.
Experimental barrier nursing techniques in a cubicled gastro-enteritis unit. *Proceedings of the Royal Society of Medicine*, Dec. 1959, p. 1017-8.

GOODNOW, MINNIE
First-year nursing: a textbook for pupils during their first year of hospital work. Philadelphia, Saunders, 1912.
2nd edn., 1916.
3rd edn., 1921.

GOULDING, FERN A., *and* TORROP, HILDA M.
The practical nurse and her patient. Philadelphia, Lippincott, 1955.

GRATION, HILDA M.
The practice of nursing. Faber, 1944.
2nd edn., 1946.
3rd edn., 1950, by H. M. Gration and D. L. Holland.
4th edn., 1954, by H. M. Gration and D. L. Holland.
5th edn., 1956, by H. M. Gration and D. L. Holland.
6th edn., 1959, by H. M. Gration and D. L. Holland.

GRATION, HILDA M.
A ward pocket-book for the nurse. Faber, 1946.
2nd edn., 1949.
3rd edn., 1951, by H. M. Gration and D. L. Holland.
4th edn., 1955, by H. M. Gration and D. L. Holland.

GREMP, ZELLA VON, *and* BROADWELL, LUCILLE
Practical nursing review: questions and situations. Philadelphia, Lippincott, 1959.

GROVES, E. W. HEY, *and* FORTESCUE-BRICKDALE, J. M.
Textbook for nurses: anatomy, physiology, surgery and medicine. Frowde and Hodder & Stoughton, 1912.
2nd edn., 1917.
3rd edn., 1925.
4th edn., 1930.
5th edn., 1936.
6th edn., 1940, by E. W. Hey Groves and J. A. Nixon, published by O.U.P.
7th edn., 1948, revised by J. A. Nixon and Sir Cecil Wakeley.

GULLAN, M. A.
Theory and practice of nursing. Lewis, 1920.
2nd edn., 1925.
3rd edn., 1930.
4th edn., 1935.
5th edn., 1946.
6th edn., 1952.
7th edn., 1956.

HAMPTON, ISABEL ADAMS
Nursing: its principles and practice for hospital and private use. 2nd edn. The Scientific Press, 1898.

HANBURY, —
The good nurse, or hints on the management of the sick and lying-in chamber and the nursery. 2nd edn. Longman, 1828.

HANSEN, HELEN F.
A review of nursing, with outlines of subjects, questions and answers. Philadelphia, Saunders, 1934.
2nd edn., 1937.
3rd edn., 1940.
4th edn., 1943.
5th edn., 1946.
6th edn., 1949.
7th edn., 1952.
8th edn., 1956.

HANSEN, HELEN F.
Study guide and review of practical nursing: with outlines of subjects and integrated situation-type questions and answers. Philadelphia, Saunders, 1955.

HARDY, GLADYS M.
Nursing. Foyle, 1949.

HARMER, BERTHA
Textbook of the principles and practice of nursing. New York, Macmillan, 1922.
2nd edn., 1928.
3rd edn., 1934.
4th edn., 1939, by B. Harmer and Virginia Henderson.
5th edn., 1955, rev. by V. Henderson.

HAWES, ALFRED TAYLOR
Care of the patient, a book for nurses. Philadelphia, Blakiston, 1911.

HAWES, ALFRED TAYLOR
Talks to first-year nurses. Boston, Whitcomb & Barrows, 1907.

HAWKINS-DEMPSTER, H.
Explanatory lectures for nurses and their teachers. Bristol, Wright, 1913.

HECTOR, WINIFRED
Modern nursing: theory and practice. Heinemann, 1960.

HENDERSON, LOUISE
Practical nursing: an elementary condensed textbook for trained attendants and for use in practical home nursing. New York, Macmillan, 1921.
2nd edn., 1929.

HENDERSON, VIRGINIA
Basic principles of nursing care. International Council of Nurses, [1960].

HENDERSON, VIRGINIA
Medical and surgical asepsis: the development of asepsis and a study of current practice with recommendations in relation to certain aseptic nursing methods in hospitals. New York, Columbia University Teachers' College, Dept. of Nursing Education, Nursing Education Bulletin, June 1935.

HILL, DOROTHY DIX
Textbook of nursing procedures; Bellevue School of Nursing. New York, Macmillan, 1923.

HITCH, MARGARET
Aids to medical nursing. Bailliere, Tindall & Cox, 1941.
2nd edn., 1943.
3rd edn., 1946.
4th edn., 1952.
5th edn., 1956, revised by Katharine F. Armstrong and E. Joan Bocock.
[Later published as "Aids to medical nursing" by Marjorie Houghton and Mary Whittow.]

HOUGHTON, MARJORIE
Aids to practical nursing. Bailliere, Tindall & Cox, 1938.
2nd edn., 1940.
3rd edn., 1941.
4th edn., 1942.
5th edn., 1947.
6th edn., 1948.
7th edn., 1952.
8th edn., 1956.
9th edn., 1960.

HOUGHTON, MARJORIE
Aids to tray and trolley setting. Bailliere, Tindall & Cox, 1941.
2nd edn., 1942.
3rd edn., 1946.
4th edn., 1948.
5th edn., 1952.
6th edn., 1960.

HULL, EDGAR, and PERRODIN, CECILIA M.
Medical nursing. Philadelphia, Davis, 1940.
2nd edn., 1941.
3rd edn., 1943.
4th edn., 1945.
5th edn., 1954.
6th edn., 1960.

HUMPHRY, LAURENCE
A manual of nursing: medical and surgical. Philadelphia, Griffin, 1889.
2nd edn., 1890.
9th edn., 1893.
11th edn., 1894.
17th edn., 1898.
18th edn., 1898.
28th edn., 1905.
29th edn., 1905.

HUMPHRY, LAURENCE, and REYNOLDS, W. MYRON
Nurses' service digest: a manual of nursing. New York, Menzies, 1918.

INGLES, THELMA
What is good nursing. American Journal of Nursing, Sept. 1959, p. 1246-9.

JACKSON, J. C.
How to nurse the sick. Dansville, New York, 1868.

JAMME, ANNA C.
Textbook of nursing procedures. New York, 1921.

JENSEN, DEBORAH MacLURG, editor
Practical nursing: a textbook for students and graduates. St. Louis, Mosby, 1958.

JENSEN, DEBORAH MacLURG, and others
The principles and practice of ward teaching: a discussion of clinical teaching in nursing. Kimpton, 1942.
2nd edn., 1946, called "Principles and practice of clinical instruction in nursing".
3rd edn., 1952, called "Clinical instruction and its integration in the curriculum".

JENSEN, DEBORAH MacLURG
Students' handbook on nursing care studies. New York, Macmillan, 1929.
2nd edn., 1932.
3rd edn., 1940, called "Nursing care studies".

JOHNSON, ROBERT WALLACE
Friendly cautions to the heads of families and others, very necessary to be observed in order to preserve health and long life; with ample directions to nurses who attend the sick, women in childbed, etc. 3rd edn. Philadelphia, Humphreys, 1804.

JOSEPH, RUTH RHODES
Nursing-arts guide. Philadelphia, Davis, 1951.

KELLY, IRENE VIRGINIA
Textbook of nursing technique. Philadelphia, Saunders, 1926.
3rd edn., 1935.

LAURENCE, E. C.
Modern nursing in hospital and home: a short course of lectures to probationers. Scientific Press, 1907.

LEAKE, MARY J.
A manual of simple nursing procedures. Philadelphia, Saunders, 1951.

LEWIS, PERCY G.
The theory and practice of nursing: a textbook for nurses. Scientific Press, 1890.
7th edn., 1893.
11th edn., 1900, called "Nursing; its theory and practice: being a complete textbook of medical, surgical and monthly nursing".

LILLY, JOSEPH L., compiler
Manual of the Ladies of Charity, 1926.

LONG, JAMES
Lectures to the nurses of the Liverpool Royal Infirmary. Liverpool, Mawdsley, Printers, 1878.

LONGSHORE, JOSEPH SKELTON
The principles and practice of nursing, or a guide to the inexperienced. Philadelphia, Merrihew & Thompson, 1842.

LUCKES, EVA C. E.
Lectures on general nursing delivered to the probationers of the London Hospital Training School for Nurses. Kegan Paul, 1884. [Subsequent editions, much enlarged, called "General Nursing".]
2nd edn., 1898.
3rd edn., 1899.
4th edn., 1902.
5th edn., 1905.
6th edn., 1906.
7th edn., 1908.
8th edn., 1910.
9th edn., 1914.

MCCLAIN, M. ESTHER
Scientific principles in nursing. Kimpton, 1950.
2nd edn., 1953.
3rd edn., 1958.

MCCRAE, ANNABELLA
Procedure in nursing: preliminary and advanced. Boston, Whitcomb & Barrows, 1923.

MCCULLOUGH, WAVA
Illustrated handbook of simple nursing. New York, McGraw-Hill, 1949.

MCGOLRICK, BETTY, and SUTHERLAND, DOROTHY
Handbook for nursing aides in hospitals . . . under the direction of Margaret G. Arnstein. Chicago, American Hospital Association, [1956?].

MCISSAC, ISABEL
Primary nursing: technique for first-year pupil nurses. New York, Macmillan, 1908.

MANNING, ANNE R.
First principles of nursing. Boston, 1901.

MARTINEAU, HARRIETT
Life in the sick room. Boston, Bowles, 1844.

MATTHEWS, F.
Sterilisation of syringes by the hot-air method. *Nursing Mirror*, Dec. 4, 1953, p. x-xii.

MAXWELL, ANNA CAROLINE, and POPE, AMY ELIZABETH
Practical nursing: a textbook for nurses. New York, Putnam, 1907.
2nd edn., 1910.
3rd edn., 1914, revised and enlarged by A. E. Pope.

MIDGLEY, R. L.
Collection and disposal of sputum. *Nursing Times*, May 23, 1958. D. 591-2.

MINISTRY OF HEALTH
Manual of nursing procedures: infection in hospitals, memoranda nos. N.P.I-N.P.VI. Ministry of Health, [1951?].
N.P.I. The method of bed isolation nursing.
N.P.II. The prevention of infection in surgical cases.
N.P.III. Masks.
N.P.IV. Disinfection.
N.P.V. The common use of articles of clothing by patients; nursing procedures.
N.P.VI. The procedure for nursing tubercular patients.

MINISTRY OF HEALTH
Manual of nursing procedures: infection in hospitals, memoranda nos. N.P.IA, N.P.IIA, N.P.VII, N.P.VIII. Ministry of Health, [195?].
N.P.IA. The method of bed isolation; nursing; modifications for children's wards.
N.P.IIA. The prevention of infection in surgical cases; modifications for children's wards.
N.P.VII. Preparation of infants' feeds; methods employed in sick children's hospitals.
N.P.VIII. Precautions to be observed when changing an infant's napkin or sundry.

MINISTRY OF HEALTH
Procedural memoranda for hospitals: infection in hospitals, nos. P.M.1, P.M.2, P.M.3. Ministry of Health, [1951?].
P.M.1. The administrative aspects of cross infection.
P.M.2. The common use of articles of clothing by patients: administrative matters.
P.M.3. The nursing of tuberculous patients.

MINISTRY OF HEALTH
Procedural memoranda for hospitals: infection in hospitals, nos. P.M.IA, P.M.IV, P.M.V. Ministry of Health, [195?].
P.M.IA. The administrative aspects of cross infection: additional measures to meet the special requirements of sick children's wards.
P.M.IV. The prevention of bed sores: hospital patients.
P.M.V. The preparation of infants' feeds: methods used in sick children's hospitals.

MINNESOTA UNIVERSITY SCHOOL OF NURSING
Nursing procedures. Minneapolis, The University, 1929.
2nd edn., 1935. A textbook of nursing techniques.
3rd edn., 1937. A textbook of nursing techniques.
4th edn., 1941. A manual of nursing procedures, pub. by Burgess.
5th edn., 1945.

MONTAG, MILDRED L., and FILSON, MARGARET
Nursing arts. Philadelphia, Saunders, 1948.
2nd edn., 1953.
[For later edition see Mildred L. Montag and Ruth P. Stewart Swenson, Fundamentals in nursing care.]

MONTAG, MILDRED L., and SWENSON, RUTH P. STEWART
Fundamentals in nursing care. 3rd edn. Philadelphia, Saunders, 1959.
[For earlier editions see Mildred L. Montag and Margaret Filson, Nursing Arts.]

MUNRO, AENEAS
The science and art of nursing the sick. Glasgow, 1872.

NATIONAL COUNCIL OF TRAINED NURSES OF FINLAND
Nursing care during long-term illness. *International Nursing Review*, Aug. 1960, p. 50-61.

NATIONAL FEDERATION OF BELGIAN NURSES
Medical nursing. *International Nursing Review*, April 1958, p. 71-85.

NEWSOME, EDITH
Everywoman a nurse: health and nursing notes. . . . O.U.P., 1927.

NEW YORK CITY. DEPARTMENT OF HOSPITALS.
COMMITTEE ON NURSING STANDARDS
Standard nursing procedures of the Department of Hospitals, City of New York; prepared by the Committee on Nursing Standards, Division of Nursing, Department of Hospitals, Mary Ellen Manley, director. New York, Macmillan, 1943.

NIGHTINGALE, FLORENCE
The art of nursing. Morris, 1946.

NIGHTINGALE, FLORENCE
Notes on nursing: what it is, and what it is not. Harrison, [1859].
New edn., 1860.
New edn., 1868, called "Notes on nursing for the labouring classes."
New edn., 1924, based on the 1861 edn.
New edn., 1952, based on the 1861 edn., with some additional chapters, pub. by Duckworth.

NORDMARK, MADELYN TITUS, and ROHWEDER, ANNE E.
Science principles applied to nursing: a reference for nurse educators. Philadelphia, Lippincott, 1959.

NORTON, FELICIE
"Preliminary" questions and answers: model answers to questions set at the preliminary state examination in nursing. 7th edn. Faber, 1941.

NUFFIELD PROVINCIAL HOSPITALS TRUST
Present sterilizing practice in six hospitals. The Trust, 1958.

NURSING MIRROR
Non-touch technique: two new ideas versus cross-infection. *Nursing Mirror*, Jan. 15, 1960, p. xiv.

OLSON, LYLA M.
A nurse's handbook for hospital, school and home. Philadelphia, Saunders, 1905.
2nd edn., 1908.
3rd edn., 1913.
4th edn., 1919.
5th edn., 1924.
6th edn., 1929.
7th edn., 1932.
8th edn., 1934.
9th edn., 1941.
10th edn., 1960.

O'NEILL, H. C., and BARNETT, EDITH A.
Our nurses, and the work they have to do. Ward, Lock [1888].

ORBISON, KATHERINE TUCKER
A handbook for nurses' aides. New York, Devin-Adair, 1945.

OXFORD, M. N.
A handbook of nursing. Methuen, 1900.
2nd edn., 1903.
3rd edn., 1906.
4th edn., 1907.
5th edn., 1909.
6th edn., 1912.
7th edn., 1916, revised by F. Sheldon.

PEABODY, FRANCES WELD
The care of the patient. Cambridge, Mass., Harvard University Press, 1927.

PEARCE, EVELYN CLARE
A general textbook of nursing: a comprehensive guide to the final state examinations. Faber, 1937.
2nd edn., 1938.
3rd edn., 1939.
4th edn., 1940.
5th edn., 1941.
6th edn., 1942.
7th edn., 1942.
8th edn., 1943.
9th edn., 1945.
10th edn., 1949.
11th edn., 1950.
12th edn., 1952.
13th edn., 1953.
14th edn., 1956.

PERRY, ALAN, and HARVEY, DOROTHY
General nursing: a textbook for the state examination. Arnold, 1932.

PIPER, PHYLLIS M.
Data book for nurses. Caxton, 1956.

POPE, AMY ELIZABETH, and YOUNG, VIRNA M.
The art and principles of nursing. New York, Putnam, 1934.

POPE, AMY ELIZABETH
Pope's manual of nursing procedure. New York, Putnam, 1919.

POWELL, N. W.
Practical preparations, mainly medical. Faber, 1933.
[Later issued as P. J. Cunningham's "Practical preparations in common use", 1953.]

PRESTON, ANN
Nursing the sick and the training of nurses. An address delivered at the request of the Board of Managers of the Women's Hospital at Philadelphia. Philadelphia, 1863.

PRICE, ALICE L.
The art, science and spirit of nursing. Philadelphia, Saunders, 1954.

PRICE, ALICE L.
A handbook and charting manual for student nurses. 2nd edn., St. Louis, Mosby, 1958.

PRICE, ALICE L.
Vocational nursing for home, school and hospital. St. Louis, Mosby, 1948.

PRIOR, PEARL L.
Practical nursing procedures. United Society for Christian Literature, 1950.

PUGH, W. T. GORDON
Practical nursing, including hygiene and dietetics. Edinburgh, Blackwood, 1904.
2nd edn., 1906.
3rd edn., 1910.
4th edn., 1915.
5th edn., 1919.
6th edn., 1921.
7th edn., 1927.
8th edn., 1933.
9th edn., 1934.
10th edn., 1936.
11th edn., 1937.
12th edn., 1940.
13th edn., 1943.
14th edn., 1943.
15th edn., 1945.
16th edn., 1949.
17th edn., 1953.
18th edn., 1955.

RAKICH, JENNIE H., THOMAS, MARGARET W., and LESTER, MARY
Nurses are asking about staphylococcal infections. *American Journal of Nursing*, Dec. 1960, p. 1766-9.

REDMOND, M. M.
The nurse as a clinical specialist. *Military Medicine*, Nov. 1957, p. 297-300.

REID, E. PRISCILLA, and others
A manual of nursing procedures by E. Priscilla Reid, Mabel E. Hoffman, Hazel L. Jennings and William A. Read. Philadelphia, Saunders, 1923.

RHODE ISLAND TRAINING SCHOOL FOR NURSING
Lessons in nursing. Philadelphia, 1911.

RIDDELL, MARGARET S.
A first year nursing manual. Faber, 1931.
2nd edn., 1934.
3rd edn., 1936.
4th edn., 1937.
5th edn., 1939.

RIDDELL, MARGARET S.
Lectures to nurses: being a complete series of lectures to probationary nurses in their first, second and third years of training. Scientific Press, [1914].
2nd edn., 1925.
3rd edn., 1928.
4th edn., 1931.
5th edn., 1933.
6th edn., 1936.
7th edn., 1938.
8th edn., 1942.
New edn., rev. by Margaret E. Hitch 1948.

ROBERTS, G. W.
Preventing bedsores. *Nursing Times*, Sept. 18, 1959, p. 866-7.

ROBERTS, G. W., and WILLIAMS, F. M.
Silicone barrier cream in the prevention of bedsores in patients nursed at home. *Nursing Times*, Oct. 25, 1957, p. 1206-7.

ROBERTS, R. LAWTON
Illustrated lectures on nursing and hygiene. 3rd edn. Lewis, 1900.

ROSS, JANET S., and WILSON, KATHLEEN J. W.
Foundations of nursing. Edinburgh, Livingstone, 1956.
2nd edn., 1957.

ROTHWEILER, ELLA L., and others
The science and art of nursing, with sections on physical therapy by John S. Coulter and a section on bandaging . . . and first aid by Felix Jarvey. Philadelphia, Davis, 1938.
[Later edns. called "The art and science of nursing", by Ella L. Rothweiler and Jean Martin White.]
2nd edn., 1941.
3rd edn., 1947.
4th edn., 1950.
5th edn., 1954.
6th edn., 1959.

SANDERS, GEORGIANA JANE
Modern methods in nursing. Philadelphia, Saunders, 1912.
2nd edn., 1916.
3rd edn., 1922.
4th edn., 1927.

SCHROTH, RUDOLPH GEORGE
Instructions for nurses: with an explanation concerning all branches of the profession. Chicago, Post-graduate Training School for Nurses, 1913.

The science and art of nursing; a guide to the various branches of nursing, theoretical and practical, by medical and nursing authorities. Cassell, n.d., 4 vols.

SCOTT, DOUGLAS HAY
Modern professional nursing. Caxton, 1936. 4 vols.

SCOTT, JOSEPHINE
Illustrated practical nursing procedures for hospital assistants. Heinemann, 1955.

SCOTT, R. J. E., editor
Pocket cyclopedia of nursing. New York, Macmillan, 1923.
2nd edn., 1924.
3rd edn., 1931.

SHEPARD, KATHERINE, and LAWRENCE, CHARLOTTE
Textbook of attendant nursing. New York, Macmillan, 1935.
2nd edn., 1942.
3rd edn., 1948, by Shepard: called "Textbook of attendant and practical nursing".
4th edn., 1955, by Helen Z. Gill: called "Basic nursing".

SMITH, C. L.
The dangers of bed blocking. *Nursing Times*, Aug. 31, 1956, p. 841-2.

SMITH, E. MAUDE
Notes on practical nursing. Faber & Gwyer, 1929.

SMITH, MARTHA RUTH, editor
An introduction to the principles of nursing care. Philadelphia, Lippincott, 1937.
2nd edn., 1939.

SMITH, WILLIAM ROBERT
Lectures on nursing. Churchill, 1878?

SOUTH, J. F.
Facts relating to hospital nurses. Richardson, 1857.

STEWART, ISLA
Practical nursing. Edinburgh, Blackwood, 1909.

STEWART, ISLA, and CUFF, HERBERT E.
Practical nursing, vols. I and II. Edinburgh, Blackwood, 1899 and 1903.

STORER, H. R.
On nurses and nursing: with especial reference to the management of sick women. Boston, Lee & Shepard, 1868.

SWIRE, MARY E.
A handbook for the assistant nurse. Bailliere, Tindall & Cox, 1949.
2nd edn., 1953, ed. and rev. by Ruby Thora Farnol.
3rd edn., 1956.
4th edn., 1959.

THOMAS, D. L.
Sterilization of instruments and dressings. *Nursing Times*, June 5, 1954, p. 603-4.

THOMAS, MARGARET W.
Aseptic nursing techniques; a survey of maternity departments in thirteen medical centers. Atlanta, Ga., U.S. Dept. of Health, Education, and Welfare, Public Health Service, Communicable Disease Center, 1960.

THOMPSON, ANTHONY TODD
The domestic management of the sick room—necessary in aid of medical treatment for the cure of diseases. Longmans, 1841.

THOMPSON, M. E.
Sterilization and ward dressing technique at Sunderland Royal Infirmary. *Nursing Times*, July 22, 1960, p. 896-9.

THORNDIKE, AUGUSTUS
A manual of bandaging, strapping and splinting. Kimpton, 1941.
2nd edn., 1950.
3rd edn., 1959.

TRACY, MARGARET A., and others
Nursing, an art and a science; by Margaret A. Tracy and collaborators. St. Louis, Mosby, 1938.
3rd edn., 1949.

TREMO, I.
How to prepare a nursing procedure manual. *Modern Hospital*, Oct. 1957, p. 69-74.

VANNIER, MARION L., and THOMPSON, BARBARA A.
A textbook of nursing technique: a manual used in the associated hospitals in the University of Minnesota School of Nursing. 2nd edn. Minneapolis, University of Minnesota Press, 1935.

VICTORIAN ORDER OF NURSES FOR CANADA
The nurse's manual. Ottawa, The Order, 1942.

VIVIAN, M.
Lectures to nurses in training. Scientific Press, [1920].

VOYSEY, MARY H. ANNESLEY
Nursing: hints to probationers on practical work. Scientific Press, [1901].

WATSON, J. K.
A handbook for nurses; with examination questions based on the contents of the chapters. Scientific Press, 1899.
5th edn., 1912.
7th edn., 1926.
8th edn., 1928, pub. Faber & Gwyer.
9th edn., 1931.
10th edn., 1934.
11th edn., 1940.
12th edn., 1946.

WATSON, J. K.
A handbook for senior nurses and midwives. O.U.P., 1926.
2nd edn., 1931.

WEEKS-SHAW, CLARA S.
A textbook of nursing for the use of training schools, families and private students. New York, Appleton, 1885.
3rd edn., 1904.

WELHAM, S.
A manual for nurses. London, 1910
2nd edn., 1916.

WESSEX REGIONAL HOSPITAL BOARD
Twenty-two nursing procedures. Winchester, The Board, 1960.

WHEELER, MARY C.
Nursing technic. 32 specially prepared illustrations under the personal supervision of the author. Philadelphia, Lippincott, 1918.
2nd edn., 1923.

WHITE, JEAN MARTIN
Practical nursing. Philadelphia, Davis, 1953.

WHITE, T. H.
Notes on injections for nurses. Bristol, John Wright, 1959.

WHYTE, VICTORIA
Manual of nursing for home and hospital, including monthly nursing and the nursing of sick children. Glasgow, Thomas D. Morison, 1886.

WILLIAMS, RACHEL, and FISHER, ALICE
Hints for hospital nurses. Edinburgh, MacLachlan & Stewart, 1877.

WISE, P. M.
A textbook for training schools for nurses—including physiology and hygiene and the principles and practice of nursing. 2nd edn. New York, ... 1896.

WOOD, CATHERINE JANE
A handbook of nursing for the home and the hospital. Cassell, [1888].

WYATT, HURLEY T.
Sterilization: a handbook for physicians, hospital executives and nurses. Madison, Wisconsin, Scanlan-Morris, 1930.
2nd edn., 1936.

YOUNG, HELEN
Essentials of nursing, edited by Eleanor Lee. New York, Putnam, 1942.
2nd edn., 1948.
3rd edn., 1953, by H. Young and E. Lee.

YOUNG, HELEN, and others, editors
Lippincott's quick reference book for nurses: compiled and arranged from various sources by Helen Young, with the assistance of Georgia A. Morison and Margaret Eliot: Philadelphia, Lippincott, 1933.
2nd edn., 1935.
3rd edn., 1937.
4th edn., 1939.
5th edn., 1943.
6th edn., 1950.
7th edn., 1955.

INTENSIVE CARE

BEAL, J. M.
Intensive nursing care. American Journal of Surgery, July 1960, p. 1-3.

BRIGH, M., and AMADEUS, SISTER
Intensive care: effective care. Hospital Progress, Dec. 1958, p. 64-6.

DE BACKER, D.
A new approach to intensive care. Hospital Progress, Mar. 1960, p. 81-3.

HARDAWAY, R. M.
Special-care ward for critically ill surgical and post-operative patients. United States Armed Forces Medical Journal, Sept. 1957, p. 1258-60.

LAMB, R. J.
How to plan intensive care. Modern Hospital, July 1958, p. 51-5

MAGEE, RICHARD B., and SKINNER, RICHARD W.
The special care unit in the Altoona hospital. Pennsylvania Medical Journal, April 1958, p. 497-500.

MILLER, J. D., JR.
The critical care unit in a 134-bed hospital. Hospitals, Oct. 16, 1956, p. 46-7.

MOSENTHAL, WILLIAM T.
The special care unit. Journal of the Maine Medical Association, Nov. 1957, p. 396-9.

MOSENTHAL, WILLIAM T., and BOYD, D. D.
Special unit saves lives, nurses and money. Modern Hospital, Dec. 1957, p. 83-6.

SALISBURY, P. F.
An intensive treatment centre meets special needs. Hospital Progress, May 1959, p. 92-4.

STURDAVANT, MADELYNE, and others
Comparisons of intensive nursing service in a circular and a rectangular unit, Rochester Methodist Hospital, Rochester, Minn. Chicago, American Hospital Association, [c. 1960].

WAGNER, R. A.
How does the intensive care unit affect nursing morale and utilization? Nursing Outlook, May 1958, p. 286-8.

WILLIAMS, L. W.
An intensive nursing care unit. Hospital Management, Oct. 1958, p. 106, and Nov. 1958, p. 94-5.

WOOLEVER, G. M.
An intensive care unit. Nursing Outlook, Dec. 1958, p. 690-1.

PATIENT CARE

ABDELLAH, FAYE G., and LEVINE, EUGENE
Developing a measure of patient and personnel satisfaction with nursing care. Nursing Research, Feb. 1957, p. 100-8.

ABDELLAH, FAYE G., and LEVINE, EUGENE
Patients and personnel speak. Washington, Govt. Printing Office, 1957.

ABDELLAH, FAYE G., and LEVINE, EUGENE
Polling patients and personnel.
    I. What patients say about their nursing care. Hospitals, Nov. 1, 1957, p. 44-8.
    II. What factors affect patients' opinion of their nursing care? Hospitals, Nov. 16, 1957, p. 61-2.
    III. What personnel say about nursing care. Hospitals, Dec. 1, 1957, p. 53-7.
    IV. What hospitals have done to improve patient care. Hospitals, Dec. 16, 1957, p. 43-4.

ABDELLAH, FAYE G., and others
Patient-centered approaches to nursing. New York, Macmillan, 1960.

ABERG, HARRIET L.
The nurse's role in hospital safety. Nursing Outlook, Mar. 1957, p. 160-2.

ALLEMANG, M.
An analysis of the experiences of eight cardiac patients during a period of hospitalization in a general hospital. Canadian Nurse, Aug. 1959, p. 702-11.

ANNIS, J. W.
Working together. Journal of the Florida Medical Association, Dec. 1958, p. 670-2.

AYDELOTTE, MYRTLE KITCHELL, *and* TENER, MARIE E.
An investigation of the relation between nursing activity and patient welfare, prepared by the Nurse Utilization Project Staff, State University of Iowa. The University, 1960.

BARTON, J.
Round-the-clock nursing or self-service: patient care is based on the medical need. *Modern Hospital*, June 1957, p. 51-6.

BELCHER, C. D.
Integrated care of patients. *Delaware State Medical Journal*, Jan. 1959, p. 13-16.

BENNALLACK, F. M.
Hospital follow-up. *Nursing Times*, Jan. 28, 1955, p. 83-4.

BIETSCH, E. M.
Changing concepts. *Canadian Nurse*, April 1957, p. 281-2.

BLUESTONE, E. M.
Hospital-home pattern. *Nursing Times*, Aug. 4, 1951, p. 758-9.

BLUESTONE, E. M.
Integrating acute and chronic in a combined hospital-home pattern. *Lancet*, Dec. 8, 1951, p. 1078-80.

BODINE, W.
The value of visitors. *Hospital Management*, Aug. 1957, p. 54-6.

BOJAR, S.
The psychotherapeutic function of the general hospital nurse. *Nursing Outlook*, Mar. 1958, p. 151-3.

BOURNE, P. J.
Home care and nursing service: Cambridge scheme to relieve pressure on hospital beds. *Nursing Mirror*, Sept. 18, 1953, p. ii-v.

BOWE, A. B.
Beyond procedures: incidental teaching. *Nursing Outlook*, Nov. 1958, p. 628-31.

BRIDGES, D. C.
The patient, the present and progress. *Canadian Nurse*, July 1958, p. 619-23.

BROWN, E. L.
The social sciences and improvement of patient care. *Canadian Nurse*, Mar. 1956, p. 175-9.

CHAMBERS, L.
The patient as an individual. *Hospital Progress*, Feb. 1960, p. 70-2.

CHIGA, D. E.
Planning the care of patients with long-term illness. *Nursing Outlook*, Nov. 1957, p. 666-8.

COLQUHOUN, DOROTHY R.
Improving patient care through nursing education. *Canadian Hospital*, April 1957, p. 48-9.

CONNOLLY, MARY GRACE
What acceptance means to patients. *American Journal of Nursing*, Dec. 1960, p. 1754-7.

COOMBE, M. E.
Night-time noise in hospital. *Nursing Mirror*, Aug. 31, 1956, p. 1567-8.

CORNELL UNIVERSITY—NEW YORK HOSPITAL.
SCHOOL OF NURSING
Toward better nursing care of patients with long-term illness: a project developed . . . in co-operation with the National League for Nursing; under the direction of Edna L. Fritz. New York, National League for Nursing, 1956.

COWLES, EDWARD
On the treatment of the sick in tents and temporary hospitals. Boston, Mead & Springfield, 1874.

DALEY, A.
Co-operation with other services in treating the patient. *Hospital*, July 1954, p. 417-24.

DERHAM, ROSALIE F.
Nursing care in long-term illness; a study in patient care conducted by the Nursing Department of the Hospital for Special Surgery. New York, [The Hospital, 195?].

DODGE, JOAN S.
Age of nurse helps determine her attitude toward patients. *Modern Hospital*, Nov. 1960, p. 116.

EDWARDS, M. M.
The patient and his needs. *Nursing Times*, Mar. 23, 1957, p. 948-52.

FAIR, ERNEST W.
Visitors are important. *Hospital Management*, Mar. 1957, p. 6-8.

FIELD, MINNA
Patients are people: a medical-social approach to prolonged illness. New York, Columbia University Press, 1953. 2nd edn., 1958.

FORTIN, DENISE
The patient comes to hospital. *Canadian Nurse*, Jan. 1960, p. 40-1.

FOX, JOSEPH
The chronically ill. Vision Press, 1958.

FOX, V., *and* SPAIN, R. W.
The long-term patient: a new challenge to nursing. *Nursing Outlook*, Oct. 1956, p. 559-61.

GARDNER, K. E.
The patient's team. *Journal of the Medical Society of New Jersey*, Jan. 1959, p. 3-8.

GEORGE, FRANCES L., *and* KUEHN, RUTH P.
Patterns of patient care: some studies of the utilization of nursing service personnel; edited by Josephine Nelson. New York, Macmillan, 1955.

GOLDMAN, F., *and* FRAENKEL, M.
Patients on home care: their characteristics and experience. *Journal of Chronic Diseases*, Jan. 1960, p. 77-87.

GRUENER, JENNETTE R., *and* JENSEN, DEBORAH MACLURG
Community problems. St. Louis, Mosby, 1954.

HART, BETTY L., *and* ROHWEDER, ANNE W.
Support in nursing. *American Journal of Nursing*, Oct. 1959, p. 1398-401.

HAYMAN, C. R., *and* PERKINS, L. D.
Home care of the sick in relation to other nursing programmes. *Nursing Outlook*, Sept. 1954, p. 472-4.

HESLIN, H. LORRAINE
A good patient care committee means good patient care. *Nursing Outlook*, Sept. 1958, p. 526-7.

INDIANA STATE BOARD OF HEALTH *and*
INDIANA UNIVERSITY MEDICAL CENTER
Basic factors; what do we mean—improvement of patient care and how do we implement it? Indianapolis, The Board, n.d.

INTERNATIONAL HOSPITAL FEDERATION
The mental well-being of patients in the general hospital. *Nursing Times*, June 17, 1955, p. 666-8; June 24, 1955, p. 693-4; July 8, 1955, p. 747-8.

JENKINSON, V. M.
Case assignment method of nursing, as practised in Williams Ward, St. George's Hospital, London, from March 1948. *Nursing Mirror*, Dec. 18, 1953, p. ii-iv and 754.

KENNAWAY, E.
Some notes on nursing from a patient's point of view. *British Medical Journal*, Dec. 21, 1957, p. 1485.

Koos, Earl Lomon
The sociology of the patient: a textbook for nurses. New York, McGraw-Hill, 1950.
2nd edn., 1954.
3rd edn., 1959.

Kranock, A., Siegel, E. L., and Mabry, J. H.
A method for the study of social interaction on the hospital ward. *Nursing Research*, Summer 1959, p. 172-6.

Lancet
Relatives in hospital. *Lancet*, May 11, 1957, p. 975-6.

Leone, Lucile Petry
Wanted: good nursing. *Nursing Outlook*, Oct. 1957, p. 576-8.

Lindsay, J.
The patient and his needs. *Nursing Mirror*, Jan. 29, 1960, p. 1487-8.

McCabe, Gracia S.
Cultural influences on patient behaviour. *American Journal of Nursing*, Aug. 1960, p. 1101-4.

MacGregor, Frances Cooke
Social science in nursing: applications for the improvement of patient care. New York, Russell Sage Foundation, 1960.

Marsh, Edith Lucile
Nursing care in chronic disease. Philadelphia, Lippincott, 1946.

Mary Crown of Thorns, Sister
Christo-therapy; in a modern Catholic mental hospital. *Hospital Progress*, Jan. 1957, p. 46-8.

Mauksch, H. O.
Nursing dilemmas in the organisation of patient care. *Nursing Outlook*, Jan. 1957, p. 31-3.

Maule, H. G.
Correspondence courses for hospital patients. *Medical Officer*, Sept. 20, 1957, p. 169-71.

Melanie, M.
Better patient care; co-ordination of functions of head nurse and clinical teacher. *Canadian Nurse*, Feb. 1957, p. 113-6.

Mickey, J. E.
Studying extra-hospital nursing needs: a preliminary report. *American Journal of Public Health and the Nation's Health*, July 1958, p. 880-7.

Mill, C. R.
Patients' attitudes toward hospital care. *Virginia Medical Monthly*, Mar. 1960, p. 159-62.

Morgan, J.
A challenge to the apostolate of care. *Hospital Progress*, Nov. 1958, p. 68-70.

Murrell, T. W., and Williams, J. B.
Visiting the sick. *Virginia Medical Monthly*, Aug. 1958, p. 440-2.

Myers, R. S.
A technique for evaluating professional activities. *Hospital Progress*, Aug. 1957, p. 42-4.

National League for Nursing. Department of Hospital Nursing and Department of Public Health Nursing
Hospitals and public health nursing services plan better patient care. New York, The League, 1957.

Norris, Catherine N.
The nurse and the dying patient. *American Journal of Nursing*, Oct. 1955, p. 1214-7.

O'Malley, M.
Utilizing new graduates for better patient care. *Hospital Progress*, Feb. 1957, part I, p. 64-7.

Ottley, L. J.
One service—the integration of hospital and domiciliary care. *Nursing Times*, May 8, 1954, p. 496-7.

Parrish, H. M., Weil, T. P., and Wolfson, B.
Accidents to patients can be avoided. *American Journal of Nursing*, May 1958, p. 679-82.

Redman, P. W.
Grouping patients: colour tabs to indicate degree of patients' dependence. *Nursing Times*, Dec. 16, 1960, p. 1559-60.

Reynolds, J.
Is nursing at the service of patients. *Canadian Nurse*, June 1959, p. 513-5.

Richardson, Henry B.
Patients have families. New York, Commonwealth Fund, 1945.

Robinson, G. Canby
The patient as a person: a study of the social aspects of illness. New York, Commonwealth Fund, 1939.

Rochester Regional Hospital Council
Average nursing hours per patient in member hospitals, Nov. 10-23, 1952. Rochester, Minnesota, The Council, 1952.

Rourke, A. J.
The impact of the hospital on the patient. *Hospital Management*, Dec. 1956, p. 52 *passim*.

Schwartz, Doris
Uncooperative patients? *American Journal of Nursing*, Jan. 1958, p. 75-7.

Schwartz, Doris, Ullman, A., and Reader, G.
The nurse, social worker and medical student in a comprehensive care program. *Nursing Outlook*, Jan. 1958, p. 39-41.

Singeisen, F.
Hospitals need more patience with patients. *Modern Hospital*, Dec. 1960, p. 79-81.

Sisler, G. C.
The nurse and the emotional needs of the patient. *Canadian Nurse*, April 1958, p. 314-7.

Speroff, B. J.
Empathy is important in nursing. *Nursing Outlook*, June 1956, p. 326-8.

Stark, S. B.
The patients' viewpoint. *Hospital Management*, July 1958, p. 42-3.

Statham, Cecily
Noise and the patient in hospital: a personal investigation. *British Medical Journal*, Dec. 5, 1959, p. 1247-8.

Stuart-Clark, A. C.
The nursing of adolescents in adult wards. *Lancet*, Dec. 26, 1953, p. 1349.

United States Public Health Service and Commission on Chronic Illness
Guide to making a survey of patients receiving nursing and personal care, by J. A. Solon, W. Roberts and E. Krueger. Washington, Govt. Printing Office, [195?].

Walker, Virginia H.
Patients, personnel and therapy. *Nursing Outlook*, Mar. 1960, p. 136-8.

Weinschreider, M. M., and Beauclair, R. R.
Patient morale mirrors nursing morale. *Hospitals*, Sept. 1, 1956, p. 44-6.

West, G. M.
Family centred nursing at the Cassel Hospital, Ham Common, Richmond. *Nursing Mirror*, Nov. 25, 1960, p. ii-iv and xvi.

Winter, Kenton E., and Metzner, C. A.
Institutional care for the long-term patient: a study of hospitals and nursing facilities in Michigan. Ann Arbor, School of Public Health, University of Michigan, 1958.

WOHL, MICHAEL G., *editor*
Long-term illness: management of the chronically ill patient . . . with the collaboration of seventy-nine contributing authorities. Philadelphia, Saunders, 1959.

ZIMMERMAN, M. W.
Instructions cards allay patients' fears. *Modern Hospital*, April 1958, p. 59-61.

PROGRESSIVE PATIENT CARE

ABDELLAH, FAYE G., *and others*
Nursing patterns vary in progressive care. *Modern Hospital*, Aug. 1960, p. 85-91.

ABDELLAH, FAYE G.
Progressive patient care: a challenge for nursing. *Hospital Management*, June 1960, p. 102-6.

ABDELLAH, FAYE G., *and* STRACHAN, E. J.
Progressive patient care. *American Journal of Nursing*, May 1959, p. 649-55.

AGNEW, G. H.
Progressive patient care. *Canadian Hospital*, Aug. 1959, p. 39-40.

CADMUS, R. R.
Progressive patient care. *North Carolina Medical Journal*, June 1960, p. 233-5.

DONOVAN, A. C., *and* MEYER, B.
Dietary service in progressive patient care. *Journal of the American Dietetic Association*, Nov. 1960, p. 448-54.

FELTON, B. L.
What administrators want to know about progressive patient care. *Modern Hospital*, Aug. 1959, p. 71-2.

FORD, L. C.
The five elements of progressive patient care. *Nursing Outlook*, Aug. 1960, p. 436-9.

HALDEMAN, J. C., *and* ABDELLAH, FAYE G.
Concepts of progressive patient care. *Hospitals*, May 16, 1959, p. 38-42 and 142-4, and June 1, 1959, p. 41-6.

HALDEMAN, J. C.
Progressive patient care: a challenge to hospitals and health agencies. *Public Health Reports*, May 1959, p. 405-8.

HUESTON, R. M.
Progressive patient care; experience of Chicago Wesley Memorial Hospital. *Hospital Management*, Sept. 1959, p. 101-2.

KENNEDY, R. B.
Progressive patient care: cure for sick hospitals? *Journal of the Mississippi Medical Association*, Aug. 1960, p. 442-6.

LANCET
Progressive patient care. *Lancet*, Aug. 29, 1959, p. 223.

LOCKWARD, H. J., GIDDINGS, L., *and* THOMS, E. J.
Progressive patient care. A preliminary report. *Journal of the American Medical Association*, Jan. 9, 1960, p. 132-7.

LONNI, L. J.
Progressive patient care: an analysis of the implementation, costs and behaviour factor. *Hospital Management*, Nov. 1960, p. 66-77.

MODERN HOSPITAL
How to determine costs of progressive care. *Modern Hospital*, Aug. 1959, p. 67-70.

Patients vote for progressive patient care. *Modern Hospital*, July 1960, p. 75-9.

REGAN, W. A.
A legal look at progressive patient care.
I. *Hospital Progress*, May 1959, p. 121-2.
II. *Hospital Progress*, June 1959, p. 80-1.
III. *Hospital Progress*, July 1959, p. 90-1.

Symposium on progressive patient care. *Hospitals*, Jan. 16, 1959, p. 42-56.

THOMS, E. J.
Progressive patient care. *Nursing World*, Feb. 1960, p. 10-13.

THOMS, E. J.
Progressive patient care: planning and research. *New York State Journal of Medicine*, July 15, 1959, p. 2777-81.

THOMS, E. J., GIDDINGS, L., *and* LOCKWOOD, H. J.
Report on progressive care: it works. *Modern Hospital*, May 1958, p. 73-8.

Three ways to plan for progressive care. *Modern Hospital*, Dec. 1960, p. 82-5.

QUALITY OF CARE

CARLISLE, B.
Quality care: an analysis of nursing care. *Hospital Management*, Oct. 1959, p. 88 *passim*.

DECARY MANCE, SISTER
The relationship between the quality of nursing care and its cost. *Canadian Nurse*, June 1959, p. 521-2.

GASS, F.
Using hospital resources effectively to maintain high quality patient care: necessary nursing. *Canadian Hospital*, Nov. 1958, p. 41-2.

INGLES, THELMA
What is good nursing? *American Journal of Nursing*, Sept. 1959, p. 1246-9.

KREUTER, F. R.
What is good nursing care. *Nursing Outlook*, May 1957, p. 302-4.

RUSSELL, E. K.
The quest for satisfactory nursing. *Canadian Journal of Public Health*, Nov. 1957, p. 454-7.

SAFFORD, BEVERLY J., *and* SCHLOTFELDT, ROZELLA M.
Nursing service staffing and quality of patient care. *Nursing Research*, Summer 1960, p. 149-54.

SIMON, J. RICHARD
Patient activity as a measure of patient welfare. *Hospital Management*, Sept. 1960, p. 95-100.

WATKIN, B.
Factors affecting the standard of nursing care in hospitals. *Nursing Times*, Mar. 27, 1959, p. 393.

WRIGHT, MARION J.
Improvement of patient care: a study at Harper Hospital. Sponsored by the American Hospital Association. New York, Putnam, 1954.

TEAM NURSING

CHRISTMAN, LUTHER, *and* BOYLES, ELLOWEEN R.
The working team plan in a psychiatric hospital. *Nursing Outlook*, Jan. 1956, p. 53-4.

COLUMBIA UNIVERSITY. TEACHERS' COLLEGE.
DIVISION OF NURSING EDUCATION
Nursing team organization and functioning: results of a study . . . [by] Eleanor C. Lambertsen. New York, Columbia University, 1953.

FIELD, M.
The nurse and the social worker on the hospital team. *American Journal of Nursing*, June 1955, p. 694-6.

FREY, M.
Preparing to introduce the team plan. *Hospitals*, Dec. 1954, p. 83-4 and 150.

HAUG, C. H.
Team planning in the Veterans' Administration Nursing Service. *Military Medicine*, June 1960, p. 403-4.

HENKE, H. F.
A team approach for total patient care. *Hospitals*, Nov. 1955, p. 80-2.

JENKINSON, V. M.
Group or team nursing. Report on a 5-year experiment at St. George's Hospital, London. *Nursing Times*, Jan. 17, 1958, p. 62-4, and Jan. 24, 1958, p. 92-3.

KELMAN, R. J.
Team or group care in nursing. *Nursing Times*, Nov. 8, 1957, p. 1268-70.

LAMB, M. N. C.
The nursing team in action in two U.S. hospitals. *Nursing Mirror*, Dec. 25, 1953, p. 811-12 and 817.

MCARTHUR, A. C.
We plan together. *Canadian Services Medical Journal*, Feb. 1957, p. 113-6.

NEWCOMB, DOROTHY PERKINS
The team plan: a manual for nursing service administrators. New York, Putnam, 1953.

PATMORE, E.
The staff nurse's part in the ward team. *Nursing Mirror*, April 26, 1957, p. 253-4.

ROSS, C. F.
Preparation for team work. *American Journal of Nursing*, Jan. 1957, p. 72-5.

VOGEL, M. A.
Team nursing. *Nursing World*, July 1955, p. 11-13.

WATKIN, B. V.
Team or group care in nursing. *Nursing Mirror*, May 24, 1957, p. 549-51.

WOOD, M. M., *and others*
Supervising the team program. *Nursing World*, May 1960, p. 18 and 33.

ZABOLI, C.
Nurse-team survey in an Italian hospital. *Nursing Times*, April 10, 1959, p. 428-30.

WAR AND DISASTER NURSING

AMERICAN NURSES' ASSOCIATION
Report of a work conference on disaster nursing of February 20-24, 1956. New York, The Association, 1956.

BURBRIDGE, D. H. D.
Sustained treatment of thermo-nuclear casualties. Teaching nursing procedures to untrained personnel. *Nursing Mirror*, Nov. 1, 1957, p. iv-v.

CAMPBELL, P. E., *and* JONES, R. M.
Experiences in the handling of a disaster in a small hospital. *Hospital Management*, June 1957, p. 52-5.

COOCH, J. W.
The role of the army health nurse in the preventive medicine program. *Military Medicine*, Nov. 1956, p. 312-6.

COWARD, R.
How the legal considerations apply to the army nurse. *Military Medicine*, June 1957, p. 426-9.

DUNSTAN, E. M.
The civil defence emergency hospital for disasters; the basic training unit, and hospital bed reservoir. *Hospital Management*, Jan. 1959, p. 38-9.

EDWARDS, M. A. F.
Atomic warfare—the nurse's part in the prevention of injuries and treatment of casualties. The nursing care of radiation casualties. *Nursing Mirror*, Nov. 4, 1960, p. x-xi and xiv.

ELLIMAN, V. B.
Nursing service in disasters. *Hospital Progress*, Nov. 1959, p. 84-5.

GARDINER, L. A.
Public health nursing in time of disaster. *American Journal of Nursing*, June 1958, p. 861-3.

GARMON, B. L.
Training of army nurses in preparation for care of mass casualties. *Medical Bulletin of the U.S. Army, Europe*, Dec. 1957, p. 279-80.

GATES, KERMIT H., *and* WEINER, LEONA
Health nursing service at an army hospital. *U.S. Armed Forces Medical Journal*, Dec. 1955, p. 1773-9.

GOODNOW, MINNIE
War nursing: a text book for the auxiliary nurse. Philadelphia, Saunders, 1918.

GRAY, J. I. L.
Atomic warfare: the nurse's part in prevention of injuries and treatment of casualties.
1. Nature of atomic and thermo-nuclear weapons.
2. The effects of atomic weapons.
Nursing Mirror, Sept. 23, 1960, p. ii-iv and xii, and Sept. 30, 1960, p. v-vii.

HAGGART, A.
Nursing care of radiation sickness. *Canadian Nurse*, May 1957, p. 408-11.

HASSARD, E. M., *and* HASSARD, A. R.
Practical nursing for male nurses in the R.A.M.C. and other forces. Hodder & Stoughton, 1910.
2nd edn., 1927.

HAUGE, CECILIA H.
Organization and management of mass casualties—the role of the nurses. *Military Medicine*, April 1956, p. 390-2.

HAYNES, INEZ
Army nurse corps role in national defense. *Army Information Digest*, April 1958, p. 55-60.

HOLGATE, W.
Atomic warfare: the nurse's part in prevention of injuries and treatment of casualties. 4. Hazards of internal radiation. *Nursing Mirror*, Oct. 21, 1960, p. xi-xii.

HOWELL, L. N.
A state-wide disaster training programme. *Nursing Outlook*, Mar. 1957, p. 144-6.

JOHNSON, P. V.
Developing volunteer nursing resources in an army community. *Medical Bulletin of the U.S. Army, Europe*, Feb. 1957, p. 41-5.

KINCH, ALICE
Bellevue responds when disaster strikes in New York City. *American Journal of Nursing*, April 1959, p. 504-9.

LUETH, HAROLD G.
Meeting disaster. *American Journal of Nursing*, Sept. 1956, p. 1135-8.

LUETH, HAROLD G.
What is a good hospital disaster plan? *Pennsylvania Medical Journal*, July 1960, p. 977-82.

MACKINTOSH, J. M., *editor*
War-time nurse: an anthology of ideas about the care and nursing of war casualties. Oliver & Boyd, 1940.

MAGNUSSEN, A. K.
Nursing in disaster. I. Red Cross Service. *American Journal of Nursing*, Oct. 1956, p. 1290-1.

MITCHINER, PHILIP HENRY, *and* MACMANUS, EMILY ELVIRA PRIMROSE
Nursing in time of war. Churchill, 1939.
2nd edn., 1943.

NABBE, FRANCES CROUCH
Disaster nursing. Paterson, N.J., Littlefield, Adams, 1960.

NATIONAL LEAGUE FOR NURSING
Nursing during disaster: a guide for instructors. New York, The League, 1951.
2nd edn., 1957.

NEW YORK CITY
MAYOR'S COMMITTEE OF WOMEN ON NATIONAL DEFENCE,
STANDING COMMITTEE ON NURSING
A study of the nursing situation in New York as of July-August, 1917. New York, The Committee, 1917.

NORTON, IRENE, *and* NEAL, MARY V.
Faculty inservice preparation for disaster nursing at the Massachusetts General Hospital School of Nursing. New York, National League for Nursing, 1960.

Nursing in disasters. *American Journal of Nursing*, Aug. 1960, p. 1130-3.

NURSING MIRROR
Atomic warfare: the nurse's part in prevention of injuries and treatment of casualties. *Nursing Mirror*, [1953?].

POOLE, D.
Preparing hospital nursing staffs for disaster service. *Nursing Outlook*, Oct. 1958, p. 586-9.

RAYNER, JEANNETTE F.
Report of studies of medical service personnel in disaster with emphasis on reactions of nurses. Washington, Walter Reed Army Institute of Research, 1957.

ROWLEY, M.
Nursing in-service programs in USAREVR hospitals. *Medical Bulletin of the U.S. Army, Europe*, April 1958, p. 82-6.

RUSSELL, C. M.
Nursing in disaster. *Hospital Progress*, Sept. 1960, p. 82-5.

SCHAFER, M. K.
Nursing in disaster. II. Civil Defence Service. *American Journal of Nursing*, Oct. 1956, p. 1291-2.

SEIFERT, V. D., *and* GERBER, W.
In this disaster plan student nurses are the link between the patients and the treatment team. *Modern Hospital*, Feb. 1957, p. 64-7.

SLOANE, AMANDA
Disaster nursing in the curriculum. *Nursing Outlook*, Feb. 1957, p. 75-7.

STEWART, B. L.
Civil defense nursing. *Military Medicine*, Sept. 1958, p. 198-201.

SULLIVAN, C. M.
The civil defense role of nurses. *Journal of the American Medical Association*, Jan. 24, 1959, p. 388-9.

TATE, BARBARA L., *and* UREY, BLANCHE
Nursing and the military medical technician. *Nursing Outlook*, Aug. 1956, p. 470-1.

THURSTON, VIOLETTA
A textbook of war nursing. New York, Putnams, 1917.

U.S. FEDERAL CIVIL DEFENSE
The nurse in civil defense. Washington, Govt. Printing Office, 1954.

VIRGINIA, SISTER
Nursing care of thermal injuries. *Canadian Nurse*, May 1957, p. 416-9.

WEDD, G. D.
Atomic warfare: the nurse's part in prevention of injuries and treatment of casualties. 3. Atomic bomb effects on the body (part 1). *Nursing Mirror*, Oct. 7, 1960, p. iv-vi.

WEDD, G. D.
Atomic warfare and the nurse: treatment of radiation casualties (part 5). *Nursing Mirror*, Oct. 28, 1960, p. x-xi.

WERLEY, H. H.
The nurse's role in nuclear disaster. *American Journal of Nursing*, Dec. 1956, p. 1580-2.

WILSON, M. J.
Inservice education and standardization of facilities and techniques in the Seventh U.S. Army nursing services: progress report. *Medical Bulletin of the U.S. Army, Europe*, April, 1958, p. 92-6.

SPECIALITIES OF KNOWLEDGE AND PRACTICE

ALLERGIES

DAVIES, J. B. M., *and* WARIN, J. F.
Penicillin sensitivity in district nurses. *Medical Officer*,
April 4, 1953, p. 143.

FRANKLAND, A. W.
Penicillin sensitivity. *Nursing Times*, July 11, 1953, p. 692-4.

GREAT BRITAIN. MINISTRY OF HEALTH
Sensitisation of nursing staffs to antibiotics. *Lancet*,
July 4, 1953, p. 33-5.

HOWELLS, G.
Prevention of streptomycin dermatitis in nurses. *Lancet*,
May 26, 1956, p. 780-1.

O'DRISCOLL, B. J.
Desensitization of nurses allergic to penicillin; report of a
case. *British Medical Journal*, Aug. 20, 1955, p. 473-5.

PINES, A.
Desensitization of a nurse to streptomycin under cortico-
steroid cover. *British Medical Journal*, July 27, 1957, p. 202.

WILSON, H. T. H.
Nurses and streptomycin dermatitis. *Nursing Times*,
Nov. 28, 1958, p. 1394-6.

ANATOMY AND PHYSIOLOGY

ASHDOWN, A. MILLICENT, *and* BLEAZBY, E.
Anatomy, physiology and hygiene: a text book for nurses.
Dent, 1935.
2nd edn., 1937.
3rd edn., 1939.
5th edn., 1953.

BENNETT, BETHINA A.
Preparatory anatomy and physiology: a textbook for
assistant nurses. Faber, 1944.
2nd edn., 1955.

BOCOCK, E. J., *and* HAINES, R. WHEELER
Applied anatomy for nurses. Edinburgh, Livingstone,
1951.
2nd edn., 1959.

BUNDY, E. R.
Textbook of anatomy and physiology for nurses. 2nd edn.
Philadelphia, 1913.

BURDON, IAN M., *and* MACDONALD, S., *editors*
Anatomical atlas for nurses and students. Faber, 1938.
2nd edn., 1941.
3rd edn., 1951.

CAIRNEY, JOHN, *and* CAIRNEY, JOHN
First studies in anatomy and physiology. Christchurch,
New Zealand, Peryer, 1956.
2nd edn., 1959.

DAVIES, D. V.
Anatomy for nurses. E.U.P., 1957.

DAWSON, P. M.
Elements of anatomy and physiology for nurses. New
York, 1917.

ECCLES, W. MCADAM
Elementary anatomy and surgery for nurses: a series of
lectures delivered to the nursing staff of the West London
Hospital. Scientific Press, 1896.

FITZGERALD, CHARLES EGERTON
Lectures on physiology, hygiene, etc., for hospital and
home nursing. 2nd edn. Bell, 1892.

FLITTER, HESSEL H., *and* ROWE, HAROLD R.
Teaching physiology and anatomy in nursing: signposts
for science teachers; with special reference to the textbook
"Physiology and Anatomy", 7th edn., by Esther M.
Greisheimer. Philadelphia, Lippincott, 1955.

FRANCIS, CARL C., *and others*
Textbook of anatomy and physiology. Kimpton, 1943.
Cover title of 1st edn., "Textbook of anatomy and physio-
logy for nurses", joint authors G. Clinton Knowlton and
W. W. Tuttle.
2nd edn., 1950, by C. C. Francis and G. C. Knowlton.

GIBSON, JOHN
Human biology: an elementary anatomy and physiology
for students and nurses. Faber, 1960.

GOWLAND, W. P., *and* CAIRNEY, JOHN
Anatomy and physiology for nurses. Christchurch, New
Zealand, Peryer, 1941.
2nd edn., 1946.
3rd edn., 1949.
4th edn., 1955.
5th edn., 1958.

HAMILTON-PATERSON, J. L.
Anatomy and physiology for nurses. Lewis, 1946.

JAMIESON, E. B.
Illustrations of anatomy for nurses. Edinburgh, Livingstone, [1938].
2nd edn., 1946.
3rd edn., 1950.

JENSEN, KATHRYN
An analysis of the content of anatomy and physiology as
taught first-year students in schools of nursing. New York,
Catholic University of America, 1936.

LAKELAND, K.
Atlas of anatomy for nurses. Sydney, Angus & Robertson,
1951.

LITTLEWOOD, C. M.
Teaching anatomy from the living angle. *Nursing Mirror*,
April 5, 1957, p. 39-40.

LODGE, P. M.
Elementary anatomy and physiology for nurses. Churchill,
1929.

NORTON, FELICIE
Anatomy and physiology for junior nurses. Faber, 1922.
6th edn., 1942.
7th edn., 1948.
8th edn., 1951.
9th edn., 1954, revised by V. M. Lake.

PEARCE, EVELYN CLARE
Anatomy and physiology for nurses: a complete textbook
for the preliminary state examinations. Faber, 1929.
2nd edn., 1931.
3rd edn., 1934.
4th edn., 1935.
5th edn., 1940.
6th edn., 1941.
7th edn., 1942.
8th edn., 1943.
9th edn., 1948.
10th edn., 1949.
11th edn., 1950.
12th edn., 1951.
13th edn., 1956.

RAEBURN, JANET K., *and* RAEBURN, HUGH ADAIR
Anatomy, physiology and hygiene for part I of the
preliminary state examination for nurses, in collaboration
with Hilda M. Gration. John Murray, 1940.
2nd edn., 1957.

RAEBURN, JANET K.
Practical anatomy, physiology and hygiene for part I of the preliminary state examination for nurses. John Murray, 1958.

ROBINS, R. A.
Textbook of anatomy and physiology for nurses and masseuses. Faber & Gwyer, 1928.

ROWE, JOYCE W., *and* WHEBLE, VICTOR H.
A concise textbook of anatomy and physiology applied for orthopaedic nurses. Edinburgh, Livingstone, 1959.

SEARS, WILLIAM GORDON
Anatomy and physiology for nurses. Arnold, 1941.
2nd edn., 1951.
3rd edn., 1958.

SPENCER, A. M.
The nurse's textbook of anatomy and physiology: a complete textbook for the preliminary state examination, incorporating over fifty model answers to questions set at previous examinations. Faber, 1946.
2nd edn., 1958.

ARITHMETIC FOR NURSES

BUTTON, DOROTHY
Mathematics for nurses, a course for pre-nursing students. Faber, 1956.

FREAM, WILLIAM C.
Aids to arithmetic in nursing. Bailliere, Tindall & Cox, 1956.
2nd edn., 1959.

JESSEE, RUTH W.
Self-teaching tests in arithmetic for nurses. 2nd edn. Kimpton, 1945.
3rd edn., 1949.
5th edn., 1958.

JONES, B. R.
A guide to calculations for student nurses. *Nursing Mirror*, May 23, 1958, p. 573-4, and June 6, 1958, p. 727-8.

McCLAIN, M. ESTHER
Simplified arithmetic for nurses. Philadelphia, Saunders, 1952.

SMITH, D. E.
Mathematics for nurses . . . with the assistance of C. B. Lipton and Nina D. Gage. New York, . . . 1915.

WARWICK HOSPITAL
A guide to calculations for student nurses, compiled at the Dispensary, Warwick Hospital. . . . [The Hospital], 1958.

WHITTET, T. D.
Changing to the metric system. *Nursing Times*, Mar. 25, 1960, p. 372-6.

BACTERIOLOGY

BOCOCK, E. JOAN, *and* ARMSTRONG, KATHERINE F.
Aids to bacteriology for nurses. Bailliere, Tindall & Cox, 1959.

BOLDUAN, CHARLES FREDERICK, *and* BOLDUAN, NILS WILLIAM
Applied microbiology and immunology for nurses. Philadelphia, Saunders, 1913.
2nd edn., 1916.
3rd edn., 1919.
4th edn., 1923.
5th edn., 1927.
6th edn., 1930.
7th edn., 1935.
8th edn., 1940.

BROADHURST, JEAN, *and* GIVEN, LELIA J.
Bacteriology applied to nursing: a combined textbook and laboratory guide in microbiology. Philadelphia, Lippincott, 1930.
2nd edn., 1934.
3rd edn., 1936, called "Microbiology applied to nursing".
4th edn., 1939.
5th edn., 1945.

CAREY, HARRY W.
Introduction to bacteriology for nurses. Philadelphia, Davis, 1915.
2nd edn., 1920.
3rd edn., 1930, called "Handbook of bacteriology for nurses".

CLARK, E. IRENE
Bacteriology and pathology for nurses. Faber, 1933.
2nd edn., 1949.

DUKES, CUTHBERT ESQUIRE
Bacteria in relation to nursing. Lewis, 1946.
2nd edn., 1953, revised by Stanley Marshall.
3rd edn., 1958.

FERRIS, ELVIRA A.
Bacteriology for the practical nurse. Albany, Delmar, 1959.

FISHER, ANNE M., *and* LEWIS, LUCIA ZYLAK
Laboratory exercises and outlines in microbiology for nurses. Philadelphia, Lippincott, 1951.

MARSHALL, STANLEY
Elementary bacteriology and immunity for nurses. Lewis, 1940.
2nd edn., 1950.
3rd edn., 1958.

MEACHEN, G. NORMAN
Elementary bacteriology for nurses. Scientific Press, 1914.
2nd edn., 1924.

MORSE, MARY ELIZABETH, *and* FROBISHER, MARTIN
Microbiology for nurses. Philadelphia, Saunders, 1919.
2nd edn., 1924.
3rd edn., 1928.
4th edn., 1932.
5th edn., 1937.
6th edn., 1941.
7th edn., 1946.
8th edn., 1951, by Morse, Frobisher and Sommermeyer.
9th edn., 1956, by Martin Frobisher and Lucille Sommermeyer.
10th edn., 1960.

NETER, ERWIN, *and* EDGEWORTH, DOROTHA RAE
Medical microbiology for nurses. Philadelphia, Davis, 1949.
2nd edn., 1950.
3rd edn., 1954.

PIETTE, E. C., *and* WHITE, J. M.
Microbiology and nursing. 2nd edn. Philadelphia, Davis, 1945.

ROGERS, HERBERT
Notes on bacteriology and clinical pathology for nurses. Lewis, 1938.

SOMMERMEYER, LUCILLE
Laboratory manual and workbook in microbiology for students of nursing. Philadelphia, Saunders, 1956.
2nd edn., 1960.

UNITED STATES. COMMUNICABLE DISEASE CENTER
Staphylococcal disease and related subjects: selected materials on nursing aspects. Washington, Govt. Printing Office, 1960.

WITTON, CATHERINE JONES
Microbiology with applications to nursing. New York, McGraw-Hill, 1950.
2nd edn., 1956.

BIOLOGY

MARTIN, MARJORIE F.
An introduction to human biology for students in schools of nursing, physiotherapy and physical education. E.U.P., 1956.

CANCER NURSING

AITKEN-SWAN, J.
Nursing the late cancer patient at home: the family's impressions. *Practitioner*, July 1959, p. 64-9.

AMERICAN CANCER SOCIETY
A cancer source book for nurses. New York, The Society, 1950, repr. 1960.

BARKLEY, VIRGINIA
What can I say to the cancer patient? *Nursing Outlook*, June 1958, p. 316-8.

BOOTH, STELLA, *and* HANISCH, VERNA K.
A clinical experience in cancer nursing for public health nurses. *Nursing Outlook*, Mar. 1960, p. 142-3.

CHANDLER, E. M.
Educating the nurse in cancer care. *Canadian Nurse*, Nov. 1958, p. 1016-7.

CHANDLER, E. M.
Nursing care in radiation therapy. *Canadian Nurse*, Nov. 1958, p. 1023-8.

FERGUSON, M.
Nursing the cancer patient. *Canadian Nurse*, Nov. 1958, p. 1020-2.

FOWLER, D.
The public health nurse in the cancer program. *Canadian Nurse*, Nov. 1958, p. 1029-30.

HEIL, LOUIS M., *and* CAVAGLIERI, NORMA
An investigation of student nurse achievement in nurse-patient relations and problem solving in emotional aspects of cancer nursing. [Bethesda, Md., National Cancer Institutes, 1956.]

HILKEMEYER, R.
Nursing care of cancer patients in hospital and home. *Bulletin of Cancer Progress*, July-Aug. 1958, p. 122-5.

HISLOP, R.
Nursing care of patients with mouth or throat cancer. *American Journal of Nursing*, Oct. 1957, p. 1317-9.

LEE, M. M.
The nurse in cancer epidemiology. *Nursing Outlook*, Mar. 1958, p. 160-2.

LOFTHOUSE, E. M., *and* STOKES, G. M.
Nursing care of children with cancer. *American Journal of Nursing*, April 1953, p. 415-8.

MARIE CURIE MEMORIAL *and* QUEEN'S INSTITUTE OF DISTRICT NURSING
Joint National Cancer Survey Committee. Report on a national survey concerning patients with cancer nursed at home. Marie Curie Memorial, 1952.

MICHIGAN UNIVERSITY SCHOOL OF PUBLIC HEALTH
Proceedings of in-service training course on cancer services for health directors and public health nurses. Ann Arbor, Michigan, The University, 1948.

RAVEN, RONALD W., *editor*
Cancer, vol. VI . . . part xi: Public health and nursing aspects of cancer. Butterworth, 1959.

RAVEN, RONALD W.
A handbook on cancer for nurses and health visitors. Butterworth, 1953.

UNITED STATES. NATIONAL CANCER INSTITUTE *and* NEW YORK STATE DEPARTMENT OF HEALTH
Cancer nursing: a manual for public health nurses, [by Margaret Knapp]. Albany, New York, State Department of Health, 1955.

UNITED STATES PUBLIC HEALTH SERVICE *and others*
Tools for evaluation of cancer nursing for nursing instructors, [prepared by the] . . . Public Health Service, National Institute of Health, National Cancer Institute. [Washington, Govt. Printing Office, 1957].

CARDIAC NURSING

DENHAM, M., ABRAHAM, S., *and* GRAVES, L. M.
Nursing services outside the hospital for cardiovascular disease patients. *Public Health Reports*, Jan. 1959, p. 21-7.

FORDHAM, M. E.
Nursing in the Cardiac Intensive Care Unit at the Mayo Clinic, St. Mary's Hospital, Rochester, Minnesota, U.S.A. 1. Planning and equipment. *Nursing Mirror*, May 20, 1960, p. ii.

HANSON, L. M., *and* DENHAM, M.
Public health nursing in a cardio-vascular disease program. *Nursing Outlook*, Feb. 1958, p. 96-8.

McLAUGHLIN, A. I. G.
Diseases of the heart and lungs: a handbook for nurses. Faber & Gwyer, 1926.

MATTINGLY, CAPITOLA B. *editor*
Cardiovascular disease nursing. Washington, Catholic University of America Press, 1960.

MODELL, WALTER
Handbook of cardiology for nurses: the disease, the patient, modern concepts of treatment. New York, Springer, 1952.
2nd edn., 1954.
3rd edn., 1958.

SMITH, B. F., *and* BROWN, J. P.
Nursing care of patients with Cushing's syndrome. *American Journal of Nursing*, Aug. 1957, p. 1036-7.

WICKENSHEIMER, V.
Nursing care for patients treated by open intra-cardiac surgical procedures. *Military Medicine*, Aug. 1960, p. 537-43.

WOOD, E. C.
Understanding the patient with heart disease. *Nursing Outlook*, Feb. 1959, p. 90-2.

WOODEN, H. E.
Patient-centered cardiac care. *Hospital Progress*, Dec. 1958, p. 80-2.

CHEMISTRY

BIDDLE, HARRY CLARENCE
Chemistry for nurses. Philadelphia, Davis, 1931.
2nd edn., 1940.
3rd edn., 1946.
4th edn., 1951.

MORSE, EDNA CURTISS
College chemistry in nursing education, ed. by I. M. Stewart. New York, Macmillan, 1947.

NEAL, RAYMOND E.
Chemistry in nursing. New York, McGraw-Hill, 1948.

PETERS, F. N.
A textbook of chemistry for nurses. St. Louis, . . . 1919.

CIRCULATORY AND GLANDULAR DISEASES

COOKE, R. V.
The treatment and nursing care of thyrotoxicosis. *Nursing Mirror*, Aug. 23, 1957, p. ii, and Aug. 30, 1957, p. iii.

DALLY, J. F. HALLS
Blood pressure: a manual for nurses, hygienists and social workers. Faber, 1931.

ELLIOTT, JOYCE T.
Nursing care in adrenal hyperfunction. *Canadian Nurse*, Feb. 1960, p. 116-7.

FOOTE, R. ROWDEN
The physical treatment of varicose ulcers; a practical manual for the physiotherapist and nurse, with a section on electrical adjuncts treatment, by T. Wareham. Edinburgh, Livingstone, 1958.

MARPLE, C. D., *and* McINTYRE, M. J.
Anticoagulant therapy.
1. Medical aspects, by C. D. Marple.
2. Nursing care, by M. J. McIntyre.
American Journal of Nursing, July 1956, p. 875-9.

WEINER, W.
Duties of the nursing staff in transfusion treatment. *Nursing Mirror*, Nov. 7, 1952, p. ii, and Nov. 14, 1952, p. i.

DENTAL NURSING

COULTAS, ROMA, *compiler*
Dental nurses' digest. Leyland, Lancs., British Dental Nurses and Assistants Society, [195?].

CULLWICK, H. RONALD
A handbook for dental nurses. Bale, Sons & Curnow, 1938.

FULTON, JOHN T.
Experiment in dental care: results of New Zealand's use of school dental nurses. Geneva, W.H.O., 1951.

GREAT BRITAIN. MINISTRY OF HEALTH *and others*
New Zealand school dental nurses: report of United Kingdom Dental Mission, Feb.-Mar. 1950. H.M.S.O., 1950.

HARLAN, H. R.
Nursing in dental health programmes. *Nursing Outlook*, Feb. 1957, p. 80-1.

HICKEY, F. C.
The nurse in an industrial dental program. Harrisburg, Pennsylvania Department of Health, Bureau of Industrial Hygiene, 1952.

LEVISON, H.
Textbook for dental nurses. Oxford, Blackwell, 1960.

MARKOWITZ, A.
A program of dental health education for nurses. *Journal of the American Dental Association*, July 1959, p. 127-9.

SALTER, K.
School dental nursing in New Zealand. *International Nursing Review*, Feb. 1960, p. 62-7.

SENIOR, W. G.
The role of the public health nurse in preventive dentistry. *Royal Society for the Promotion of Health Journal*, Dec. 1956, p. 754-7.

DERMATOLOGY

BULKLEY, L. DUNCAN
Nurses' manual of the skin in health and disease. Philadelphia, Saunders, 1921.

DOWLING, G. B.
Some common skin diseases and their nursing care. *Nursing Mirror*, Jan. 29, 1960, p. 1485-6 and 1488, and Feb. 5, 1960, p. ii-iv.

GOLDMAN, L.
Pyogenic skin infections: preliminary report, an outline of some medical and nursing care technics after a control program of eighteen months. *Medical Times*, Jan. 1959, p. 56-8.

INGRAM, J. T.
Nursing care of psoriasis. 1 and 2. *Nursing Mirror*, July 1, 1955, p. ii-iv, and July 8, 1955, p. ii-iv.

MEACHEN, G. NORMAN
Skin diseases: their nursing and general management. Scientific Press, 1923.

PERCIVAL, F. H., *and* TODDIE, ELIZABETH
Dermatology for nurses. Edinburgh, Livingstone, 1947.

RATTNER, HERBERT
Dermatology: a textbook for nurses. Philadelphia, Saunders, 1953.

STOKES, JOHN HINCHMAN
Dermatology and syphilology for nurses, including social hygiene. Philadelphia, Saunders, 1930.
3rd edn., 1940.
4th edn., 1948, by J. H. Stokes and Jane Barbara Taylor, entitled "Dermatology and venereology for nurses".

WILKINSON, D. S.
The nursing and management of skin diseases. Faber, 1958.

DIABETES

CATES, J. E.
A survey of diabetics visited by district nurses in Bristol. *Medical Officer*, Mar. 2, 1956, p. 107.

LAWRENCE, ROBERT DANIEL
The diabetic ABC: a practical book for patients and nurses. Lewis, 1929.
2nd edn., 1932.
3rd edn., 1935.
4th edn., 1936.
5th edn., 1937.
6th edn., 1939.
7th edn., 1940.
8th edn., 1944.
9th edn., 1946.
10th edn., 1948.
11th edn., 1955.
12th edn., 1960.

MARTIN, MARGUERITE M.
Diabetes mellitus: a handbook for nurses. Philadelphia, Saunders, 1960.

WALKER, JOAN B.
The nurse and the diabetic. Iliffe, 1958.

DIGESTIVE SYSTEM

WAKELY, C.
Nursing care and treatment of hernia.
1. External hernia.
2. The treatment of femoral hernia.
3. Umbilical hernia.
Nursing Mirror, Sept. 6, 1957, p. iii-iv; Sept. 13, 1957, p. iii-iv; Sept. 20, 1957, p. ii-iii.

EAR NOSE AND THROAT

ADAMS, W. STIRK, *and* STRANG, R. R. S., *editors*
Treatment of ear, nose and throat conditions: a series of articles by various contributors. *Nursing Mirror*, [1954].

DENISON, ABBY HELEN
Textbook of eye, ear, nose and throat nursing. New York, Macmillan, 1929.
2nd edn., 1937?

HOLLENDER, ABRAHAM R., *and* SNITMAN, MAURICE F.
Nursing in eye, ear, nose and throat. Philadelphia, Davis, 1946.

KORKIS, F. BOYES
Ear, nose and throat nursing. Churchill, 1955.

KORKIS, F. BOYES
Post-laryngectomy nursing care. *Nursing Mirror*, Oct. 7, 1955, p. vi-vii.

MARSHALL, SUSANNA
Aids to ear, nose and throat nursing. Bailliere, Tindall & Cox, 1953.

NEIL, JAMES HARDIE, *and* NEIL, T. HARDIE
Ear, nose and throat nursing. 4th edn. Auckland, Auckland Service Printery, 1948.

NEW YORK CITY, MANHATTAN EYE, EAR AND THROAT HOSPITAL
Nursing in diseases of the eye, ear, nose and throat. Philadelphia, Saunders, 1910.
2nd edn., 1915.
3rd edn., 1922.
4th edn., 1927.
5th edn., 1931.
6th edn., 1937.
7th edn., 1942.
8th edn., 1948.
10th edn., 1958.

PARKINSON, ROY H.
Eye, ear, nose and throat manual for nurses. Kimpton, 1925.
2nd edn., 1931.
5th edn., 1944.
6th edn., 1949.
8th edn., 1959.

ROBERTS, JOY G.
Eye, ear, nose and throat for nurses. Philadelphia, Davis, 1931.

ROTTER, KENNETH
The ear, nose and throat for nurses. Faber, 1956.

SHEPARD, MARY ESTELLE
Nursing care of patients with eye, ear, nose and throat disorders. New York, Macmillan, 1958.

SMITH, HARMON
Nursing in diseases of the eye, ear, nose and throat. Philadelphia, Saunders, 1931.

VLASTO, MICHAEL
The nursing of diseases of the nose, ear and throat. Faber, 1926.
2nd edn., 1938, entitled "The nose, ear and throat for nurses and dressers".
3rd edn., 1945.

GENETICS

DUTTON, G.
Genetics for nurses. *Nursing Mirror*, Nov. 20, 1959, p. 641.

GENITO-URINARY SYSTEM

ANDERSON, THOMAS
Urine examination for nurses, with notes on the collection of specimens for laboratory examination. Glasgow, Macdougall, 1936.

CARLSON, HJALMAR E.
Urology for nurses. Minneapolis, Burgess, 1955.

DAVIS, DAVID
Urological nursing. Philadelphia, Saunders, 1929.
2nd edn., 1936.
3rd edn., 1941.
4th edn., 1946.
5th edn., 1953.
6th edn., 1959, by David Davis and Kenneth C. Warren.

DWYER, SHEILA MAUREEN
Modern urology for nurses. Philadelphia, Lea & Febiger, 1940.

LOWSLEY, OSWALD SWINNEY, *and* KIRWIN, THOMAS JOSEPH
Urology for nurses. Philadelphia, Lippincott, 1936.
2nd edn., 1948.

ROCHE, A. E.
Treatment and nursing care of the urological patient. *Nursing Mirror*, Mar. 22, 1957, p. v.-vi, and Mar. 29, 1957, p. iii-iv.

SAYER, JOHN
Aids to male genito-urinary nursing. Bailliere, Tindall & Cox, 1948.
2nd edn., 1953.
3rd edn., 1958.

TOLLEFSON, D. M.
Nursing care of the patient with an ileac diversion of the urine. *American Journal of Nursing*, April 1959, p. 534-6.

GERIATRICS

AKESTER, J.
The health visitor's contribution to the care of the aged. *Royal Society of Health Journal*, Nov.-Dec. 1958, p. 834-7.

AUSTIN, CATHERINE L.
The basic six needs of the aging. *Nursing Outlook*, Mar. 1959, p. 138-41.

BROWN, FRANCES GOLD
Gerontology and geriatrics for practical nursing students. *Nursing Outlook*, Dec. 1959, p. 720-1.

BROWN, J. R.
New concepts in geriatric nursing. *Canadian Nurse*, April 1957, p. 289-93.

BROWN, J. R., *and* KIRK, T. E.
Some new concepts in geriatric nursing. *Canadian Services Medical Journal*, July-Aug. 1957, p. 449-55.

GEFFEN, D.
The nurse in the domiciliary geriatric team: successful scheme at St. Pancras. *Nursing Mirror*, Nov. 6, 1959, p. vii-ix.

GOLDMANN, F.
Nursing service in homes for the aged. *Public Health Reports*, Dec. 1960, p. 1124-32.

GROUSE, G.
Nursing the senile patient.
1. Problems and aims.
2. Reorientation and rehabilitation.
Nursing Mirror, Mar. 25, 1960, p. iii-iv, and April 1, 1960, p. xiv-xv.

HALPIN, J.
Where are the geriatric nurses of the future. *Nursing Mirror*, June 5, 1959, p. v.

HOWELL, T. H.
Tell me, sister: an analysis of questions arising in geriatric ward rounds. *Nursing Times*, Nov. 4, 1960, p. 1369-71.

NEWTON, KATHLEEN
Geriatric nursing. St. Louis, Mosby, 1950.
2nd edn., 1954.
3rd edn., 1960.

NORTON, DOREEN
The place of geriatric nursing in training. *Nursing Times*, July 6, 1956, p. 621-4.

RANDALL, O. A.
Nursing care of the aged. *Nursing World*, April 1956, p. 10-12.

ROUTHIER, A. M., *and* BERNADETTE DE LOURDES, SISTER
Gerontology in the basic curriculum. *Nursing Outlook*, May 1957, p. 276-8.

RUDD, T. N.
The nursing of the elderly sick: a practical handbook of geriatric nursing. Faber, 1953.
2nd edn., 1954.
3rd edn., 1960.

RUDD, T. N.
Senile confusion—and the nurse. *Nursing Mirror*, Oct. 18, 1957, p. 209-10.

SARGENT, EMILIE G., *and* CORLEY, CATHERINE
Health and welfare of the aged—nursing contributions. *American Journal of Nursing*, Nov. 1960, p. 1616-9.

TAIETZ, P., *and* ELLENBOGEN, B. L.
Recruiting the professional nurse to the nursing home setting. *Geriatrics*, Jan. 1957, p. 62-5.

GYNAECOLOGY

BERKELEY, COMYNS
Gynaecology for nurses. Faber, 1910.
4th edn., 1925.
5th edn., 1929.
6th edn., 1934.
7th edn., 1937.
8th edn., 1941.
9th edn., 1943.
10th edn., 1945.

CAIRNEY, JOHN
Gynaecology for senior students of nursing. Christchurch, N.Z., Peryer, 1954.

CAMPBELL, A. D., *and* SHANNON, MABEL A.
Gynecology for nurses. Philadelphia, Davis, 1946.

CLYNE, D. G. WILSON
A handbook of obstetrics and gynaecology for nurses. Bristol, Wright, 1958.

COWAN, M. CORDELIA
Nursing manual of gynaecology and obstetrics. Philadelphia, Lippincott, 1931.

CROSSEN, HARRY STURGEON
Gynaecology for nurses. St. Louis, Mosby, 1927.
2nd edn., 1936.
3rd edn., 1946, by Robert James Crossen and Frances W. Hoffert, called "Gynaecologic nursing".
4th-5th edns., by Robert James Crossen and Ann Campbell.
(5th edn., 1956.)

DICKINSON, DOROTHY M.
Gynaecology explained to nurses. Faber, 1933.

DODDS, GLADYS H.
Gynaecology: a handbook for nurses. Faber, 1946.
2nd edn., 1952.
3rd edn., 1957.

FALLS, FREDERICK HOWARD, *and* McLAUGHLIN, JANE R.
Obstetrics and gynecologic nursing. St. Louis, Mosby, 1937.

FULLERTON, ANNA MARTHA
Nursing in abdominal surgery and diseases of women. Philadelphia, 1891.
2nd edn., 1893.
[A computation of the lectures upon abdominal surgery and gynaecology, and general surgical conditions and procedures—delivered to the classes in the training school for nurses connected with the Women's Hospital in Philadelphia. 1893.]

GARLAND, GORDON W., *and* QUIXLEY, JOAN M. E.
Obstetrics and gynaecology for nurses. E.U.P., 1956.

GERMAN NURSES' FEDERATION
Gynaecological nursing, a paper prepared on behalf of the German Nurses' Federation at the request of the Nursing Service Committee of the International Council of Nurses. I.C.N., 1960.

GRATION, HILDA M., *and* HOLLAND, DOROTHY L.
Aids to gynaecological nursing. Bailliere, Tindall & Cox, 1939.
2nd edn., 1941.
3rd edn., 1944.
4th edn., 1947.
5th edn., 1952.

HAWKINS-AMBLER, GEORGE ARTHUR
Gynaecological nursing. Scientific Press, [1900].

HECTOR, WINIFRED E., *and* HOWKINS, JOHN
Modern gynaecology with obstetrics for nurses. Heinemann, 1956.
2nd edn., 1960.

HELLIER, JOHN B.
Notes on gynaecological nursing. Churchill, 1892.

MILLER, NORMAN F., *and* BRYANT, VIRGINIA
Gynecology and gynecologic nursing: with a chapter on the gynecology operating room, by Molly Kowal. Philadelphia, Saunders, 1944.
2nd edn., 1949.
3rd edn., 1954, by N. F. Miller and Hazel Avery.
4th edn., 1959.

NORTON, FELICIE
Notes on gynaecological nursing. Faber, 1922.
2nd edn., 1927.

OAKES, LOIS
Essentials of gynaecology for nurses: a brief course of questions and answers for examination candidates. Putnam, 1928.

STEWART, NETTA
Gynaecological nursing. Edinburgh, Oliver & Boyd, 1903.

HYGIENE

CHARLES, E.
Hygiene without tears for the student nurse. *Nursing Mirror*, Sept. 7, 1956, p. 1635-6, and Sept. 14, 1956, p. 1707-8.

COOPER, YVONNE V., *and* DAVIES, HELENA V.
Aids to practical hygiene for nurses. Bailliere, Tindall & Cox, 1951.

DARLING, H. C. RUTHERFORD
Elementary hygiene for nurses: a handbook for nurses and others. Churchill, 1917.
2nd edn., 1924.
3rd edn., 1926.
4th edn., 1929.
5th edn., 1932.
6th edn., 1935.
7th edn., 1940.
8th edn., 1944.
9th edn., 1947.
10th edn., 1952, ed. H. C. R. Darling and John Denis Murphy.

DIEHL, HAROLD SHEELY, *and* BOYNTON, RUTH
Healthful living for nurses. New York, McGraw-Hill, 1944.

FUNNELL, EDITH M.
Aids to hygiene for nurses. Bailliere, Tindall & Cox, 1938.
2nd edn., 1940.
3rd edn., 1948.
4th edn., 1950.
5th edn., 1956.

GIBSON, JOHN
Health personal and communal: a short hygiene for nurses. Faber, 1959.

GUY, JOHN, *and* LINKLATER, G. J. I.
Hygiene for nurses. Edinburgh, Livingstone, 1930.
2nd edn., 1933.
3rd edn., 1935.
4th edn., 1937.
5th edn., 1940.
6th edn., 1943.
7th edn., 1948.

McISAACS, ISABEL
Hygiene for nurses. New York, 1908.

MURREY, N.
Hygiene for nurses. St. Louis, Mosby, 1915.

NIGHTINGALE, FLORENCE
Rural hygiene: health teaching in towns and villages. Spottiswoode, 1894.

PAVEY, AGNES
Hygiene for nursing students. Faber, 1939.
2nd edn., 1942.
3rd edn., 1946.
4th edn., 1948.
6th edn., 1954.
7th edn., 1956.
8th edn., 1958.

PEARCE, EVELYN CLARE
Aids to elementary hygiene: a guide to the preliminary state examination. Faber, 1934.
2nd edn., 1939.
3rd edn., 1942, entitled "A complete handbook of hygiene in questions and answers".
4th edn., 1943.
5th edn., 1944.
6th edn., 1945.
7th edn., 1947.
8th edn., 1951.
9th edn., 1956

PRIEST, M. A.
Modern hygiene for nurses: including bacteriology and the principles of asepsis. Heinemann, 1960.

ROBERTS, R. LAWTON
Illustrated lectures on nursing and hygiene. Lewis, 1892.

SMITH, FRED J.
Domestic hygiene for nurses: with so much of chemistry and physics as are necessary to the reasonable understanding thereof. Churchill, 1911.
2nd edn., 1915.

WHITBY, L. E. H.
The nurses' handbook of hygiene. Faber, 1925.
2nd edn., 1929.
3rd edn., 1931.
4th edn., 1932.
5th edn., 1934.
6th edn., 1938.
7th edn., 1941.

INFECTIOUS DISEASES

ACLAND, SIR HENRY WENTWORTH
Memories of the cholera at Oxford in the year 1854.
[Contains an account of the arrangements made for nursing cholera patients in this epidemic.]

ANDERSON, GAYLORD WEST, and ARNSTEIN, MARGARET G.
Communicable disease control: a volume for the health officer and public health nurse. New York, Macmillan, 1941.
2nd edn., 1948.
3rd edn., 1953.

BOWER, ALBERT G., and PILANT, EDITH P.
Communicable diseases for nurses. Philadelphia, Saunders, 1929.
2nd edn., 1932.
3rd edn., 1935.
4th edn., 1939.
5th edn., 1943, with the assistance of Wilton J. Halverson.
6th edn., 1948.
7th edn., 1953, entitled "Communicable diseases: a textbook for nurses".
8th edn., 1958, by A. G. Bower, E. P. Pilant and Nina B. Craft.

BREEN, GERALD E.
Fevers for nurses. Edinburgh, Livingstone, 1938.
2nd edn., 1944.
3rd edn., 1950.

BROWER, JACOB VREDENBURG
A popular treatise; containing observations concerning the origin of yellow fever; together with practical rules of conduct for preventing that disease, and the best methods of nursing fever patients. New York, printed for the author by Geo. Forman, 1805.

CAREY, MATHEW
A short account of the malignant fever, lately prevalent in Philadelphia: with a statment of the proceedings that took place on the subject in different parts of the United States. Philadelphia, printed by the author, 1793.
2nd edn., 1793.
3rd edn., 1793.
4th edn., 1794.
[Remarks reflect upon the conduct of negro nurses in the yellow fever epidemic.]

CHANG, R. K.
The responsibility of the professional nurse in the prevention and control of infections. *Hawaii Medical Journal and Inter-Island Nurses' Bulletin*, May-June 1960, p. 558-62.

DARCY, RUTH, LUNDBLAD, ELEANOR, and SACHS, GERTRUDE
A comparison of isolation technics as taught in 17 selected general hospitals with schools of nursing in North America. New York, Columbia University, Teachers' College, 1954.

DRAKARD, M.
The nurse in fever hospitals.
See
NURSING TIMES
The nurse and the nation: a survey of her position in the State today. *Nursing Times*, Nov. 5, 1910, p. 904-31.

DUNDAS, GRACE H. G.
Textbook for fever nurses. Edinburgh, Bruce, 1923.

ENSWORTH, HERBERT, and GREENWOOD, LILA
Pneumonia and its nursing care. Philadelphia, Lippincott, 1940.

GORDON, A. KNYVETT
Asepsis and fever nursing. *British Journal of Nursing*, May 9, 1914, p. 407-9, and May 16, 1914, p. 431-3.

HARDING, WILLIAM
Fevers and infectious diseases—their nursing and practical management. London, . . . 1907.

HASENJAEGER, ELLA
Asepsis in communicable-disease nursing. Philadelphia, Lippincott, 1940.

JOHNSTONE, F.
Lessons on the prevention of the spread of fevers delivered to the Ladies' Educational Society of Hastings and St. Leonard's in November, 1873, with additions. 2nd edn. St. Leonards-on-Sea, [1876].

LESTER, MARY R.
Challenge of communicable disease today: nursing opportunities. *American Journal of Public Health and the Nation's Health*, July 1959, p. 857-61.

LESTER, MARY R.
Every nurse an epidemiologist. *American Journal of Nursing*, Nov. 1957, p. 1434-5.

LYNCH, THERESA I.
Communicable disease nursing. St. Louis, Mosby, 1942.
2nd edn., 1949.

MITMAN, M., and COUZINS, E. M.
Fever training in a general hospital. *Nursing Mirror*, Mar. 13, 1953, p. xi-xiii.

PEARCE, EVELYN CLARE
Fevers and fever nursing. Faber, 1930.
2nd edn., 1932.
3rd edn., 1934.
4th edn., 1940.
5th edn., 1943.
6th edn., 1944.
7th edn., 1949, called "Communicable diseases and their nursing care".

PILLSBURY, MARY ELIZABETH
Nursing care of communicable diseases: prophylactic technics for the prevention and control of disease. Philadelphia, Lippincott, 1929.
2nd edn., 1931.
3rd edn., 1934.
4th edn., 1936.
5th edn., 1938.
6th edn., 1942.
7th edn., 1952, by M. E. Pillsbury and Elizabeth J. Sachs.

RICHARDSON, D. C.
Infectious diseases and aseptic nursing technic. Philadelphia, Saunders, 1927.

THORP, EUSTACE
Infectious diseases for nurses. Bailliere, Tindall & Cox, 1929.

WATSON, JOYCE M.
Aids to fever nursing. Bailliere, Tindall & Cox, 1939.
2nd edn., 1945, called "Aids to fevers for nurses".
3rd edn., 1949.
4th edn., 1955, rev. by Clara Bell and Katharine F. Armstrong.

WILSON, J. C.
Practical lessons in nursing: fever nursing, designed for the use of professional and other nurses, and especially as a textbook for nurses in training. Philadelphia, . . . 1888.

WOOLLACOTT, F. J.
Lectures upon the nursing of infectious diseases. Scientific Press, [1906].

POLIOMYELITIS

BULLOUGH, J.
Nursing care of patients suffering from bulbar respiratory poliomyelitis. *Nursing Mirror*, Aug. 22, 1958, p. vii and p. x.

CAMPION, F. L.
Nursing care of patients with poliomyelitis. *Canadian Nurse*, June 1954, p. 454-61.

HARDY, GLADYS M.
Nursing and treatment of acute anterior poliomyelitis. Faber, 1954.

KENNY, ELIZABETH
My battle and victory: history of the discovery of poliomyelitis as a systemic disease. Hale, 1955.

KENNY, ELIZABETH
Infantile paralysis and cerebral diplegia: methods used for the restoration of function. Sydney, Angus & Robertson, 1937.

NATIONAL ORGANIZATION FOR PUBLIC HEALTH NURSING *and* THE NATIONAL LEAGUE OF NURSING EDUCATION.
JOINT ORTHOPAEDIC NURSING ADVISORY SERVICE
A guide for nurses in the nursing care of patients with infantile paralysis. New York, The National Foundation for Infantile Paralysis, 1946.

NATIONAL ORGANIZATION FOR PUBLIC HEALTH NURSING *and* NATIONAL LEAGUE FOR NURSING EDUCATION.
JOINT ORTHOPAEDIC NURSING ADVISORY SERVICE
Nursing for the poliomyelitis patient. New York, The Service, 1948.

SMITH, H. G.
Special methods and respirators in the treatment of poliomyelitis. *Nursing Times*, June 26, 1954, p. 677-8.

STEVENSON, JESSIE
The nursing care of patients with infantile paralysis. New York, the National Foundation for Infantile Paralysis, 1940.

WESTON, E. M. A.
Nursing treatment of poliomyelitis patients.
1. Signs and symptoms of spinal and bulbar types of acute anterior poliomyelitis. *Nursing Mirror*, Aug. 21, 1953, p. ii-iv.

2. Personnel and equipment in a poliomyelitis unit. *Nursing Mirror*, Aug. 28, 1953, p. v-vi.
3. The nursing care. *Nursing Mirror*, Sept. 4, 1953, p. v-vii.
4. The nursing care. *Nursing Mirror*, Sept. 11, 1953, p. v and 1544.

WESTON, E. M. A.
Psychological considerations in the care of poliomyelitis patients. *Nursing Mirror*, June 4, 1954, p. 629-30.

LOCOMOTOR SYSTEM

ARTHRITIS AND RHEUMATISM FOUNDATION
Arthritis and related disorders: manual for nurses, physical therapists and medical social workers. New York, The Foundation, 1952.

FASH, BERNICE
Body mechanics in nursing arts. New York, McGraw-Hill, 1946.

FASH, BERNICE
Kinesiology in nursing: laboratory manual. New York, McGraw-Hill, 1952.

GOLDRING, D., BEHRER, M. R., *and* McQUATER, F.
Rheumatoid arthritis in children. *American Journal of Nursing*, Nov. 1956, p. 1437-9.

KENNEDY, P. E.
Posture for nurses. *Nursing Mirror*, April 26, 1957, p. 255; *Nursing Times*, May 3, 1957, p. 488-90.

LIVINGSTON, M. C.
"Body mechanics" applied to the nurse's work. *Nursing Mirror*, April 12, 1957, p. ii-iv.

NEIL, C. A.
Body management in nursing. *Nursing Times*, Feb. 6, 1959, p. 163-4 and 170.

SADLER, SABRA
Rheumatic fever: nursing care in pictures. Philadelphia, Lippincott, 1949.

STEVENSON, JESSIE L.
Posture and nursing. New York, Joint Orthopaedic Nursing Advisory Service of the National Organization for Public Health Nursing and the National League of Nursing Education, 1942.
2nd edn., 1948.

WEBER, S.
Posture and the nurse. *Public Health Nursing*, June 1951, p. 325-30.

WINTERS, MARGARET CAMPBELL
Protective body mechanics in daily life and nursing: a manual for nurses and their co-workers. Philadelphia, Saunders, 1952.

MEDICINE

AIKENS, CHARLOTTE A.
Clinical studies for nurses: a textbook for second- and third-year pupil nurses and a handbook for all who are engaged in caring for the sick. Philadelphia, Saunders, 1909.
2nd edn., 1912.
3rd edn., 1916.
4th edn., 1920.

ALMA, SISTER
Clinical laboratory manual for nurses and technicians. Kimpton, 1932.

ANDERSON, JAMES
Notes given on medical nursing from the lectures given to the probationers at the London Hospital . . ., edited by Ethel F. Lamport, with introductory biographical notice by Sir Andrew Clark. Lewis, 1894.
3rd edn., 1897.

ASHER, PATRIA
An introduction to medicine for nurses, with a chapter on mental ill health by Portia Holman. Heinemann, 1948.
2nd edn., 1951.
3rd edn., 1954, entitled "Modern medicine for nurses".
4th edn., 1957.

BAILEY, HAMILTON
101 clinical demonstrations to nurses. Edinburgh, Livingstone, 1944.
2nd edn., 1946.

BIRCH, C. ALLEN
Common symptoms described and explained for nurses. Edinburgh, Livingstone, 1953.

BIRCH, C. ALLEN
Hazards of medical procedures.
1. Emergencies and the nurse.
2. The unconscious patient.
Nursing Times, Sept. 2, 1960, p. 1072-3, and Sept. 9, 1960, p. 1104-6.

BREDOW, MIRIAM
The medical assistant: a guide for the nurse, secretary and technician in the doctor's office. New York, McGraw Hill, 1958.

BROWN, AMY FRANCES
Medical nursing. Philadelphia, Saunders, 1945.
2nd edn., 1952.
3rd edn., 1957.

BROWN, AMY FRANCES
Medical and surgical nursing. Philadelphia, Saunders, 1959.

CABLE, JAMES VERNEY
Principles of medicine: an integrated textbook for nurses. Christchurch, New Zealand, Peryer, 1960.

CASELEY, DONALD J.
Trends in medical practice—their implications for nursing. *Nursing Outlook*, May 1957, p. 300-2.

CHAMBERLAIN, E. NOBLE
A textbook of medicine for nurses. O.U.P., 1931.
2nd edn., 1935.
3rd edn., 1938.
4th edn., 1943.
5th edn., 1949.
6th edn., 1954.

CLARK-KENNEDY, A. E.
Lectures on medicine to nurses. Edinburgh, Livingstone, 1950.

COOKE, R. GORDON
A summary of medicine for nurses for use in revision. Faber, 1945.
2nd edn., 1953, rev. by A. G. Stevenson.
3rd edn., 1957, rev. by A. G. Stevenson.

COOKE, R. GORDON
Textbook of chronic diseases: a handbook for nurses. Faber, 1936.

CUFF, HERBERT
A course of lectures on medicine to nurses. Churchill, 1896.
2nd edn., 1898.
3rd edn., 1900.
4th edn., 1903.
5th edn., 1907.
6th edn., 1913.
7th edn., 1920.

EMERSON, CHARLES PHILLIPS
Essentials of medicine: the basis of nursing care. Philadelphia, Lippincott, 1908.
2nd edn., 1911.
3rd edn., 1915.
4th edn., 1920.
5th edn., 1923.
6th edn., 1925.
7th edn., 1926.

8th edn., 1928, by C. P. Emerson and N. G. Brown.
9th edn., 1929.
10th edn., 1931.
11th edn., 1933.
12th edn., 1936.
13th edn., 1938.
14th edn., 1940, by C. P. Emerson and J. E. Taylor.
15th edn., 1946.
16th edn., 1950.
17th edn., 1955, by C. P. Emerson and J. S. Bragdon

FADDIS, MARGENE O., *and* HAYMAN, JOSEPH M.
Care of the medical patient: a textbook. New York, McGraw-Hill, 1952.

FISHER, ESTHER
The nurse's textbook: a manual of medical and surgical nursing. Faber, 1937.

HENRY, J. N.
A nurse's handbook of medicine. Philadelphia, Lippincott, 1906.
3rd edn., 1913.

HITCH, MARGARET
Aids to medical nursing. Bailliere, Tindall & Cox, 1941.
2nd edn., 1943.
3rd edn., 1946.
4th edn., 1952.
5th edn., 1956, by K. F. Armstrong and E. J. Bocock.

HOOD, D. W. C.
Diseases and their commencement: lectures to trained nurses delivered at the West London Hospital. London, 1886.

HOUSTON, J. C., *and* STOCKDALE, MARION G.
Principles of medicine and medical nursing. English Universities Press, 1958.

HOXIE, GEORGE HOWARD
Practice of medicine for nurses: a textbook for nurses and students of domestic science . . . with a chapter on the technic of nursing by Pearl Laptad. Philadelphia, Saunders, 1908.

HULL, EDGAR, *and* PERRODIN, CECILIA M.
Medical nursing. Philadelphia, Davis, 1940.
2nd edn., 1941.
3rd edn., 1943.
4th edn., 1949.
5th edn., 1954.
6th edn., 1960.

HUNT, J.
The medical photography department and how it concerns the nurse. *Nursing Mirror*, Sept. 7, 1956, p. xiv-xvi.

JENSEN, JULIUS, *and* JENSEN, DEBORAH MACLURG
Clinical nursing in medicine. New York, Macmillan, 1941.
2nd edn., 1945.
3rd and 4th edns., called "Nursing in clinical medicine", 1949 and 1954.

JOULE, J. W.
Textbook of medicine for nurses. Lewis, 1952.
2nd edn., 1955.

LOCKET, S.
Medical cases described for nurses: an introduction to clinical medicine for nurses. Edinburgh, Livingstone, 1948.

MASON, MILDRED A.
Basic medical-surgical nursing. New York, Macmillan, 1959.

OSLER, SIR WILLIAM
Medicine and nursing. New York, 1919. *In* Essays on vocation, ed. Basil Mathews.

PAVEY, AGNES E.
Clinical procedures and their background for senior nursing students. Faber, 1944.
2nd edn., 1956.

PERRY, C. BRUCE
Medicine for nurses. Edinburgh, Livingstone, 1938.

SEARS, WILLIAM GORDON
Medicine for nurses. Arnold, 1935.
2nd edn., 1937.
3rd edn., 1939.
4th edn., 1945.
5th edn., 1949.
6th edn., 1954.
7th edn., 1957.
8th edn., 1960.

SHAFER, KATHLEEN NEWTON, *and others*
Medical-surgical nursing. St. Louis, Mosby, 1958.

STEWART, I.
A medical handbook for nurses. Faber, 1931.
2nd edn., 1934.
3rd edn., 1936.
4th edn., 1938.
5th edn., 1941.
6th edn., 1943.

TOOHEY, M.
Medicine for nurses: with a chapter on psychosomatic medicine by H. R. Rollin. Edinburgh, Livingstone, 1953.
2nd edn., 1955.
3rd edn., 1957.
4th edn., 1959.
5th edn., 1960.

WEITZMAN, DAVID
Principles of medicine for nurses. Faber, 1959.

FIRST AID—DOMESTIC MEDICINE

AMERICAN SCHOOL OF HOME ECONOMICS, CHICAGO
Handbook of health and nursing: a complete home study course comprising: Household bacteriology, by S. Maria Elliott; Personal hygiene, by Maurice M. Bosquet; Home care of the sick, by Amy E. Pope. Chicago, American School of Home Economics, 1912. 3 vols. in 1.

BRIGGS, SUSAN LENNOX
Home nursing with confidence. New York, Chester R. Heck, 1946.

BRITISH MEDICAL ASSOCIATION
First-aid in industry. B.M.A., 1939.

CAMPBELL, FRANCES
The book of home nursing: a practical guide for the treatment of sickness in the home. New York, E. P. Dutton, 1917.

CHILD, LYDIA MARIA
The family nurse or companion of the frugal housewife. Boston, 1837.

CHURCHILL, STELLA
Nursing in the home, including first-aid in common emergencies. Faber & Gwyer, 1925.

CLARKE, E. M.
An ABC of nursing in accidents and illnesses, revised and corrected by P. Barrett. Bentley, 1909.

CONNECTICUT TRAINING SCHOOL FOR NURSES
A handbook of nursing for family and general use. Philadelphia, Lippincott, 1888.
2nd edn., 1905.

CUTLER, G. E.
Care of the sick room. Cambridge, Mass., Harvard U.P. 1914.

DAVIES, MARY
The nurse's companion in the sick room. London, 1888.

DOUGLAS, GEORGE MARGARETTA
Health and home nursing. New York, Putnam, 1932.

DREW, MENA
Hints on nursing. London, 1913.

DRUMMOND, W. B.
Golden rules for sick nursing. Bristol, 1905.

FURGUSON, KATHLEEN
Sick room cookery with notes on sick nursing. Dublin, James Duffy, 1907.

GIDSEG, LUCILLE, *and* SARA, DOROTHY
Home nurses' handbook. New York, Funk, 1951.

GILBERT, NORMA S.
Home care of the sick. Philadelphia, Saunders, 1929.

GRIFFITH, JOHN QUINTIN
Helps and hints in nursing. Philadelphia, J. C. Winston, 1905.

HARRISON, E.
A textbook of home nursing: modern scientific methods for the care of the sick. New York, 1918.

HAWKINS-AMBLER, G. A.
The gentle art of nursing the sick. Scott, 18—.

HENDERSON, LOUISE
Practical home nursing: an elementary condensed textbook for trained attendants. New York, Macmillan, 1919.

HOPE, GEORGE H.
Till the doctor comes and how to help him. New York, Putnam, 1871.

HUTTON, MARY
Teach yourself home nursing. E.U.P., 1950.

JOHNSON, ROBERT WALLACE
Friendly cautions to the heads of families and others, very necessary to be observed in order to preserve health and long life: with ample directions to nurses who attend the sick, women in child-bed, etc. 1st American edn. with notes and additions, Philadelphia, James Humphreys, 1804.
[First published anonymously in London in 1767 under title "Some friendly cautions to the heads of families". 2nd American edn., Philadelphia, 1818, under title "The nurse's guide, and family assistant".]

KANE, H. H.
The sick room, a practical manual in nursing with a chapter on the dietary of the sick. New York, Nat. Pub. Co., 1879.

KEELE, K. D., *editor*
Modern home nursing and first aid: everybody's guide to the principles and practice of hygiene and nursing in the home. Odhams, [1944?].

LIPPOTT, L. C.
Personal hygiene and home nursing. Yonkers,. . . 1919.

LOWRY, EDITH BELLE
The home nurse. Chicago, Forbes, 1914.

Management of the sick room, with rules for diet, cookery for the sick and convalescent, and the treatment of the sudden illnesses and various accidents that require prompt and judicious care, with practical hints on digestion. Compiled from the latest medical authorities by a lady of New York under the supervision of Charles Aber, M.D. 2nd edn., New York, 1845.

MOHS, EMMA LOUISE
Principles of home nursing: a textbook for college students. Philadelphia, Saunders, 1923.

MOLES, CHARLOTTE L.
A guide to nursing in the home. Rider, [19?].

MORLEY, H.
A tract upon interrupted health and sick room duties. London, . . . 1847.

OAKES. LOIS, *compiler*
Illustrations of bandaging and first-aid. Edinburgh, Livingstone, 1940.
2nd edn., 1942.
3rd edn., 1944.
4th edn., 1950.
5th edn., 1956.

OVERLOCK, MELVIN GEORGE
A nurse in every home. Boston, Overlock Associates for the Protection of Health, [1913].

OVINGTON, L. H.
Helps for home nursing. Chicago, . . . 1891.

Plain directions for the care of the sick and recipes for sick people; by a Fellow of the College of Physicians, Philadelphia. New York, Mutual Life Insurance Co., [1875].

ROSSMAN, I. J., and SCHWARTZ, DORIS R.
The family handbook of home nursing and medical care. New York, Random House, 1958.

SCOTT, DOUGLAS HAY
Health and nursing in the home. Methuen, 1935.

SELBERT, NORMA
Home care of the sick. Philadelphia, Saunders, 1929.

SHIMBERG, BENJAMIN, and AIRD, ELLEN
Effectiveness of television in teaching home nursing. *Nursing Research*, June 1955, p. 28-41.

SOCIETY FOR PROMOTING CHRISTIAN KNOWLEDGE
Plain cookery, giving a variety of cheap and wholesome dishes; with cookery for the sick. The Society, 1856.
[Also contains "Plain rules to be observed in case of illness or accident", compiled by Robert Druitt.]

THOMSON, A. S.
The domestic management of the sick room, necessary in aid of medical treatment for the cure of diseases. 1st American edn. from 2nd London edn., revised with additions by R. E. Griffith. Philadelphia, 1845.

TREVETHICK, R. A.
Advanced industrial first-aid. Sheffield United Steel Co., 1947.

TROTT, LONA L.
Red Cross home nursing: American Red Cross Home Nursing Service. Philadelphia, Blakiston, 1942.

WAGNER, BETTY QUIN
The art of home nursing: simple techniques and practical procedures. Philadelphia, Davis, 1945.

WEBB, DORIS E.
Home nursing for everybody. Faber, 1939.

TROPICAL MEDICINE

ADAMS, A. R. D., and MAEGRAITH, B. G.
Tropical medicine for nurses. Oxford, Blackwell, 1955.

COCKER, DOROTHY E.
Aids to tropical nursing. Bailliere, Tindall & Cox, 1944.
2nd edn., 1944.
3rd edn., 1954.

DUNCAN, ANDREW
A guide to sick nursing in the tropics. Scientific Press, 1908.

GREGG, A. L.
Tropical nursing: a handbook for nurses and others going abroad. Cassell, 1929.
2nd edn., 1943.

JOHNSON, SIGRID C., editor
A text book for nurses in India: prepared under the direction of a Committee of the Nurses' Auxiliary of the Christian Medical Association of India. . . . Madras, Christian Literature Society for India, 1942.

LANGLEY, G.
Hints on tropical nursing.
I. Outfit. *Nursing Times*, Jan. 24, 1914, p. 85.
II. The colonial nurse and her duties. *Nursing Times*, Mar. 21, 1914, p. 353-4.

MACKIE, THOMAS TINLAY
Florence Nightingale and tropical and military medicine. American Society of Tropical Medicine, 1942.

ROBINSON, M. G.
The nursing of kwashiorkor. *Nursing Times*, Nov. 2, 1956, p. 1106-10.

TRAINED NURSES' ASSOCIATION OF INDIA
The essentials of tropical disease nursing; paper prepared by the Trained Nurses' Association of India on behalf o the International Council of Nurses. Supplement to the *International Nursing Review*, Oct. 1958. International Council of Nurses, 1958.

TROWELL, H. C.
A handbook for dressers and nurses in the tropics. Sheldon Press, 1937.
2nd edn., 1946.
3rd edn., 1953.

YOUNG, E. HILLS
Lectures on nursing for native orderlies. [1940.]
[The Arabic translation of the text is bound in with the English text.]

MENTAL HEALTH

ASHFORD, MARY E.
Home care of mentally ill patients. *American Journal of Nursing*, Feb. 1957, p. 206-7.

BEASLEY, FLORENCE A., and RHODES, WILLIAM C.
An evaluation of public health nursing service for families of the mentally ill. *Nursing Outlook*, Aug. 1956, p. 445-7.

BEASLEY, FLORENCE A., CALLAWAY, C. S., and STUBBS, T. H.
The follow-up of discharged mental patients by the public health nurse. *American Journal of Psychiatry*, Mar. 1960, p. 834-7.

CARSE, J., and others
A district mental health service. The Worthing experiment. *Lancet*, Jan. 4, 1958, p. 39-41.

CLARKE, ERIC KENT
Mental hygiene for community nursing. Minneapolis, University of Minnesota Press, 1942.

CRUICKSHANK, W. H.
Mental health for nurses. *Canadian Nurse*, Feb. 1956, p. 95-101.

DALZELL-WARD, A. J.
Mental health through human relations.
1. How the mind works.
2. Emotional security.
3. Nursing and human relations.
Nursing Times, June 29, 1956, p. 594-5; July 13, 1956, p. 653-4; July 27, 1956, p. 708-9.

GOIK, MARIE C., FOSTER, MARY L. and
WILLIAMS, FRANCES A.
Mental health in public health nursing. *Nursing Outlook*. May 1960, p. 269-73.

JEANNE, MARIE, SISTER
Mental health in the school of nursing program. *Hospital Progress*, May 1960, p. 100-1.

KINGCADE, M. E.
A training program in mental health nursing for public health nurses. *Nursing Outlook*, Jan. 1958, p. 683-5.

MACDONALD, V. MAY
Mental hygiene and the public health nurse: practical suggestions for the nurse of today. Philadelphia, Lippincott, 1923.

NATIONAL ORGANIZATION FOR PUBLIC HEALTH NURSING
Report of a conference on mental hygiene education for public health nurses. New York, The Organization, 1949.

PARMET, M.
The supervisory nurse's role in promoting mental health. *American Journal of Nursing*, March 1957, p. 328-30.

REES, M. I. H.
Nurses and mental health.
1. What is meant by health?
2. The basis of mental health.
3. The nurse and her patients.
Nursing Times, April 10, 1954, p. 391-2; April 24, 1954, p. 451-2; May 8, 1954, p. 507.

RYKKEN, MARJORIE B.
The nurse's role in preventing suicide. *Nursing Outlook*, July 1958, p. 377-8.

SIMONSON, R. E.
Variations on the theme mental health in nursing. *Public Health Reports*, July 1956, p. 700-4.

SOUTHERN REGIONAL EDUCATION BOARD, ATLANTA, GEORGIA
Nursing personnel for mental health programs; report of a conference sponsored by the Southern Regional Program in Mental Health Training and Research, March 27-29, 1957. Atlanta, The Board, 1958.

STAFFORD-CLARK, DAVID
British Red Cross Society mental health manual. The Society, 1958.

U.S. PUBLIC HEALTH SERVICE
Careers in mental health as a psychiatric nurse. Washington, Govt. Printing Office, 1957.

VINCENT, E. L.
Mental hygiene for nurses. Philadelphia, Saunders, 1938.

NEUROLOGY

BUCKLEY, A. C.
Nursing mental and nervous diseases, from the view points of biology, psychology and neurology—a textbook for use in schools for the training of nurses. Philadelphia and London, 1927.

ERNE, M. JULIE
A psychosomatic approach to the nursing care of a patient with Sydenham's Chorea. Washington, Catholic University of America Press, 1948.

FLANAGAN, EILEEN C., *and* HERDAN, IRENE M.
A preliminary study and analysis of nursing requirements in neurological nursing. *Canadian Nurse*, Nov. 1955, p. 855-62.

GOTTEN, NICHOLAS, *and* WILSON, LETITIA
Neurologic nursing. Philadelphia, Davis, 1941.
2nd edn., 1949.
3rd edn., 1957.

HABER, M. E.
Nursing care of the patient with trigeminal neuralgia. *American Journal of Nursing*, June 1958, p. 855-8.

MARSHALL, JOHN
Neurological nursing: a practical guide. Oxford, Blackwell, 1956.

MOERSCH, FREDERICK PAUL
Neurology and psychiatry for nurses. Minneapolis, Burgess, 1935.
2nd edn., 1942.
3rd edn., 1946.

PALMER, M. E.
Nursing the patient with multiple sclerosis. *American Journal of Nursing*, June 1957, p. 753-5.

RILEY, T. P.
Observations on nursing care in a paraplegic unit. *Nursing Times*, Oct. 18, 1957, p. 1178-9.

RUBIN, C.
The role of the nurse in hemiplegia. *Nursing Mirror*, Aug. 2, 1957, p. 1289-90.

RUSHTON, J. G.
Neurology for nurses. Minneapolis, Burgess, 1959.

SANDS, IRVING J.
Nervous and mental diseases for nurses. Philadelphia, Saunders, 1928.
2nd edn., 1933.
3rd edn., 1937.
4th edn., 1941.
5th edn., 1948, called "Neuro-psychiatry for nurses".

SMITH, GENEVIEVE WAMPLER
Care of the patient with a stroke: a handbook for the patient's family and the nurse. New York, Springer, 1959.

OBSTETRICS

AMERICAN COLLEGE OF NURSE-MIDWIFERY
Education for nurse-midwifery. Santa Fe, New Mexico, The College, 1958.

ANDREWS, HENRY RUSSELL
Midwifery for nurses. Arnold, 1906.
2nd edn., 1909.
3rd edn., 1911.
4th edn., 1914.
5th edn., 1920.
6th edn., 1922.
7th edn., 1934, by H. R. Andrews and Victor Lack.
8th edn., 1939.
9th edn., 1945.

AUERBACH, A. B.
New approaches to work with expectant parent groups; a report on a pilot leadership training programme for nurses. *American Journal of Public Health and the Nation's Health*, Feb. 1957, p. 184-91.

AUERBACH, A. B., *and* GOLLER, G.
How do nurses take to new ways in leading parent groups? *Nursing Outlook*, Dec. 1958, p. 674-7.

AVELING, J. H.
English midwives, their history and prospects. Churchill, 1872.

BIRDWOOD, G. T.
Advice to the expectant mother: fifty ante-natal talks; for the use of doctors, nurses and expectant mothers. Bale, Sons & Danielssohn, 1932.

BOOKMILLER, MAE M., *and* BOWEN, GEORGE LOVERIDGE
Textbook of obstetrics and obstetric nursing. Philadelphia, Saunders, 1949.
2nd edn., 1954.
3rd edn., 1958.

BOURNE, ALECK W.
Midwifery for nurses. Churchill, 1935.
2nd edn., 1939.
3rd edn., 1944.
[Continued as "Midwifery: a textbook for pupil midwives", by A. W. Bourne and Mary Williams].

BREAY, MARGARET
The scope of the maternity nurse. *British Journal of Nursing*, Aug. 10, 1907, p. 103-5.

BREAY, MARGARET
The training of midwives and monthly nurses. *Nursing Record*, Jan. 11, 1896, p. 28-9; Jan. 25, 1896, p. 76-7; Feb. 15, 1896, p. 128-30.

BROWNE, O'DONEL, *editor*
The Rotunda textbook of midwifery for nurses. Bristol, Wright, 1952.

BULL, THOMAS
Hints to mothers, for the management of health during the period of pregnancy, and in the lying-in room: with an exposure of popular errors in connexion with those subjects, etc., and hints upon nursing. 6th edn. Longman, 1849.
15th edn., 1864.

BULMAN, MICHAEL W.
Midwifery and obstetrical nursing. Faber, 1941.
2nd edn., 1945.
3rd edn., 1951.

CLYNE, D. G. WILSON
A handbook of obstetrics and gynaecology for nurses. Bristol, Wright, 1958.

COOKE, JOSEPH BROWN
A nurse's handbook of obstetrics. Philadelphia, Lippincott, 1903.
2nd edn., 1905.
3rd edn., 1907.
4th edn., 1909.
5th edn., 1911.
6th edn., 1913.
7th edn., 1915.
8th edn., 1917.
9th edn., 1920.
10th edn., 1926, revised by Carolyn E. Gray and Philip E. Williams.

CORBIN, H.
Maternity nursing education; yesterday, today, and tomorrow. *Nursing Outlook*, Feb. 1959, p. 82-4.

CULLINGWORTH, CHARLES J.
A short manual for monthly nurses. 6th edn., revised and enlarged. Churchill, 1907.

DAVIS, EDWARD P.
Obstetric and gynaecologic nursing. Philadelphia, Saunders, 1903.

DE LEE, JOSEPH BOLIVER, *and* CARMON, MABEL C.
Obstetrics for nurses. Philadelphia, Saunders, 1904.
2nd edn., 1906.
3rd edn., 1908.
4th edn., 1913.
5th edn., 1917.
6th edn., 1922.
7th edn., 1924.
8th edn., 1927.
9th edn., 1930.
10th edn., 1933.
11th edn., 1937.
12th edn., 1941.
13th edn., 1944.
14th edn., 1947.
15th edn., 1951.
16th edn., 1957, by M. Edward Davis and Catherine E. Sheckler.

DICK, ELISHA CULLEN
Doctor Dick's instructions for the nursing and management of lying-in women: with some remarks concerning the treatment of new-born infants. Alexandria, [D.C.]. Printed by Thomas & Westcott, 1798.

ENGELLS, A. M.
Nursing in a maternity clinic. *Nursing Outlook*, Dec. 1958, p. 702-4.

EWELL, THOMAS
Letters to ladies detailing important information, concerning themselves and infants. Philadelphia, W. Brown, 1817.
[Reissued in 1818 under title "The ladies' medical companion: containing in a series of letters, an account of the latest improvements and most successful means of preserving their beauty and health; of relieving the diseases peculiar to the sex, and an explanation of the offices they should perform to each other at births. . . . Also, the best means of nursing, preventing and curing the diseases of children."]

FALLS, FREDERICK H., *and* MCLAUGHLIN, JANE R.
Obstetric nursing. Kimpton, 1946.

FRENCH, MARGARET
Babies: a book for maternity nurses. Macmillan, 1922.

FULLERTON, ANNA MARTHA
A handbook of obstetric nursing for nurses, students and mothers. 5th edn., rev. Philadelphia, Blakiston, 1899.

GARLAND, GORDON W., *and* QUIXLEY, JOAN M. E.
Obstetrics and gynaecology for nurses. E.U.P., 1956.

GENERAL NURSING COUNCIL *and* CENTRAL MIDWIVES' BOARD
Obstetric training for student nurses. *Nursing Mirror*, Oct. 21, 1960, p. 263-4.

GOODRICH, F. W.
Modern obstetrics and the nurse. *American Journal of Nursing*, May 1957, p. 586-8.

GOW, W. J.
The education of the maternity nurse. *British Journal of Nursing*, Dec. 8, 1906, p. 447-50.

HAYDON, M. OLIVE
The midwife and maternity nurse.
See
NURSING TIMES
The nurse and the nation: a survey of her position in the State today. *Nursing Times*, Nov. 5, 1910, p. 904-31.

HUGHES, AMY
The nursing of maternity cases. *British Journal of Nursing*, Dec. 8, 1906, p. 450-1.

HUMFREY, MARIAN
A manual of obstetric nursing. Sampson Low, Marston, [1898].

JELLETT, HENRY
A short practice of midwifery for nurses, embodying the treatment adopted in the Rotunda Hospital, Dublin. Churchill, 1901.
2nd edn., 1905.
3rd edn., 1908.
4th edn., 1913.
5th edn., 1918.
6th edn., 1922.
7th edn., 1926.
8th edn., 1929.
9th edn., 1933.
10th edn., 1937.
11th edn., 1940.
12th edn., 1942.
13th edn., 1945.
14th edn., 1948, by Henry Jellett and J. Bernard Dawson.
15th edn., 1952, by J. Bernard Dawson.

LESSER, MARION S., *and* KEANE, VERA R.
Nurse-patient relationships in a hospital maternity service. St. Louis, Mosby, 1956.

MAYES, MARY
Handbook for midwives and maternity nurses. Bailliere, Tindall & Cox, 1937.
2nd edn., 1938, rev. by M. A. Gammon.
3rd edn., 1941, rev. by F. D. Thomas.
4th edn., 1953.
5th edn., 1955.

MILLER, DOUGLAS
Midwifery for nurses. Arnold, 1931.
2nd edn., 1937.
3rd edn., 1943.

MILLS, A. C.
The role of the nurse-midwife in Great Britain. *Canadian Nurse*, Nov. 1959, p. 995-9.

MUNRO, E.
Deaths in childbed and our lying-in hospitals, together with a proposal for organizing an institution for training midwives and midwifery nurses. Smith & Elder, 1879.

MYLES, M. F.
Maternity ward sister as clinical teacher. *Nursing Mirror*, July 8, 1960, p. x-xii.

NIGHTINGALE, FLORENCE
Introductory notes on lying-in institutions; together with a proposal for organising an institution for training midwives and midwifery nurses. Longmans, 1871.

PARLIAMENT
Obstetric nurses' registration bill. *Nursing Record*, July 24, 1897, p. 70-1; Aug. 7, 1897, p. 108-9; Aug. 14, 1897, p. 129-30.

PLASS, EVERETT DUDLEY
Obstetrics for nurses. New York, Appleton, 1922.

POPE, GEORGINA
Obstetric nursing.
In
HAMPTON, ISABEL A., *and others*
Nursing of the sick, 1893.

REED, C. B.
Obstetrics for nurses. St. Louis, Mosby, 1917.
2nd edn., 1923.

RIDDING, LAURA
The work of midwives and maternity nurses: its need and organization in rural districts. *Nursing Record*, Oct. 29, 1898, p. 351-3, and Nov. 5, 1898, p. 370-2.

SOLOMONS, BETHEL
Practical midwifery for nurses. O.U.P., 1930.

STATHAM, R. S. S.
An outline of practical obstetrics for nurses. Bristol, Wright, 1933.

VAN BLARCOM, CAROLYN CONANT
Obstetrical nursing. New York, Macmillan, 1922.
2nd edn., 1928.
3rd edn., 1933.
4th edn., 1957, revised by Erna Ziegel.

WARRINGTON, J.
The nurse's guide—containing a series of instructions to females who wish to engage in the important business of nursing mother and child in the lying-in chamber. Philadelphia, Cowperthwaite, 1839.

WHITRIDGE, J., JR.
Nurse-midwife fills a gap in obstetric care. *Modern Hospital*, Nov. 1959, p. 95-8.

WICKHAM, ELIZABETH
Maternity nursing in a nutshell. Philadelphia, Davis, 1924.

WIEDENBACH, ERNESTINE
Family-centred maternity nursing. New York, Putnam, 1958.

WIEDENBACH, ERNESTINE
Nurse-midwifery: purpose, practice and opportunity. *Nursing Outlook*, May 1960, p. 256-9.

WOOD, A. G.
Practical maternity nursing—commonsense in childbirth. For the use of the practical nurse in confinement cases. Chicago, 1927.

WOODWARD, HENRY L., *and* GARDNER, BERNICE
Obstetric management and nursing. Philadelphia, Davis, 1936.
2nd edn., 1940.
3rd edn., 1945.
4th edn., 1950.
5th edn., 1954, revised by Richard D. Bryant and Anne E. Overland.
6th edn., 1959, revised by R. D. Bryant.

ZABRISKIE, LOUISE
Nurse's handbook of obstetrics. Philadelphia, Lippincott, 1929.
2nd edn., 1931.
3rd edn., 1933.
4th edn., 1934.
5th edn., 1937.
6th edn., 1940.
7th edn., 1943, by L. Zabriskie and N. J. Eastman.
8th edn., 1948.
9th edn., 1952.
10th edn., 1960, called "Obstetrics for nurses", by E. Fitzpatrick and N. J. Eastman.

OCCUPATIONAL HEALTH NURSING

AMERICAN ASSOCIATION OF INDUSTRIAL NURSES
Duties and responsibilities of the industrial nurse. New York, The Association, 1949.

AMERICAN ASSOCIATION OF INDUSTRIAL NURSES
Duties and responsibilities of the professional nurse in an industrial medical service. New York, The Association, 1955.

AMERICAN ASSOCIATION OF INDUSTRIAL NURSES
Formation, structure and functions of the American Association of Industrial Nurses, Inc., by R. G. Whitfield. *American Association of Industrial Nurses' Journal*, Feb. 1960, p. 18.

AMERICAN ASSOCIATION OF INDUSTRIAL NURSES
A guide for the industrial nurse to plan a student program.
Part 1. A one-day period of observation in the Industrial Health Service.
Part 2. A one-week period of observation in the Industrial Health Service.
American Association of Industrial Nurses Journal, Sept. 1958, p. 31-5.

AMERICAN ASSOCIATION OF INDUSTRIAL NURSES
Recommended job responsibilities. The Committee on Professional Standards of the A.A.I.N. has prepared a statement on the "Recommended Job Responsibilities" for seven industrial nursing positions. *American Association of Industrial Nurses' Journal*, Dec. 1960, p. 21.

AMERICAN ASSOCIATION OF INDUSTRIAL NURSES
Industrial nursing as students see it. *American Association of Industrial Nurses' Journal*, Sept. 1958, p. 9-12.

AMERICAN BRAKE SHOE COMPANY. MEDICAL DEPARTMENT
Industrial nursing program; manual of procedures. Chicago, The Company, 1945.
4th edn., 1955.

AMERICAN MEDICAL ASSOCIATION. COUNCIL ON INDUSTRIAL HEALTH
Guiding principles and procedures for industrial nurses. Chicago, The Association, 1955.

AMERICAN NURSES' ASSOCIATION. INDUSTRIAL NURSES' SECTION
Functions, standards and qualifications for an industrial nurse in a one-nurse service in industry or commerce. New York, The Association, [1956].

ANDERSON, A.
The changing emphasis in industrial nursing. *American Journal of Nursing*, 1955, p. 35-45.

BARFIELD, K. A.
Teamwork in industry: a successful experiment. *Journal for Industrial Nurses*, Winter 1956-57, p. 181.

BARSCHAK, ERNA
Today's industrial nurse and her job: a study of the functions of nurses and their relationship to industry. New York, Putnam, 1956.

BELKNAP, E. L.
Nurse-doctor team in small industry. *Industrial Medicine and Surgery*, Sept. 1956, p. 429-30.

BOAK, E.
The work of the nurse in industry. *Nursing Times*, April 19, 1957, p. 437-9.

BRAND, M.
What labor expects from industrial nurses. *Nursing Outlook*, April 1958, p. 226-9.

BROWN, MARY LOUISE
Occupational health nursing, by Mary Louise Brown, in collaboration with John Wister Meigs. New York, Springer, 1956.

BROWN, MARY LOUISE, *and* MEIGS, JOHN WISTER
Working with, not for. *Nursing Outlook*, April 1959, p. 201-3.

CALABRO, A. M.
The industrial nurse. *American Association of Industrial Nurses' Journal*, Oct. 1959, p. 9-11.

CANDLAND, L.
How the industrial nurse contributes to accident prevention. *Nursing World*, Feb. 1957, p. 28-9.

CANDLAND, L.
Is occupational health nursing a specialty. *Nursing World*, Feb. 1960, p. 19-22 and 33.

CHARD, S. D.
The nurse in an industrial health service. *Nursing Times*, Aug. 15, 1958, p. 948-50.

CHARD, S. D.
The role of the industrial nurse. *Industrial Welfare*, May-June, 1958, p. 65.

CHARLEY, IRENE H.
The industrial nurse. *Rehabilitation*, Spring 1957, p. 12.

CONNECTICUT STATE DEPARTMENT OF HEALTH.
BUREAU OF INDUSTRIAL HYGIENE
Nursing care of eye injuries and infections in industry. Connecticut, The Bureau, [195?].

COUSENS, H. M.
The role of the nurse in industry. *Rehabilitation*, Oct.-Dec. 1960, p. 9.

CRAGG, M. J.
Nursing services in an atomic research establishment. *Nursing Times*, May 23, 1958, p. 598.

DAMART, L. M.
What an industrial nurse can accomplish. *Journal of the Iowa State Medical Society*, June 1960, p. 302-6.

DELEHANTY, M. E.
The role of the industrial nurse in the plant program. *American Association of Industrial Nurses' Journal*, Jan. 1957, p. 10-13.

DOWSON-WEISSKOPF, A. B.
Industrial nursing: its aims and practice. Arnold, 1944.

DUGGAN, MARY G.
The industrial nurse teaches health. *American Journal of Nursing*, April 1958, p. 537-40.

ELLIOTT, V.
Industrial nursing in Australia. *American Association of Industrial Nurses' Journal*, Jan. 1957, p. 22-4.

FARR, M.
The nurse in the small college. *Student Medicine*, Dec. 1958, p. 159-62.

FERGUSON, LEONA E., and MASTERS, RAYMOND E.
The occupational health nurse and atomic energy. *American Journal of Nursing*, Nov. 1958, p. 1533-5.

GRAHAM, J. C.
The part played by nurses in medical examinations. *Journal for Industrial Nurses*, Jan. 1959, p. 27-34.

GREVILLE, T.
Nursing service: the role of the industrial nurse in accident prevention. *Canadian Nurse*, Feb. 1956, p. 112-3.

HENRIKSEN, HEIDE L.
Nursing service for employees in small plants. *Nursing Outlook*, Nov. 1957, p. 658-60.

HODGSON, VIOLET H.
Public health nursing in industry. New York, Macmillan, 1933.

KILMER, ESTHER W., and RYER, ISABELLE
A health counseling program for small industries. *American Journal of Nursing*, Sept. 1959, p. 1284-7.

LANGLEY, G.
The factory matron. *Nursing Times*, Oct. 21, 1910, p. 1224.

LEE, W. R.
The industrial nurse's part in the patient's return to work. *Journal for Industrial Nurses*, Winter 1959-60, p. 208-11.

The legal scope of industrial nursing practice. *American Journal of Nursing*, July 1959, p. 996-9.

LEMBRIGHT, K. A.
The nurse in small industry. *American Journal of Nursing*, June 1959, p. 829.

MACDONALD, M. GRAY
Handbook of nursing in industry. Philadelphia, Saunders, 1944.

MACDONALD, SARAH
The industrial nurse and her possibilities. *Nursing Times*, Jan. 19, 1918, p. 69-70, and Jan. 26, 1918, p. 97-8.

MCGIRR, P. O. M.
The place of the state-enrolled assistant nurse in industry. *Journal for Industrial Nurses*, Autumn 1958, p. 133.

MCGRATH, BETHEL J.
Nursing in commerce and industry, by B. McGrath, for the National Organization for Public Health Nursing. New York, Commonwealth Fund, 1946.

MAUNDERS, S. H.
Ophthalmic training for nurses in industry. *Journal for Industrial Nurses*, Summer 1958, p. 81.

MUMFORD, ELEANOR W.
Nursing care of eyes in industry. New York, National Society for the Prevention of Blindness, 1943.

NATIONAL ORGANIZATION FOR PUBLIC HEALTH NURSING.
COMMITTEE ON PART-TIME NURSING SERVICE TO INDUSTRY
Part-time nursing in industry as provided by visiting nurse associations in the United States. New York, The Organization [195?].

PEMBERTON, D. A.
A nurse's contribution to preplacement medical examinations for a large industrial concern. *Journal for Industrial Nurses*, Winter 1956-7, p. 189.

PETHER, G. C.
The nurse in industry. *Nursing Times*, Nov. 9, 1956, p. 1145.

PIKE, C. F.
Industrial nursing: a South African experiment. *American Association of Industrial Nurses' Journal*, April 1957, p. 38.

RADWANSKI, D. M.
An industrial nurse in a general hospital occupational health unit. (Description of Central Middlesex Hospital experiment.) *Journal for Industrial Nurses*, Nov.-Dec. 1960, p. 195.

ROYAL COLLEGE OF NURSING
OCCUPATIONAL HEALTH SECTION
Nursing service to industry and commerce: salaries and conditions of service, duties and responsibilities and ethical relationships. The College, 1959.

SMITH, W. D. L.
The industrial nurse and the National Health Service. *Nursing Times*, Aug. 17, 1956, p. 786.

SMITH, WENDELL I.
The industrial nurse: an analysis of her functions. Lewisburg, Bucknell University, 1957.

STEWART, G. A.
The challenges ahead in industrial nursing. *American Association of Industrial Nurses' Journal*, Jan. 1959, p. 8.

SUTTER, R. A.
The nurse's role in health maintenance and accident prevention. *Industrial Medicine and Surgery*, May 1959, p. 238-45.

UBER, W. J.
Radiation and the industrial nurse. *American Association of Industrial Nurses' Journal*, Feb. 1959, p. 29.

WAGNER, S. P.
Industrial nursing and its future. *American Association of Industrial Nurses' Journal*, Aug. 1957, p. 4.

WEST, MARION M.
A handbook for industrial nurses. Arnold, 1941.
2nd edn., 1949.

WHEELER, M. M.
Industrial nursing—demands and scope. *American Association of Industrial Nurses' Journal*, Oct. 1957, p. 11.

WHITLOCK, OLIVE M., TRASKO, VICTORIA M., *and*
KAHL, F. RUTH
Nursing practice in industry. Washington, Govt. Printing Office, 1944.

WILLIAMS, MARGARET M.
Nurse in industry. *Nursing Times*, Feb. 26, 1960, p. 253.

WORLD HEALTH ORGANIZATION.
REGIONAL OFFICE FOR EUROPE
The nurse in industry; report of a seminar sponsored by the International Labour Organization and W.H.O. Regional Office for Europe in collaboration with the Government of the U.K. and Northern Ireland, London, 25 April-4 May 1957. Copenhagen, W.H.O., 1957.

WRIGHT, FLORENCE SWIFT
Industrial nursing for industrial, public health and pupil nurses, and for employers of labor. New York, Macmillan, 1919.

WRIGHT, FLORENCE SWIFT
The visiting nurse in industrial welfare work: an address delivered at the Congress of the National Safety Council, Detroit, 1916. [Detroit, The Council, 1916.]

ADMINISTRATION

AMERICAN ASSOCIATION OF INDUSTRIAL NURSES
Guide for the preparation of a manual of policies and procedures for the professional nurse in industry. New York, The Association, 1957.

AMERICAN ASSOCIATION OF INDUSTRIAL NURSES
Guide for the preparation of recommended personnel practices and policies for industrial nurses. New York, The Association, 1949.

AMERICAN ASSOCIATION OF INDUSTRIAL NURSES
Objectives of an industrial nursing service. New York, The Association, 1955.

AMERICAN ASSOCIATION OF INDUSTRIAL NURSES
Principles of physician-nurse relationship in industry. New York, The Association, 1957.

AMERICAN ASSOCIATION OF INDUSTRIAL NURSES
Recommendations for a professional nurse working without nursing supervision in an industrial medical service. New York, The Association, 1955.

AMERICAN ASSOCIATION OF INDUSTRIAL NURSES
COMMITTEE ON EDUCATION
A guide to interviewing and counseling for the nurses in industry. New York, The Association, 1960.

AMERICAN ASSOCIATION OF INDUSTRIAL NURSES.
MANAGEMENT ADVISORY COUNCIL
Principles of management-nurse relationships in industry. New York, The Association, 1957.

AMERICAN CONFERENCE OF GOVERNMENTAL INDUSTRIAL HYGIENISTS
The nursing consultant in occupational health. Minneapolis, Minnesota State Department of Health, 1954.

BAILEY, ELEANOR C., *and* FRASIER, ELIZABETH S.
A time study. Nursing services in small manufacturing plants. Washington, Govt. Printing Office, 1952.

BEWS, D. C.
Effective utilization of nurses in industry. *American Association of Industrial Nurses' Journal*, Oct. 1957, p. 23.

BROWN, MARY LOUISE
The educational responsibilities of the nurse consultant in occupational health. New York, National League of Nursing Education, 1956.

BROWN, MARY LOUISE
Leadership positions in occupational health nursing. *Nursing Outlook*, Mar. 1958, p. 164.

BROWN, MARY LOUISE
Occupational health nursing manpower. *Industrial Medicine and Surgery*, Dec. 1959, p. 548-50.

BUTTERLEY COMPANY. MEDICAL DEPARTMENT
Manual for nursing officers. [Derby], The Company, [1946].

CAMERON, DALE
Human relations in occupational health. *International Nursing Review*, April 1955, p. 25-8.

CANADA. DEPARTMENT OF NATIONAL HEALTH.
CIVIL SERVICE HEALTH DIVISION
Evaluating an occupational health nursing program by a work sampling study. Ottawa, Department of National Health, 1960.

EPSTEIN, CHARLOTTE
Intergroup relations in occupational health nursing. *Canadian Nurse*, Nov. 1960, p. 1010-20.

GORDON, ETHEL M., *and* HUFFMAN, VERNA M.
Evaluating an occupational health nursing program by a work sampling study. *Canadian Nurse*, April 1960, p. 314-20.

KLUTAS, EDNA MAY
Nursing supervision in industry. New York, National League for Nursing, 1958.

MINNESOTA UNIVERSITY. CENTER FOR CONTINUATION STUDY
Guide for the orientation of newly employed occupational health nurses, prepared by Minnesota occupational health nurses at the Center . . . 1955. New York, National League for Nursing, 1956.

PARKER, C.
The interview in industrial nursing. *Nursing Outlook*, June 1958, p. 345-7.

PERKINS, D. T.
Counseling in occupational health nursing. *American Journal of Nursing*, Aug. 1957, p. 1024-6.

WATSON, E.
What is the industrial nurse's role in counseling. *American Association of Industrial Nurses' Journal*, Aug. 1960, p. 30.

EDUCATION

AMERICAN ASSOCIATION OF INDUSTRIAL NURSES
Criteria for evaluation of programs of study in industrial nursing. New York, The Association, 1949.

AMERICAN ASSOCIATION OF INDUSTRIAL NURSES
Qualifications for an industrial nurse. New York, The Association, 1950.

AMERICAN ASSOCIATION OF INDUSTRIAL NURSES
Recommended qualifications for a professional nurse working with nursing supervision in an industrial medical service. New York, The Association, 1955.

AMERICAN ASSOCIATION OF INDUSTRIAL NURSES
Recommended qualifications for industrial nurses working without nursing supervision. New York, The Association, 1950.

AMERICAN ASSOCIATION OF INDUSTRIAL NURSES *and*
NATIONAL LEAGUE FOR NURSING
Guide for evaluating and teaching occupational health nursing concepts. New York, The League, 1956.

AMOR, A. J., *and* SYKES, CLARE
Training of the industrial nurse. *British Journal of Industrial Medicine*, April 1944, p. 81-9.

FELTON, J. S.
Educational trends in industrial nursing. *Nursing Outlook*, Nov. 1957, p. 655-7.

SPECIALITIES

HENRIKSEN, HEIDE L.
Curriculum study of the occupational health aspects of nursing; an adventure in co-operation. A report of an educational project in six collegiate schools of nursing in Minnesota. Minneapolis, Minnesota League for Nursing, 1959.

HENRIKSEN, HEIDE L., and NATTESTAD, L.
Education for cardiac nursing in industry. *American Journal of Nursing*, Dec. 1959, p. 1726-9.

LANE, RONALD E.
The education and function of the industrial health team. Reprinted from *British Journal of Industrial Medicine*, Oct. 1950.

SAYNAJARVI, RUTH
The professional education of the occupational health nurse in Finland. *Journal for Industrial Nurses*, Autumn 1957, p. 133-135.

SIMPSON, H. MARJORIE
Education and the occupational health nurse. *Journal for Industrial Nurses*, Autumn 1957, p. 124-132.

SIMPSON, H. MARJORIE
Education and training of industrial nurses in various European countries. *Journal for Industrial Nurses*, Nov.-Dec. 1960, p. 202-209.

SMITH, EMILY MYRTLE
Occupational health integration in the Yale University School of Nursing: a curriculum appraisal, November 1949-June 1951. New York, National League of Nursing Education, 1952.

YINGLING, D. B.
Educational opportunities for industrial nurses. *Journal of Occupational Medicine*, July 1960, p. 325-6.

OPHTHALMIC NURSING

COLE, GLADYS ELAINE
Wills Hospital eye manual for nurses. Philadelphia, Saunders, 1936.

DOGGART, JAMES HAMILTON
Children's eye nursing. Kimpton, 1948.

EDWARDS, R.
Care and management of the ophthalmic patient in hospital. *Nursing Times*, June 8, 1956, p. 511.

ELMS, JESSIE
Nursing of diseases of the eye: a simple treatise for nurses. Scientific Press, 1922.

EVANS, P. J.
Modern trends in ophthalmic surgery and nursing. *Nursing Times*, June 8, 1956, p. 506.

FARFOR, UNA C. M.
Aids to ophthalmic nursing. Bailliere, Tindall & Cox, 1956.

FOSTER, J. B.
Ophthalmic nursing. Sydney, Angus & Robertson, 1959.

GARLAND, PHYLLIS
Ophthalmic nursing. Faber, 1950.
2nd edn., 1954.
3rd edn., 1956.

GRAND, D. E.
Ophthalmic nursing. Edinburgh, Livingstone, 1938.

LEWIS, G. GRIFFIN
The ophthalmic nurse. Philadelphia, Saunders, 1920.

NATIONAL SOCIETY FOR THE PREVENTION OF BLINDNESS
Eye health; a teaching handbook for nurses. New York, The Society, 1945.

OPHTHALMIC NURSING BOARD
Diploma of ophthalmic nursing: conditions and syllabus of training. *Nursing Mirror*, May 30, 1952, p. 205.

OPHTHALMIC NURSING BOARD
The work of the Ophthalmic Nursing Board. *Nursing Times*, Feb. 14, 1958, p. 190.

STALLARD, H. B., and others
Principles and practice of ophthalmic nursing. *Nursing Mirror*, Jan. 21, 1955, p. vi; Jan. 28, 1955, p. vi; Feb. 4, 1955, p. v; Feb. 11, 1955, p. x; Feb. 18, 1955, p. v; Feb. 25, 1955, p. xiii.

WHITING, MAURICE H.
Ophthalmic nursing. Churchill, 1926.
2nd edn., 1935.
4th edn., 1945.
5th edn., 1948.
6th edn., 1951.
7th edn., 1959.

PAEDIATRIC NURSING

APLEY, J.
Cold babies and the nurse's responsibility. *Nursing Mirror*, April 15, 1960, p. 242-3.

ARLITT, ADA HART
Pediatric nursing. 2nd edn. New York, Macmillan, 1930.

ARMSTRONG, INEZ L., and BROWDER, JANE J.
The nursing care of children. Philadelphia, Davis, 1960

AUFHAUSER, T.
When comprehensive child care counts. *Nursing Outlook*, Oct. 1957, p. 601-4.

BAHIRATHI, —
Pediatric nursing. IV. *Indian Journal of Pediatrics*, Feb. 1957, p. 41-3.

BALDWIN, JOHN C.
Pediatrics for nurses. New York, Appleton, 1924.

BENZ, GLADYS S.
Pediatric nursing. St. Louis, Mosby, 1948.
2nd edn., 1953.
3rd edn., 1956.
4th edn., 1960.

BLAKE, FLORENCE
The child, his parents and the nurse. Philadelphia, Lippincott, 1954.

CADOGAN, WILLIAM
An essay upon nursing and the management of children from their birth to three years of age in a letter to one of the Governors of the Foundling Hospital. 2nd edn. Roberts, 1748.

CAPLAN, H., and DIMOCK, H. G.
The student nurse in a pediatric setting. *Canadian Nurse*, Dec. 1956, p. 959-62.

Challenges, new and old, in the nursing of children. *Journal of the Christian Medical Association of India*, Sept. 1957, p. 258-60.

CLARK, F. LE GROS
ABC of food and child feeding: a short introduction for the use of student nurses and others. National Society of Children's Nurseries, [1955?].

CRAIG, WILLIAM STEWART, and others
Nursing care of the newly born infant. Edinburgh, Livingstone, 1955.

CRAIG, WILLIAM STEWART
Trends in the nursing care of the sick child. *Nursing Mirror*, June 11, 1954, p. ii; June 18, 1954, p. ii; June 25, 1954, p. xi.

CUTLER, BESSIE INGERSOLL
Pediatric nursing: its principles and practice. New York, Macmillan, 1923. Later edns. by M. Corinne Bancroft, Elizabeth Pierce, and Bessie Cutler.
2nd edn., 1931.
3rd edn., 1938.

DESJARDINS, MARIETTE
Pediatric surgical nursing. *Canadian Nurse*, Oct. 1959, p. 896-9.

ERXLEBEN, MARGUERITE C.
Notes on children's nursing. Philadelphia, Davis, 1931.

FARROW, RAYMOND
The surgery of childhood for nurses. Edinburgh, Livingstone, 1956.

FOSTER, L. M.
Introducing pre-nursing students to pediatrics. *Nursing Outlook*, Sept. 1956, p. 502-4.

GILSON, M., and MATSON, D. D.
Care of a child after an arachnoid-ureteral shunt. *American Journal of Nursing*, Nov. 1956, p. 1424-6.

GRAHAM, —
The role of the nurse in pediatrics. *Indian Journal of Pediatrics*, July 1956, p. 245-8.

GREAT ORMOND STREET HOSPITAL FOR SICK CHILDREN
How to nurse sick children: intended especially as a help to the nurses at the Hospital for Sick Children, but containing directions which may be found of service to all who have charge of the young. New York, 1855.

HEWER, J. LANGTON
Our baby: for mothers and nurses. Bristol, Wright, 1891.
22nd edn., 1942, rev. by Margaret Scott-Brown.
23rd edn., 1945, rev. by Margaret Scott-Brown.

JACKSON, QUEENIE M.
A handbook of paediatrics for nurses in general training. Lewis, 1952.
2nd edn., 1960.

JEANS, PHILIP C., and others
Essentials of pediatrics, by Philip C. Jeans, F. Howell Wright and Florence G. Blake. Philadelphia, Lippincott, 1934.
2nd edn., 1936.
3rd edn., 1939.
4th edn., 1946.
5th edn., 1954.
6th edn., 1958.

KENNEDY, D. A.
The care and nursing of the infant for infant welfare workers and nursery nurses. Heinemann, 1930.

KESSEL, I.
The essentials of paediatrics for nurses. Edinburgh, Livingstone, 1957.

LEACH, MARGARET M.
Children in hospital: paediatrics for the general hospital nurse. Faber, 1956.

LOVELY, EVELYN M.
The nursing of sick children. Edinburgh, Livingstone, 1951.

LYON, ROBERT A., and WALLINGER, ELGIE M.
Nursing of children. Philadelphia, Saunders, 1939.
5th edn., 1959.

McCOMBS, ROBERT SHELMERDINE
Diseases of children for nurses, including infant feeding, therapeutic measures employed in childhood, treatment for emergencies, prophylaxis, hygiene and nursing. Philadelphia, Saunders, 1907.

MacNAB, G. H.
Pre- and post-operative care of intussusception in infants. *Nursing Mirror*, July 29, 1955, p. ii.

MITCHELL, ALBERT GRAEME
Mitchell's pediatrics and pediatric nursing, by E. K. Upham and E. M. Wallinger. Philadelphia, Saunders, 1939.
2nd edn., 1944, by Robert A. Lyon and Winifred Kattenbach.
3rd edn., 1949, by Robert A. Lyon and E. M. Wallinger.
4th edn., 1954.

MONCRIEFF, ALAN, editor
A textbook on the nursing and diseases of sick children for nurses and welfare workers. Lewis, 1930.
3rd edn., 1941.
4th edn., 1947.
5th edn., 1952.
6th edn., 1957, edited by A. Moncrieff and A. P. Norman.

NICKOLLS, —
Paediatric nursing curriculum. *Indian Journal of Pediatrics*, June 1958, p. 371-3.

OUELLET, FRANÇOISE MILLER
Play therapy and the nurse. *Canadian Nurse*, April 1960, p. 342-50, and May 1960, p. 444-6.

PERKINS, RUTH ALICE
Essentials of pediatric nursing. Philadelphia, Davis, 1930.
2nd edn., 1932.

POHOWALLA, J. N.
Paediatric nursing. II. *Indian Journal of Pediatrics*, Feb. 1957, p. 33-6.

PRABHU, M. B.
Pediatric nursing. I. *Indian Journal of Pediatrics*, Feb. 1957, p. 31-2.

PRITCHARD, ERIC
The new-born baby: a manual for the use of midwives and maternity nurses. Kimpton, 1934.

ROBINSON, P.
Millions of pediatric nurses. III. *Indian Journal of Pediatrics*, Feb. 1957, p. 37-40.

ROSS, A.
The pediatric setting. *Canadian Nurse*, Dec. 1956, p. 955.

SAUER, LOUIS W.
Nursery guide: a vade-mecum on infant and child care. Kimpton, 1923.
2nd edn., 1926.
3rd edn., 1933.

SCHIFF, S.
Gaining a child's confidence. *American Journal of Nursing*, Dec. 1959, p. 1748-9.

SELLEW, GLADYS
Nursing of children. Philadelphia, Saunders, 1943.
7th edn., 1953, by Gladys Sellew and Mary F. Pepper.

SELLEW, GLADYS
Pediatric nursing, including the nursing care of the well infant and child. Philadelphia, Saunders, 1926.

TODD, R. McL.
Child health and paediatrics for nurses, health visitors and social workers. Heinemann, 1958.

URBAN LIFE RESEARCH INSTITUTE
Nursing services in a premature infant center. New Orleans, Tulane University, 1953.

WATKINS, ARTHUR G.
Paediatrics for nurses. Bristol, Wright, 1947.
2nd edn., 1958.

WEST, CHARLES
How to nurse sick children, with a preface by George F. Still. Longmans, 1852.
2nd edn., 1860.
New edn., 1908.

WOOD, CATHERINE JANE
A handbook on the nursing of sick children. Cassell, 1890.

WOOD, CATHERINE JANE
The training of nurses for sick children. *Nursing Record*, Dec. 6, 1888, p. 507-10.

WORTHAM, E. D., and RITCHIE, G.
Nursing care of children after open heart surgery. *American Journal of Nursing*, Feb. 1958, p. 203-4.

YAPP, C. SEYMOUR
Children's nursing. Poor-law Publications, 1920.

CHILDREN IN HOSPITAL

CAPES, MARY
The child in hospital. *W.H.O. Bulletin*, vol. 12, no. 3, 1955.

CENTRAL HEALTH SERVICES COUNCIL
The welfare of children in hospital; report of the committee. H.M.S.O., 1959.

DIMOCK, HEDLEY, G.
The child in hospital; a study of his emotional and social well-being. Toronto, Macmillan, 1959.

ERICKSON, F.
Reactions of children to hospital experience. *Nursing Outlook*, Sept. 1958, p. 501-4.

FAUGHNAN, J. E.
The child in hospital. *Canadian Nurse*, Dec. 1956, p. 956-9.

GODFREY, ANN E.
A study of nursing care designed to assist hospitalized children and their parents in their separation. *Nursing Research*, Oct. 1955, p. 52-70.

JAMES, C. F.
The parents' point of view. *Canadian Nurse*, Dec. 1956, p. 963-6.

ROYAL COLLEGE OF PHYSICIANS OF LONDON.
PAEDIATRIC COMMITTEE
Report on the care of children in hospital. Royal College of Physicians of London, [1957].

SWIFT, A., COMPTON, D. E., and JAMES, H. M.
Symposium on children in hospital: preparation and aftercare. *Royal Society for the Promotion of Health Journal*, Sept.-Oct. 1959, p. 561-75.

HANDICAPPED CHILDREN

BURR, ANITA M.
Learning to care for mentally retarded children. *American Journal of Nursing*, July 1960, p. 1000-3.

KENNEDY, MILLICENT V., and SOMERSET, H. C. D.
Bringing up crippled children: suggestions for parents, teachers and nurses. New Zealand Council for Educational Research in association with New Zealand Crippled Children Society, 1951.

McBRIDE, EARL DUWAIN
Crippled children, their treatment and orthopaedic nursing. St. Louis, Mosby, 1931.
2nd edn., 1937, in collaboration with Winifred R. Sink.

MARTINEZ, RUTH E.
The nurse as group psychotherapist. *American Journal of Nursing*, Dec. 1958, p. 1681-2.

WEST, JESSIE STEVENSON
Congenital malformations and birth injuries: a handbook on nursing. New York, Association for the Aid of Crippled Children, 1954.

HOSPITAL HOME CARE

BIRMINGHAM CHILDREN'S HOSPITAL
Domiciilary nursing service for infants and children, by J. M. Smellie. *British Medical Journal*, May 5, 1956, p. 256, supp.

ROTHERHAM COUNTY BOROUGH COUNCIL
Nursing of sick children at home. The Rotherham plan. *Hospital and Social Service Journal*, Feb. 12, 1954, p. 177; *Nursing Times*, June 3, 1955, p. 619.

ROTHERHAM COUNTY BOROUGH COUNCIL
Nursing sick children at home. The Rotherham scheme, by V. McCarthy. *Nursing Times*, July 10, 1954, p. 735.

ROTHERHAM COUNTY BOROUGH COUNCIL
A children's home nursing unit. The Rotherham scheme, by J. A. Gillet. *Medical Officer*, Feb. 19, 1954, p. 85; *British Medical Journal*, Mar. 20, 1954, p. 684; *Mother and Child*, Nov. 1955, p. 194.

ST. MARY'S HOSPITAL, PADDINGTON
Home care scheme for sick children. *Nursing Times*, Oct. 28, 1960, p. 1337.

ST. MARY'S HOSPITAL, PADDINGTON
Nursing seriously ill children at home. Description of scheme in operation at St. Mary's Hospital, Paddington, by J. A. Davis and J. Campbell. *Nursing Mirror*, July 12, 1957, p. iii.

ST. MARY'S HOSPITAL, PADDINGTON
A London trial of home care for sick children. A description of the St. Mary's Paddington Hospital home nursing scheme, by R. Lightwood and others. *Lancet*, Feb. 9, 1957, p. 313.

ST. MARY'S HOSPITAL, PADDINGTON
The St. Mary's Hospital home-care for sick children scheme, by C. R. McClure. *Public Health*, May 1960, p. 313-7.

MATERNAL AND CHILD HEALTH

ADAMS, MARTHA L., and DISBROW, MILDRED
A method of teaching maternal child health nursing. *Nursing Outlook*, July 1960, p. 390-1.

ADAMS, M. M.
New approaches to teaching maternity and pediatric nursing. *Nursing Outlook*, Nov. 1956, p. 631-3.

CALIFORNIA STATE. DEPARTMENT OF PUBLIC HEALTH
Hospital nursing care of mothers and babies. Berkeley, California, Department of Public Health, 1957.
[Revision of "A guide to nursing care for maternity patients and newborn infants in hospitals", 1950.]

CASSIE, ETHEL
Maternity and child welfare: a textbook for public health workers. Lewis, 1929.

CRABBE, VIOLET EYRE
The nurse in schools for mothers.
See
NURSING TIMES
The nurse and the nation: a survey of her position in the State today. *Nursing Times*, Nov. 5, 1910, p. 904-31.

CRAIG, M.
Child care in the outback. *American Journal of Nursing*, Dec. 1958, p. 1696-8.

SLEDGE, MADGE, and BARTON, PAULINE HINTON
A masters program in maternal and child health nursing. *Nursing Outlook*, Aug. 1960, p. 453-5.

TAYLOR, RUTH G.
Some significant developments in maternal and child health nursing. *Nursing Outlook*, Aug. 1960, p. 442-7.

PREMATURE BABIES

DUCHESS OF YORK HOSPITAL FOR BABIES, MANCHESTER
Nursing methods in use in the Catherine Chisholm Premature Babies Unit.... Manchester, The Hospital, 1952.

GEDDES, A. K.
Premature babies: their nursing care and management. Philadelphia, Saunders, 1960.

HESS, JULIUS H., and LUNDEEN, EVELYN C.
The premature infant: its medical and nursing care. Philadelphia, Lippincott, 1941.
2nd edn., 1949.

PATHOLOGY

EDEN, A. J.
Pathology and the nurse.
1. Haematology.
2. Bacteriology.
3. Chemical pathology.
Nursing Mirror, Sept. 14, 1956, p. ii; Sept. 21, 1956, p. iii; Sept. 28, 1956, p. xi.

GOODALE, RAYMOND
Nursing pathology. Philadelphia, Saunders, 1948.
2nd edn., 1956.

RABIN, COLEMAN B.
A textbook of pathology for nurses. Philadelphia, Saunders, 1934.
2nd edn., rev., 1939.

PHYSICS

BLISS, A. R., *and* OLIVE, A. H.
A textbook of physics and chemistry for nurses. Philadelphia, 1916.
2nd edn., 1918.

FLITTER, HESSEL HOWARD
An introduction to physics in nursing. St. Louis, Mosby, 1948.
2nd edn., 1954.
3rd edn., 1958.

GOODNOW, MINNIE
Practical physics for nurses. Philadelphia, Saunders, 1919.

LEE, JULIETTE THELMA, *and* SEWALL, ANNA MAE
A manual of selected physics topics for students of nursing. Minneapolis, Burgess, 1949.

SACKHEIM, GEORGE I.
Practical physics for nurses. Philadelphia, Saunders, 1957.

WATERS, MURIEL
Elementary physics for nurses. Faber, 1939.

PSYCHIATRIC NURSING

ADAMSON, F. K.
The psychiatric nurse in the outpatient psychiatric clinic. *Nursing Outlook*, Jan. 1957, p. 24-7.

ALLAN MEMORIAL INSTITUTE OF PSYCHIATRY.
McGILL UNIVERSITY
Psychiatric nursing in general hospitals: proceedings of the first Canadian Conference on Nursing in Psychiatric Divisions of General Hospitals, Nov. 1958. Montreal, McGill University, 1958.

ALTSCHUL, A.
Aids to psychiatric nursing. Bailliere, Tindall & Cox, 1957.

AYLLON, T., *and* MICHAEL, J.
The psychiatric nurse as a behavioural engineer. *Journal of the Experimental Analysis of Behavior*, Oct. 1959, p. 323-4.

BAILEY, HARRIET
Nursing mental diseases. New York, Macmillan, 1920.
2nd edn., 1929.
3rd edn., 1937.
4th edn., 1939.

BARCKLEY, VIRGINIA
The nurse in preventive psychiatry. *Nursing Outlook*, May 1960, p. 252-4.

BARRUS, CLARA
Nursing the insane. New York, Macmillan, 1908.

BECCLE, H. C.
Psychiatry: theory and practice for nurses. Faber, 1946.
2nd edn., 1948.
3rd edn., 1953.
4th edn., 1958.

BENNETT, A. E., *and* ENGLE, B.
Psychiatric nursing and occupational therapy. *Progress in Neurology and Psychiatry*. vol. 11, 1956, p. 457-66.

BENNETT, A. E., *and* PURDY, AVIS B.
Psychiatric nursing technique. Philadelphia, Davis, 1940.

BLACK, KATHLEEN
Nursing in a psychiatric hospital. *Mental Hygiene*, Oct. 1955, p. 533-44.

BLAIR, D.
The psychoneurotic patient and the mental nurse. *Nursing Mirror*, Dec. 16, 1955, p. 749-50.

BOGIE, HAZEL
Nursing emotionally disturbed patients. 4. Nursing the new patient. *Nursing Times*, June 14, p. 659-60.

BRASS, R., *and others*
The mixed unit for long-stay regressed mental patients. *Nursing Mirror*, Oct. 11, 1957, p. vi.

BROWN, MARTHA MONTGOMERY, *and* FOWLER, GRACE R.
Psychodynamic nursing. Philadelphia, Saunders, 1954.

CARMICHAEL, F. A., *and* CHAPMAN, JOHN
A guide to psychiatric nursing. Philadelphia, Lea & Febiger, 1936.

CHADWICK, MARY
Nursing psychological patients. Allen & Unwin, 1931.

CHAPMAN, —
Asylum nursing. *Nursing Record*, June 14, 1902, p. 474-6.

COSTELLO, C. G.
The role of the nurse in a psychiatric unit. *Canadian Nurse*, May 1958, p. 411-3.

DAX, E. CUNNINGHAM
Modern mental treatment: a handbook for nurses. Faber, 1947.

EAGER, RICHARD
Hints to probationer nurses in mental hospitals: with a brief introduction to psychology with an additional chapter on the organization of occupation, recreation and amusement. Lewis, 1922.
3rd edn., 1939.

EBAUGH, FRANKLIN G.
The care of the psychiatric patient in general hospitals. Chicago, American Hospital Association, 1940.

ELLES, G. W.
Nursing emotionally disturbed patients—8. *Nursing Times*, July 12, 1957, p. 780-1.

EVANS, B. L.
Psychiatry in modern nursing. *Journal of the Christian Medical Association of India*, Mar. 1960, p. 153-8.

FISHER, J. W.
Modern methods of mental treatment: a guide for nurses. Staples Press, [1948?].

FORRER, G. R., *and* GRISELL, J. L.
Patient improvement and psychiatric nursing care. *Diseases of the Nervous System*, Aug. 1959, p. 357-63.

FRENCH, MARY ANNE
The visiting nurse in a psychiatric program. *Nursing Outlook*, Oct. 1956, p. 572-4.

FREY, L. M.
Psychiatric nursing. *American Journal of Psychiatry*, Jan. 1958, p. 630-2.

GAZDAR, E. JEANETTE
Nursing emotionally disturbed patients, 6. *Nursing Times*, June 28, 1957, p. 717-18.

GLEESON, I.
Nursing emotionally disturbed patients—7. *Nursing Times*, July 5, 1957, p. 745.

GRANT-SMITH, RACHEL
The experiences of an asylum patient. Allen & Unwin, 1922.

GRIFFITH, OLIVE F.
The present position of mental nursing in England. *British Medical Bulletin*, vol. 6, no. 3, 1949.

GROUP FOR THE ADVANCEMENT OF PSYCHIATRY.
COMMITTEE ON PSYCHIATRIC NURSING
Therapeutic use of self: a concept for teaching patient care. Topeka, Kansas, The Group, 1955.

GROUP FOR THE ADVANCEMENT OF PSYCHIATRY.
COMMITTEE ON PSYCHIATRIC NURSING *and*
COMMITTEE ON HOSPITALS
The psychiatric nurse in the mental hospital. Topeka, Kansas, The Group, 1952.

HALL, B. H.
A colleague looks at psychiatric nursing. *Nursing Outlook*, Feb. 1954, p. 66-9.

HARRIS, PAUL, *editor*
Handbook for psychiatric aides. New York, National Association for Mental Health, 1950.

HEAD, PHOEBE
The nurse in mental hospitals.
See
NURSING TIMES
The nurse and the nation: a survey of her position in the State today. *Nursing Times*, Nov. 5, 1910, p. 904-31.

HEADLEE, RAYMOND, *and* COREY, BONNIE WELLS
Psychiatry in nursing. New York, Rhinehart, 1948.

HIRD, N. G.
Re-socialisation of chronic mental patients by reciprocal interaction. *Nursing Mirror*, Feb. 6, 1959, p. iii.

HOFLING, CHARLES K., *and* LEININGER, MADELEINE M.
Basic psychiatric concepts in nursing. Philadelphia, Lippincott, [c. 1960].

HOLLANDER, BERNARD
Mental nursing. *British Journal of Nursing*, June 18, 1910, p. 487-8, and June 25, 1910, p. 508-9.

HOULISTON, MAY
The practice of mental nursing. Edinburgh, Livingstone, 1947.
2nd edn., 1955.

HYDE, ROBERT W.
Experiencing the patients' day: a manual for psychiatric hospital personnel.... New York, Putnam, 1955.

INGRAM, MADALENE ELLIOTT
Principles of psychiatric nursing. Philadelphia, Saunders, 1939.
2nd edn., 1944.
3rd edn., 1949.
4th edn., 1955, called "Principles and technique of psychiatric nursing".
5th edn., 1960.

INTERDEPARTMENTAL COMMITTEE ON NURSING SERVICES.
SUB-COMMITTEE ON MENTAL NURSING AND THE NURSING
OF THE MENTALLY DEFECTIVE
Report.... H.M.S.O., 1945.

IZZARD, W. P.
A study of therapeutic meetings in a neurosis hospital. *Nursing Mirror*, Dec. 7, 1956, p. 699.
[Belmont Hospital, Surrey, experiment in group therapy.]

JENKINS, S. B.
The use of group therapeutic methods in ward conferences with attendants: an aid to patients' ward adjustments. *Psychiatric Quarterly Supplement*, 1957, p. 312-7.

JONES, M., *and* SKELLERN, EILEEN
Social rehabilitation: a joint project of patients and staff. *Nursing Mirror*, Aug. 23, 1957, p. 1497.
[An experiment at Belmont Hospital, Surrey.]

KALKMAN, MARION E.
Interpreting psychiatric nursing to the public. *American Journal of Nursing*, Nov. 1955, p. 1359-61.

KALKMAN, MARION E.
Introduction to psychiatric nursing. New York, McGraw-Hill, 1950.
2nd edn., 1958.

KAPLAN, STANLEY M., *and* PLOGSTED, HELEN
The nurse and psychosomatic medicine. *Nursing Outlook*, April 1957, p. 207-9.

KARNOSH, LOUIS J., *and* GAGE, EDITH B.
Psychiatry for nurses. Kimpton, 1940.
2nd edn., 1944.
3rd edn., 1949.
4th edn., 1953, by Louis J. Karnosh and Dorothy Mereness.
5th edn., 1958.

LAIRD, S. LOUISE
Nursing of the insane. *Nursing Record*, Mar. 1, 1902, p. 166-8, and Mar. 8, 1902, p. 185-7.

LAMB, J. T.
Freedom for patients in mental hospitals. *American Journal of Nursing*, Mar. 1958, p. 358-60.

LANCET
Mental nursing: a new beginning. *Lancet*, Jan. 16, 1954, p. 139-41.

LANCET
Mental nursing revived? *Lancet*, July 25, 1953, p. 176-7.

LAWRENCE, B.
A psychiatric ward in a general hospital. *Nursing Times*, Oct. 18, 1957, p. 1185-7.

LEMKAU, P. V.
Follow-up services for psychiatric patients. *Nursing Outlook*, Mar. 1958, p. 148-50.

LISTON, M. F.
Psychiatric nursing. *American Journal of Psychiatry*, Jan. 1960, p. 641-4.

MACCALMAN, D. R.
Ideals in mental nursing. *Nursing Mirror*, Oct. 12, 1956, p. 111.

MACDONALD, J. M., *and* DANIELS, M. L.
The psychiatric ward as a therapeutic community. *Journal of Nervous and Mental Disease*, Aug. 1957, p. 148-55.

McGHIE, ANDREW
The role of the mental nurse.
1. Historical development.
2. The nursing attitude.
3. Differences in nursing attitude.
4. Future developments.
Nursing Mirror, May 17, 1957, p. xiii; May 24, 1957, p. xi-xii; May 31, 1957, p. xiii; June 7, 1957, p. xi.

MACDOUGALL, A. A., *and* CAMPBELL, D.
New technique in electro-convulsant therapy.
1. From the nursing point of view.
2. From the nursing point of view (cont.).
3. Old and new methods compared.
4. Use of methods in various mental diseases.
5. Use of methods in various mental diseases (cont.).
Nursing Mirror, Nov. 15, 1957, p. iii; Nov. 22, 1957, p. viii; Nov. 29, 1957, p. xi; Dec. 6, 1957, p. xi; Dec. 13, 1957, p. xi.

McGREGOR, E. M.
Is psychiatric nursing at the crossroads. *Nursing World*, April 1958, p. 29-33.

MADDOX, H.
The work of mental nurses. *Nursing Mirror*, April 19, 1957, p. 189-90.

MANCHESTER REGIONAL HOSPITAL BOARD AND
MANCHESTER UNIVERSITY
The work of the mental nurse: a survey organized by a joint committee of the Manchester R.H.B. and the University of Manchester. Manchester University Press, 1955.

MANDELBROTE, B.
Development of a comprehensive psychiatric community service around the mental hospital. *Mental Hygiene*, July 1959, p. 368-77.

MARCHESINI, E. H.
The widening horizon in psychiatric nursing. *American Journal of Nursing*, July 1959, p. 978-81.

MARTIN, D. V.
The mental hospital as a therapeutic community: the role of the nurse. *Nursing Mirror*, Aug. 15, 1958, p.v.

MARWICK, I. I.
General and psychiatric nursing—why they should be integrated. *Nursing Times*, Sept. 26, 1958, p. 1117-9.

MATHENEY, RUTH V., and TOPALIS, MARY
Psychiatric nursing. St. Louis, Mosby, 1953.
2nd edn., 1957.

MEIR, E.
The role of the student nurse in a mental hospital. *Nursing Times*, Feb. 14, 1958, p. 183-4 and 189-90.

MILLS, C. K.
Practical lessons in nursing. The nursing and care of the nervous and the insane. Philadelphia, . . . 1887.

MINSKI, LOUIS
A practical handbook of psychiatry for students and nurses. Heinemann, 1946.
2nd edn., 1950.
3rd edn., 1956.
4th edn., 1959.

MITCHELL, S. D.
Use of music in psychiatry. *Nursing Mirror*, Mar. 27, 1953, p. vi.

MONTREAL ROYAL VICTORIA HOSPITAL and
MCGILL UNIVERSITY
Nursing in psychiatric divisions of general hospitals. *Canadian Nurse*, Mar. 1959, p. 250-54.

MORRISON, L. J.
One approach to psychotherapeutic nursing. *Nursing World*, Aug. 1956, p. 9-13.

MULLER, THERESA GRACE, editor
Mental health in nursing: psychological approach. Washington, Catholic University of America Press, 1949.

MULLER, THERESA GRACE
The nature and direction of psychiatric nursing: the dynamics of human relationships in nursing. Philadelphia, Lippincott, 1950.

NORTH CAROLINA UNIVERSITY.
INSTITUTE FOR RESEARCH IN SOCIAL SCIENCE
Patterns of psychiatric nursing: a survey of psychiatric nursing in North Carolina; [by] Harry W. Martin and Ida Harper Simpson. North Carolina, [Chapel Hill], 1956.

NOYES, ARTHUR P.
Textbook of psychiatry. New York, Macmillan, 1927.
2nd edn., 1936.
3rd edn., 1940, by A. P. Noyes and Edith M. Haydon.
4th edn., 1946, by A. P. Noyes and E. M. Haydon, called "Textbook of psychiatric nursing".
5th edn., 1957, by A. P. Noyes, E. M. Haydon and Mildred van Sickel.

NURSING TIMES
Psychiatric nursing—a challenge and an invitation. *Nursing Times*, June 24, 1950, p. 650-2 and 657.

PEARN, O. P. NAPIER
Mental nursing (simplified). Bailliere, Tindall & Cox, 1931.
2nd edn., 1936.
3rd edn., 1942.
4th edn., 1956, rev. by Edward S. Stern and Violet A. Spratley.

PEPLAU, HILDEGARDE E.
Present-day trends in psychiatric nursing. *Neuropsychiatry*, Spring 1956, p. 190-204.

PIERCE, BEDFORD, editor
Addresses to mental nurses: a series of fifteen lectures delivered to the nursing staff of the Retreat, York, by various authorities. Bailliere, Tindall & Cox, 1924.

POLLARD, J. C.
The psychiatric nurse and the adolescent; the problem of testing. *Canadian Nurse*, May 1958, p. 417-9.

POTTER, H. W., and KLEIN, H. R.
On nursing behaviour. *Psychiatry*, Feb. 1957, p. 39-46.

REES, T. P.
The important role of the nurse in modern mental treatment. *Nursing Mirror*, Sept. 5, 1952, p. 495-6.

REGISTRATION OF ASYLUM ATTENDANTS AS NURSES
Report of a public meeting held on Jan. 7th at St. Martin's Town Hall to consider the resolution—"that this meeting condemns the suggestion accepted by the General Council of the R.B.N.A. to admit to membership, and to place upon the register of trained nurses, asylum attendants who have not been trained in general hospitals, and who do not conform to the regulations for membership and registration. And this meeting considers that such a course would be both injurious to the nursing profession and dangerous and misleading to the public." *Nursing Record*, Jan. 16, 1897, p. 50-5.

RENDER, HELENA WILLIS
Nurse-patient relationships in psychiatry. New York, McGraw-Hill, 1947.
2nd edn., 1959.

RICHARDS, ESTHER LORING
Introduction to psycho-biology and psychiatry: a textbook for nurses. St. Louis, Mosby, 1941.
2nd edn., 1946.

ROBERTSON, G. M.
Observations on the introduction of hospital nurses to asylums, and the hospitalisation of asylums. [Abridged.] *British Journal of Nursing*, Dec. 15, 1906, p. 467-70.

ROBINSON, ALICE M.
The psychiatric aide: his part in patient care. Philadelphia, Lippincott, 1954.
2nd edn., 1959.

RODEMAN, CHARLOTTE R.
A guide for psychiatric aides. New York, Macmillan, 1956.

ROYAL COLLEGE OF NURSING
WARD AND DEPARTMENTAL SISTERS SECTION
A comprehensive mental nursing service: the part of the ward sister and charge nurse. R.C.N., 1960.

ROYAL MEDICO-PSYCHOLOGICAL ASSOCIATION
Handbook for mental nurses (handbook for attendants on the insane). Bailliere, Tindall & Cox, 1885.
8th edn., 1954.

RUSSELL, WILLIAM L.
A survey of the nursing of mental diseases. *British Journal of Nursing*, Aug. 13, 1910, p. 124-6; Aug. 20, 1910, p. 147; Sept. 3, 1910, p. 183-4.

SADLER, WILLIAM S., and others
Psychiatric nursing. St. Louis, Mosby, 1937.

SATCHWELL, —
Mental nursing. *British Journal of Nursing*, Dec. 15, 1906, p. 470-1.

SCHWARTZ, CHARLOTTE GREEN
Rehabilitation of mental hospital patients, Washington, Govt. Printing Office, 1953.

SCHWARTZ, MORRIS S., and SHOCKLEY, EMMY LANNING
The nurse and the mental patient: a study in inter-personal relations. New York, Russell Sage Foundation, 1956.

SCHWARTZ, MORRIS S.
Patient demands in a menta lhospital context. *Psychiatry*, Aug. 1957, p. 257-91.

SCLARE, I. M.
Mental nursing in observation wards. Edinburgh, Livingstone, 1938.

SMITH, H.
The changing role of the psychiatric nurse. *Nursing Mirror*, Sept. 11, 1959, p. 1231-2.

SOMMER, ROBERT
Working effectively with groups. *American Journal of Nursing*, Feb. 1960, p. 223-6.

STEARNS, L.
A therapeutic community: as a nurse sees it. *Military Medicine*, Aug. 1957, p. 121-4.

STEELE, KATHARINE MCLEAN, and MANFREDA, MARGUERITE LUCY
Psychiatric nursing. Philadelphia, Davis, 1937.
2nd edn., 1941.
3rd edn., 1943.
4th edn., 1951.

THOMAS, B.
Nursing emotionally disturbed patients—5. *Nursing Times* , June 21, 1957, p. 687.

TUDBURY, MARY A.
The psychiatric nurse in the general hospital. Springfield, Illinois, Thomas, 1959.

TYSON, J.
Case assignment in a mental hospital. *Nursing Mirror*, June 6, 1958, p. v, and June 13, 1958, p. vi.

WEDDELL, DOREEN
Nursing emotionally disturbed patients—1. *Nursing Times*, May 24, 1957, p. 580-2.

WEDDELL, DOREEN
Nursing emotionally disturbed patients—2. *Nursing Times*, May 31, 1957, p. 609-10.

WEDDELL, DOREEN
Nursing emotionally disturbed patients—3. *Nursing Times*, June 7, 1957, p. 630-1.

WEISS, MADELINE OLGA
Attitudes in psychiatric nursing care. New York, Putnam, 1954.

WORLD HEALTH ORGANIZATION.
EXPERT COMMITTEE ON PSYCHIATRIC NURSING
First report. Geneva, W.H.O., 1956.

WORLD HEALTH ORGANIZATION.
REGIONAL OFFICE FOR EUROPE
The nurse in the psychiatric team: report of a seminar organized by the Regional Office for Europe of the W.H.O., in collaboration with the Government of the Netherlands, Noordwijk, 4-15 November, 1957. Copenhagen, W.H.O., 1959.

ADMINISTRATION

ADAMS, H.
The psychiatrist and the nurse: a working partnership. I. The sharing of responsibility. *Mental Hospitals*, Jan. 1959, p. 7-8.

BIRMINGHAM REGIONAL HOSPITAL BOARD.
MENTAL HEALTH SERVICES COMMITTEE
Report of a working party appointed to advise on standards of staffing in mental deficiency hospitals. The Board, [1956].

BIRMINGHAM REGIONAL BOARD.
MENTAL HEALTH SERVICES COMMITTEE
Report of a working party appointed to advise on standards of staffing in mental hospitals. The Board, 1954.

BURKE, CHRISTIANA, and others
A time study of nursing activities in a psychiatric hospital. *Nursing Research*, June 1956, p. 27-35.

CAVEY, M.
Nursing needs in Virginia state mental institutions. *Virginia Medical Monthly*, Sept. 1957, p. 467-8.

GREAT BRITAIN. BOARD OF CONTROL
Departmental Committee on Nursing in County and Borough Mental Hospitals. Report. . . . H.M.S.O., 1924.

GREAT BRITAIN. BOARD OF CONTROL
The nursing service in mental hospitals: report of the proceedings of the conference convened by Sir Frederick Willis . . . to consider the nursing service in mental hospitals, with special reference to the recommendations made in the Report of the Departmental Committee, set up by the Board of Control in 1922. H.M.S.O., 1925.

GREAT BRITAIN.
INTERDEPARTMENTAL COMMITTEE ON NURSING SERVICES
Subcommittee on Mental Nursing and the Nursing of the Mentally Defective. Report. H.M.S.O., 1945.

HEDMAN, L. L.
The psychiatrist and the nurse: a working partnership. II. The common goal of treatment. *Mental Hospitals*, Jan. 1959, p. 8-10.

LIVERPOOL UNIVERSITY. DEPARTMENT OF SOCIAL SCIENCE
Deva Hospital: the work and status of mental nurses. Liverpool University, 1954.

MANCHESTER REGIONAL HOSPITAL BOARD
Report of the working party on standards of nursing staff for mental hospitals and mental deficiency hospitals. Manchester, The Board, [1959].

MIDDLETON, AGNES B.
Staffing a psychiatric research unit. *Nursing Outlook*, Sept. 1957, p. 519-21.

MISHLER, E. G.
The nursing service and the aims of a psychiatric hospital: orientations of ward personnel to the care and rehabilitation of psychiatric patients. *American Journal of Psychiatry*, III, 1955, p. 664-72.

AFTER-CARE

GELBER, IDA
Released mental patients on tranquillizing drugs, and the public health nurse. New York, New York University Press, 1959.

FRASER, R. D., and KENNEDY, M. E.
Psychiatric day hospital in Glasgow. *Nursing Times*, Sept. 16, 1960, p. 1138-40.

FRIEDMAN, T. T., ROLFE, P., and PERRY, S. E.
Home treatment of psychiatric patients. *American Journal of Psychiatry*, Mar. 1960, p. 807-9.

ROGERS, D. L. M.
Outpatient psychiatric nursing at St. Thomas's Hospital. *Nursing Times*, Sept. 20, 1957, p. 1056-60.

EDUCATION

ACKNER, B., and others
Training the psychiatric nurse on the ward. *Lancet*, Sept. 17, 1955, p. 606-8; *Nursing Times*, Oct. 14, 1955, p. 1154-7.

ALTSCHUL, A.
New concepts in psychiatric nursing education. *Nursing Mirror*, April 18, 1958, p. 181-2, and April 25, 1958, p. 269-70.

CHASE, R. H.
Mental medicine and nursing: for use in training schools for nurses. Philadelphia and London, 1914.

CLANCEY, I. L., CUMMING, J., and CUMMING, E.
Training psychiatric nurses; a re-evaluation. *Canadian Psychiatric Association Journal*, Jan. 1957, p. 26-33.

COOPER, M., and BLACKER, H.
Re-orientation to mental nursing. *Nursing Mirror*, Oct. 25, 1957, p. vii.

CRAWFORD, ANNIE LAURIE, and KILANDER, VIRGINIA CURRY
Nursing manual for psychiatric aides designed to assist the psychiatric aide in giving better nursing care. Philadelphia, Davis, 1954.

FITZSIMMONS, LAURA W.
Manual for training attendants in mental hospitals. New York, American Psychiatric Association, 1945.

FITZSIMMONS, LAURA W.
Textbook for psychiatric attendants. New York, Macmillan, 1947.

GILLIS, L.
A South African inservice program: Tara Hospital's way of teaching new methods of dealing with emotional problems is effective not only for psychiatric nurses but for other nurses as well. *American Journal of Nursing*, Feb. 1959, p. 210-12.

HALL, B. H., and others
Psychiatric aide education. New York, Grune & Stratton, 1952.

JONES, ROBERT ARMSTRONG
The necessity of hospital training for mental nurses. *British Journal of Nursing*, July 3, 1920, p. 2-3, and July 10, 1920, p. 17-18.

KIMBALL, LEONORE
Psychiatric nursing: syllabus and workbook for student nurses. New York, Kimpton, 1952.

KRUSH, T. P.
A teaching experience in a state mental hospital. *Nursing World*, April 1954, p. 23-4 and 40.

MACAULAY, ELIZABETH L.
A textbook for mental nurses. Faber, 1930.

McCABE, GRACIA S.
Some role experiences of nursing students in psychiatric nursing—and some parallels with other clinical areas. *Nursing Outlook*, June 1960, p. 338-42.

MEDICO-PSYCHOLOGICAL ASSOCIATION OF GREAT BRITAIN AND IRELAND
The nursing examination of the Medico-Psychological Association of Great Britain and Ireland. *Nursing Record*, Sept. 11, 1897, p. 206-8.

NATIONAL LEAGUE OF NURSING EDUCATION
Descriptive criteria for evaluation of advanced programs of study in psychiatric nursing and mental hygiene. New York, The League, 1949.

Notes for the mental nurse in training, by a medical officer of a mental hospital: a complete series of lectures. . . . Manchester, National Asylum Workers' Union, 1927.

OPPENHEIM, A. N.
The function and training of mental nurses: an analysis of the work and training of nurses in the Bethlem Royal Hospital and the Maudsley Hospital. Chapman & Hall, for the Hospitals, 1955.

ROBERTS, T.
New mental training syllabus. *Nursing Mirror*, Aug. 9, 1957, p. 1357.

ROWE, P. R. M.
An experimental scheme for training in mental nursing prepared by the Middlesex Hospital and Shenley Hospital. *Nursing Times*, Sept. 27, 1952, p. 952-55.

ROYAL MEDICO-PSYCHOLOGICAL ASSOCIATION
The state registration of mental nurses. 1. Extract from the annual report of the Council, 1928. 2. Report on questionnaire. 3. The training and examination of those nursing mental defectives. Adlard, 1928.

ROYAL MEDICO-PSYCHOLOGICAL ASSOCIATION
Training of psychiatric nurses (mental illness and mental deficiency). Royal Medico-Psychological Association, [1956].

STERN, EDITH M.
The attendant's guide. New York, Commonwealth Fund, 1945.

TOKUHATA, GEORGE K.
A behavioral analysis of the practical nurse psychiatric affiliation program. *Nursing Research*, Summer 1960, p. 141-8.

MENTAL DEFICIENCY

GIBSON, JOHN, and FRENCH, THOMAS
Mental deficiency nursing. Faber, 1958.

HALLAS, CHARLES H.
The nursing of mental defectives. Bristol, Wright, 1958.

HILLIARD, L. T.
Recent changes in mental deficiency nursing.
1. Working of new Mental Health Act.
2. Future of psychiatric nursing.
3. Categories of patients.
Nursing Mirror, Oct. 23, 1959, p. 309-10, Oct. 30, 1959, p. 385-6, and Nov. 6, 1959, p. 463-4.

INTERNATIONAL COUNCIL OF NURSES
Mental deficiency nursing. *Nursing Mirror*, Feb. 28, 1958, p. iv; Mar. 7, 1958, p. iii; Mar. 14, 1958, p. xi.

JARRETT, R. FITZROY, and others
The shortage of mental deficiency nurses. *Lancet*, 1954.

KASSLER, R.
Planning resident care; professional nursing personnel and their functions. *American Journal of Mental Deficiency*, Jan. 1958, p. 597-600.

MICHAL-SMITH, HAROLD
The mentally retarded patient. Philadelphia, Lippincott, 1956.

PEARN, E. O. NAPIER
Mental deficiency nursing (simplified). Bailliere, Tindall & Cox. 1934.

ROYAL MEDICO-PSYCHOLOGICAL ASSOCIATION
Manual for mental deficiency nurses. Bailliere, Tindall & Cox. 1931.

RESEARCH

GORHAM, D. R.
An evaluation of attitudes towards psychiatric nursing care. *Nursing Research*, June 1958, p. 71-6.

MELLOW, JUNE, and others
Research in psychiatric nursing. Part 2. Nursing therapy with individual patients. *American Journal of Nursing*, May 1955, p. 572-5.

NAHM, HELEN
Research in psychiatric nursing. *Nursing Outlook*, Feb. 1957, p. 89-91.

ROBINSON, ALICE M.
Research in psychiatric nursing. Part 1. The role of one nurse-therapist in a large public mental hospital. *American Journal of Nursing*, April 1955, p. 441-4.

ROBINSON, ALICE M.
Research in psychiatric nursing. Part 3. The psychiatric head nurse. *American Journal of Nursing*, June 1955, p. 704-7.

PSYCHOLOGY

AIKIN, R. CATHERINE
Psychology for student nurses. *Canadian Nurse*, July 1953, p. 555-9, and Aug. 1953, p. 625-30.

SPECIALITIES

AVERILL, LAWRENCE AUGUSTUS, *and* KEMPF, FLORENCE C.
Psychology applied to nursing. Philadelphia, Saunders, 1930.
2nd edn., 1942.
3rd edn., 1946.
4th edn., 1951.
5th edn., 1956.

CHADWICK, MARY
Psychology for nurses: introductory lectures for nurses upon psychology and psycho-analysis. Heinemann, 1925.

COSTELLO, CHARLES G., *and* ANDERSON, MARIAN E.
The vocational and personal preferences of psychiatric and general nurses. *Nursing Research*, Summer 1960, p. 155-6.

CROW, LESTER D., *and others*
Psychology in nursing practice, by Lester D. Crow, Alice Crow and Charles E. Skinner. New York, Macmillan, 1954.

CRUZE, WENDELL W.
Psychology in nursing. New York, Blakiston Division, McGraw-Hill, 1955.
2nd edn., 1960.

CUNNINGHAM, BESS V.
Psychology for nurses: designed and written for student nurses. New York, Appleton-Century-Crofts, 1946.
2nd edn., 1951.

DALE, BETH
The work of the church nurse. *Canadian Nurse*, Dec. 1958, p. 1119-20.

DENNIS, LORRAINE BRADT
Psychology of human behaviour for nurses. Philadelphia, Saunders, 1957.

DWYER, SISTER M. THEOPHANE
A sociometric study among a selected group of students in nursing. Washington, Catholic University of America Press, 1947.

EYRE, MARY B.
Psychology and mental hygiene for nurses. New York, Macmillan, 1922.

FISHER, J. W.
Psychology and mental disorders for nurses. Arnold, 1941.

GILBERT, J. G., *and* WEITZ, R. D.
Psychology for the profession of nursing. New York, Ronald Press, 1949.

HARRIMAN, PHILIP LAWRENCE, GREENWOOD, LELA LORENE, *and* SKINNER, CHARLES EDWARD
Psychology in nursing practice. New York, Macmillan, 1942.

HIGGINS, AILEEN CLEVELAND
The psychology of nursing. New York, Putnam, 1921.

HIGHLEY, BETTY L., *and* NORRIS, CATHERINE M.
When a student dislikes a patient. *American Journal of Nursing*, Sept. 1957, p. 1163-6.

HOLMAN, PORTIA
Psychology and psychological medicine for nurses. Heinemann, 1957.

HURD, ARCHER WILLIS
Man and his sociological and psychological environment: a textbook for nurses. Richmond, Bureau of Educational Research and Service, Medical College of Virginia, 1950.

JOSEPH OVIDE, SISTER
Illness and applied psychology. *Canadian Nurse*, Mar. 1960, p. 213-5.

KIMBER, W. J. T.
Practical psychology for nurses and other workers in mental hospitals. O.U.P., 1937.

LAIRD, DONALD A.
Applied psychology for nurses: an introduction. Philadelphia, Lippincott, 1923.

MCGHIE, ANDREW
Psychology as applied to nursing. Edinburgh, Livingstone, 1959.

MACKENZIE, NORAH
Aids to psychology for nurses. Bailliere, Tindall & Cox, 1951.

MULLER, THERESA GRACE
The foundations of human behaviour: dynamic psychology in nursing. New York, Putnams, 1956.

MUSE, MAUDE BLANCHE
A textbook of psychology for nurses. Philadelphia, Saunders, 1925.
2nd edn., 1930.
4th edn., 1939.

NICOLE, J. ERNEST
Normal and abnormal psychology: a precis for junior students, nurses, occupational therapists, welfare workers and others. Allen & Unwin, 1948.

ODLUM, DORIS
Psychology, the nurse and the patient. *Nursing Mirror*, 1952.
2nd edn., 1954.
3rd edn., 1959.

O'HARA, FRANK J.
Psychology and the nurse. Philadelphia, Saunders, 1939.
2nd edn., 1943.
4th edn., 1954.

PARLOFF, MORRIS B.
The impact of ward-milieu philosophies on nursing-role concepts. *Psychiatry*, vol. 23, no. 2, May 1960.

PORTER, E.
He learned how patients really felt. *Modern Hospital*, July 1957, p. 51-4.

PORTER, MARY F.
Applied psychology for nurses. Philadelphia, Saunders, 1921.

RAUTH, J. E., *and* SHEEHY, SISTER M. M.
Principles of psychology for the basic course in nursing. Milwaukee, Bruce, 1945.

ROBINSON, E. S., *and* KIRK, V.
Introduction to psychology. New York, Macmillan, 1935.

SHERMAN, MANDEL
Psychology for nurses. New York, Longmans Green, 1947.

SODDY, KENNETH
Importance of social psychology in modern nursing. *Nursing Mirror*, Oct. 21, 1955, p. 191-2; Oct. 28, 1955, p. 261-2; Nov. 5, 1955, p. 331-2; Nov. 11, 1955, p. 399-400; Nov. 18, 1955, p. 475.

SOMMER, ROBERT
The role of the nurse in psychological testing. *Journal of Clinical Psychology*, April 1958, p. 200-2.

WEDDELL, DOREEN
Psychology applied to nursing. *Nursing Times*, Sept. 4, 1954, p. 959-60; Sept. 18, 1954, p. 1009-10; Oct. 1, 1954, p. 1066-8; Oct. 15, 1954, p. 1138-9; Oct. 29, 1954, p. 1191-2; Nov. 12, 1954, p. 1249-50; Nov. 26, 1954, p. p. 1317-18; Jan. 14, 1955, p. 41-2; Jan. 28, 1955, p. 85-6; Feb. 25, 1955, p. 194-5; Mar. 11, 1955, p. 263-4.

WILLIAMS, JESSIE
Psychology for student nurses. Methuen, 1954.
2nd edn., 1957.

WILSON, ISABEL G. H.
Psychology in general nursing. Arnold, 1931.

PUBLIC HEALTH NURSING

GENERAL WORKS

ALLWOOD-PAREDES, J.
The health administrator views the role of the nurse in the health programme. *Journal of the Christian Medical Association of India*, Mar. 1957, p. 95-8.

AMERICAN NURSES' ASSOCIATION *and* THE NATIONAL ORGANIZATION FOR PUBLIC HEALTH NURSING.
COMMITTEE ON NURSING IN MEDICAL CARE PLANS
Guide for the inclusion of nursing service in medical care plans. New York, The Committee, 1950.

BEARD, MARY
The nurse in public health. New York, Harper, 1929.

BLACK, I.
Public health nursing in a changing environment. *Canadian Journal of Public Health*, Feb. 1960, p. 57-61.

BOWERS, HELEN G.
Women's work in public health departments. *British Journal of Nursing*, Jan. 11, 1908, p. 23-4.

CAMERON, C. M., JR.
Cherokee Indian health survey. *Public Health Reports*, Nov. 1956, p. 1086-8.

COULTER, PEARL PARVIN
The nurse in the public health program. New York, Putnam, 1954.

GORDON, ETHEL M.
Nursing counsellors of the Federal Employee Health Service. *Canadian Nurse*, Feb. 1957, p. 109-13.

GRUNDY, FRED
A handbook of social medicine written especially for midwives, but also suitable for nurses, health visitors, etc. Luton, Leagrave Press, 1945.
2nd edn., 1945.
3rd edn., 1945.
4th edn., 1947.
5th edn., 1948.

GRUNDY, FRED
The new public health: an introduction for midwives, health visitors and social workers. Luton, Leagrave Press, 1949.
3rd edn., 1952.
4th edn., 1957.

MANNIN, E.
Home nursing versus the hospital. *Medical World*, Sept. 1958, p. 268.

MAYNARD, EDITH L.
Women in the public health service. Scientific Press, 1915.

MINER, L.
Public health nursing implications. *Canadian Journal of Public Health*, Feb. 1959, p. 53-7.

NATIONAL LEAGUE FOR NURSING.
DEPARTMENT OF PUBLIC HEALTH NURSING
Communications between nursing services. New York, The League, 1957.

NATIONAL LEAGUE FOR NURSING.
DEPARTMENT OF PUBLIC HEALTH NURSING
Guide in personnel policies for employers of public health nurses. New York, The League, 1957.

NATIONAL ORGANIZATION FOR PUBLIC HEALTH NURSING
A study of combination services in public health nursing, by D. Rusby. New York, The Organization, 1950.

PEARSE, H. L.
The nurse as a social worker. *British Journal of Nursing*, Sept. 3, 1910, p. 186-7.

PEEBLES, ALLON
Nursing services and insurance for medical care in Brattleboro, Vermont: a study of the activities of the Thomas Thompson Trust, by A. T. and Valeria V. McDermott, with an evaluation of the nursing programme by Violet H. Hodgson . . . and Katherine Tucker. Chicago, University of Chicago Press, 1932.

SINDLINGER, ELIZABETH, *and* FARIS, MILDRED
Nurse and social worker collaborate in a milieu program. *Nursing Outlook*, May 1955, p. 296-8.

VINES, H. W. C.
Can nurses promote health. *Nursing Times*, Aug. 19, 1955, p. 912-4.

WILLIAMS, ROSA L.
The social work of the coloured nurse. *British Journal of Nursing*, Nov. 23, 1912, p. 412-3.

WOOD, A.
A comprehensive community nursing service. *Royal Society for the Promotion of Health Journal*, Aug. 1956, p. 496-7.

DISTRICT NURSING

General Works

AHLA, ANNIKI MERVI MASIA
Referred by visiting nurse: a study of co-operation between the visiting nurse and the social case worker. Cleveland, Ohio, Western Reserve University Press, 1950.

ASSOCIATED HOSPITAL SERVICE OF NEW YORK
Report of a study concerning the feasibility of providing visiting nurse service following hospitalization for Blue Cross subscribers. New York, The Service, 1957.

BAKST, H. J.
Observations on home care program in the United States. *B.M.Q.*, June 1958, p. 46-8.

BLACKWOOD, HERMIONE
The nursing of the poor in their own homes. *British Journal of Nursing*, Sept. 7, 1907, p. 183-5.

BÖGE, ELSE
The nurse on the district.
See
NURSING TIMES
The nurse and the nation: a survey of her position in the State today. *Nursing Times*, Nov. 5, 1910, p. 904-31.

BRADY, KATHLEEN
Planning and implementation of a nursing referral program. *Canadian Nurse*, Sept. 1957, p. 795-9.

BREAY, MARGARET
County Nursing Association. *British Journal of Nursing*, Oct. 15, 1904, p. 306-7.

CANADA. DOMINION BUREAU OF STATISTICS
Statistics of home nursing services (Victorian Order of Nurses for Canada), 1957. Ottawa, Dominion Bureau of Statistics, 1958.

CHALONER, L.
Foster parents and the visiting nurse's opportunity. *Nursing Times*, Dec. 20, 1957, p. 1444-5.

COPE, ZACHARY
District nursing—a challenge. *Nursing Times*, Jan. 9, 1959, p. 42 and 47.

CRAVEN, MRS. DACRE
On district nursing.
In
HAMPTON, ISABEL A., *and others*
Nursing of the sick, 1893.

DALZELL-WARD, A. J.
The district nurse as a health educator. *District Nursing*, April 1960, p. 8-10.

110

EDMAN, HULDA
The practical nurse in the visiting nurse service. *Nursing Outlook*, Aug. 1958, p. 446-8.

ELDER, A. T.
The National Health Service and the home nurse. *Nursing Times*, Dec. 28, 1956, p. 1336-7.

ESSEX-CATER, A. J.
The changing pattern of domiciliary care: the younger generation. *Royal Society for the Promotion of Health Journal*, Sept.-Oct. 1959, p. 590-3.

FOLEY, EDNA LOUISE
Visiting nurse manual, prepared for the Visiting Nurse Association of Chicago and other public health nurses. Chicago, National Organization for Public Health Nursing of Chicago, 1916.

FRANCIS, H. W. S., and MORRIS, I. H.
Trends in home nursing. The Birmingham service, 1950-57. *Lancet*, April 11, 1959, p. 774-6.

FRENCH, M. A.
The visiting nurse in a psychiatric program. *Nursing Outlook*, Oct. 1956, p. 572-4.

GIBSON, R. M.
Domiciliary care in the Newcastle district. *Medical Journal of Australia*, Oct. 5, 1957, p. 485-9.

GILLETT, J. A.
The changing pattern of domiciliary care: the older citizen. *Royal Society for the Promotion of Health Journal*, Sept.-Oct. 1959, p. 593-7.

GRAZIER, G. M.
An edge-punched district nursing record card. *Medical Officer*, Mar. 8, 1957, p. 137.

HORNER, C. M.
Home nursing service by public health nurses. *Canadian Journal of Public Health*, Feb. 1959, p. 57-9.

HUGHES, AMY
Practical hints on district nursing. Scientific Press, [1897].

JACQUES, MABEL
District nursing. New York, 1911.

KAARIAINEN, H.
Home care scheme in Helsinki. *Nursing Mirror*, April 19, 1957, p. viii.

KAARIAINEN, H., and LARTIO, M.
Visiting nurse in Helsinki. *American Journal of Nursing*, June 1958, p. 866-7.

KITCHING, R. L.
The home nursing service; a plea for district assistant nurses. *Practitioner*, Feb. 1957, p. 234-6.

LEES, FLORENCE S.
A guide to district nurses and home nursing. Macmillan, 1890.

LESSON, G.
Changing pattern of district nursing. *Hospital and Social Service Journal*, June 7, 1957, p. 613.

LESSON, G.
Trends in district nursing. *Hospital and Social Service Journal*, Feb. 11, 1955, p. 133.

LOANE, M.
The incidental opportunities of district nursing. Women's Printing Society, 19?

LOANE, M.
Outlines of routine in district nursing: drawn up for the use of district probationers and private nurses. Scientific Press Ltd., 1905.

LOANE, M.
Thoughts on the final training of district probationers. *British Journal of Nursing*, Oct. 22, 1904, p. 329-31; Oct. 29, 1904, p. 349-50; Nov. 5, 1904, p. 369-71; Nov. 12, 1904, p. 390-2.

LONDON COUNTY COUNCIL
A survey of district nursing in the administrative county of London (prepared by Margaret Hogarth and submitted by the County Medical Officer of Health). L.C.C., 1931.

MACLEOD, CHARLOTTE
District nursing in Canada. *British Journal of Nursing*, July 26, 1902, p. 76-8.

MANSELL, E. M.
District nurses and their work. *Nursing Record*, Dec. 20, 1888, p. 540-1.

MERRY, ELEANOR JEANETTE, and IRVIN, IRIS DUNDAS
District nursing: a handbook for district nurses and for all concerned in the administration of a district nursing service. Bailliere, Tindall & Cox, 1948.
2nd edn., 1955.
3rd edn., 1960.

MERRY, ELEANOR JEANETTE
Problems in the home nursing and care of elderly people today. *Practitioner*, April 1957, p. 473-6.

MORROW, J. T.
Mental health in the visiting nurse program. *Nursing Outlook*, Sept. 1958, p. 505-7.

NATIONAL LEAGUE FOR NURSING.
DEPARTMENT OF PUBLIC HEALTH NURSING
Report of a conference on public health nursing care of the sick at home. New York, The League, 1953.

NATIONAL ORGANIZATION FOR PUBLIC HEALTH NURSING
Public health nursing care of the sick. New York, National League for Nursing, 1943.

NIGHTINGALE, FLORENCE
Rural hygiene: health teaching in towns and villages. Spottiswoode, 1894.

PRACTITIONER
Home care and nursing. *The Practitioner*, July, 1956.

QUEEN'S INSTITUTE OF DISTRICT NURSING
Handbook for Queen's Nurses: by some Queen's Superintendents. Scientific Press, 1924.
2nd edn., Faber, 1932.
3rd edn., 1943.

QUEEN'S INSTITUTE OF DISTRICT NURSING
Lectures to nurses. The Institute, [193?].

QUEEN'S INSTITUTE OF DISTRICT NURSING
Outline of district nursing technique for Queen's Nurses. Queen's Institute of District Nursing, [19?].
2nd edn., 1954.

QUEEN'S INSTITUTE OF DISTRICT NURSING
Report of special study on the future scope of the District Nursing Service and the personnel needed (undertaken by E. A. B. Davis . . .). Queen's Institute of District Nursing, 1955.

QUEEN'S INSTITUTE OF DISTRICT NURSING
Survey of district nursing in England and Wales: information obtained and compiled by the Queen's Institute of District Nursing. The Institute, [193?].

QUEEN'S INSTITUTE OF DISTRICT NURSING SECRETARIES' ASSOCIATION
The domiciliary nursing services: an account of British district nursing, midwifery and health visiting, with a comparative review of the Canadian system of home nursing. Leicester, Taylor & Bloxham, 1942.
2nd edn., 1943.

REID, MABEL
Changing patterns in visiting nurse service. *Nursing Outlook*, Sept. 1959, p. 534-5.

ROBERTS, DOROTHY I.
A psychiatric service policy for visiting nurses. *Nursing Outlook*, Sept. 1956, p. 510-12.

ROBERTS, L., and McWATT, F.
The work of a district nurse. *Medical Officer*, Feb. 10, 1956, p. 69.

SOMERVILLE, C. E. M.
District nursing.
In
HAMPTON, ISABEL A., *and others*
Nursing of the sick, 1893.

STEVENSON, E. A.
The equality of rich and poor in sickness: the relation of cottage nurses to the nursing profession. *British Journal of Nursing*, Sept. 19, 1908, p. 223-5.

WATERS, ISABELLA
Visiting nursing in the United States. Containing a directory of the organizations employing visiting nurses. New York, Charities Publication Committee, 1909. 2nd edn., 1912.

WESTMORLAND, J. E.
Psychiatric district nurse? *Nursing Times*, Nov. 25, 1960, p. 1472-3.

WILLIAMS, D. M.
The changing pattern of domiciliary care: the years between. *Royal Society for the Promotion of Health Journal*, Sept.-Oct. 1959, p. 597-603.

Administration

HURRY, JAMIESON B.
District nursing on a provident basis. Scientific Press, 1898.

WOFINDEN, R. C., *and* EMBLEM, R. G.
District nursing records. *Medical Officer*, Jan. 3, 1953, p. 5.

WOOD, CATHERINE JANE
Co-ordination in rural nursing. *Nursing Times*, June 12, 1909, p. 480-1.

Education

BLACK, AUGUSTA
The training of a district nurse. *Nursing Times*, Sept. 16, 1955, p. 1031-2.

ILLING, MARGARET
District nurse training. *Nursing Times*, Aug. 12, 1960, p. 988-9.

MINISTRY OF HEALTH
Training of district nurses: report of the Advisory Committee. H.M.S.O., 1959.

MINISTRY OF HEALTH AND SCOTLAND DEPARTMENT OF HEALTH.
WORKING PARTY ON THE TRAINING OF DISTRICT NURSES
Report. H.M.S.O., 1955.

QUEEN'S INSTITUTE OF DISTRICT NURSING
The training of district nurses. *Nursing Times*, Aug. 7, 1954, p. 846-7.

QUEEN'S INSTITUTE OF DISTRICT NURSING
The training and work of district nurses. Queen's Institute of District Nursing, [195?].

ROBERTSON, J. D.
Syllabus of lectures on home nursing given at the Chicago training school for home and public health nursing. Chicago, 1920.

WITTING, M.
Preparation for district nursing. *Nursing Times*, Oct. 14, 1955, p. 1169-71.

HEALTH VISITORS

General Works

AKESTER, JOYCE M.
The duties and responsibilities of health visitors. The Royal Sanitary Institute, 1954.

AKESTER, JOYCE M.
The health visitor and health education. *Nursing Mirror*, May 31, 1957, p. iii.

AMERICAN NURSES' ASSOCIATION
Preparing an economic brief for public health nurses. New York, The Association, 1959.

AMERICAN NURSES' ASSOCIATION.
PUBLIC HEALTH NURSES SECTION
Functions, standards and qualifications for public health nurses. New York, The Association, [1955].

ARMITAGE, C. PHYLLIS
Health visiting, the new profession; a handbook for health visitors and school nurses, and for all who are interested in maternity and child welfare. Bale, Sons & Danielssohn, 1927.

ARNSTEIN, MARGARET G.
Forward with public health nursing. *Nursing Outlook*, May 1958, p. 261-3.

ARNSTEIN, MARGARET G.
Priorities in public health nursing. *Public Health Reports*, July 1958, p. 577-81.

ASHBY, LUCY E., *and* EARP, KATE ATHERTON
Health visitor's guide. Faber & Gwyer, 1926.

BANNINGTON, B. G.
The health visitor from a sanitary inspector's point of view. *Nursing Times*, Jan. 13, 1917, p. 33-4.

BEATTIE, I. T.
Towards the all-purpose health visitor. *Nursing Mirror*, Dec. 30, 1960, p. vii and x.

BRODY, WILLIAM
Position classification in public health nursing. *Nursing Outlook*, Nov. 1959, p. 637-40.

BRODY, WILLIAM
Recruiting public health nurses. *Nursing Outlook*, Dec. 1959, p. 696-9.

BROWN, ESTHER LUCILLE
Role of the public health nurse in mental health. *American Journal of Public Health*, June 1956, p. 745-7.

BRYAN, EDITH S.
The art of public health nursing. Philadelphia, Saunders, 1935.

BYRNE, A.
Is your health visitor really necessary. *Medical World*, Jan. 1960, p. 77-81.

CARPENTER, HELEN M.
An analysis of home visits to newborn infants made by public health nurses in the East York Leaside Health Unit, Ontario. *Canadian Nurse*, Sept. 1959, p. 809-25.

CARTER, DOROTHY
Volunteers and other auxiliary workers in public health nursing. New York, National Organization for Public Health Nursing, 1943.

CATTO, I. M.
Public health visiting. *British Journal of Nursing*, Mar. 14, 1914, p. 225-6.

CENTRAL HANOVER BANK & TRUST CO., NEW YORK
The public health nurse—New York Department of Philanthropic Information. New York, The Bank, 1937.

COBURN, EDNA P.
An evaluation of graduates of baccalaureate basic programs employed in public health nursing settings. New York, National League for Nursing, 1959.

CRANDALL, ELLA P.
The municipal nurse in relation to public health. New York, 1916.

CREELMAN, LYLE
Trends in nursing and in public health; having implications for health visitors. *Royal Society for the Promotion of Health Journal*, Aug. 1955, p. 602-4.

CREW, F. A. E.
The health visitor. *Nursing Times*, July 31, 1954, p. 814-6.

DANIELLS, N. C.
The health visitor's preparation for health education. *Nursing Times*, April 25, 1958, p. 477-80.

DANIELLS, N. C.
Health visiting: the challenge of 1960. Meeting the challenge of change. *Royal Society of Health Journal*, July-Aug. 1960, p. 356-9.

DAVIES, M. E.
The consultant health visitor. *Nursing Mirror*, Aug. 12, 1955, p. 1327-8.

DAVIS, EVELYN K.
The volunteer in public health nursing. New York, National Organization for Public Health Nursing, 1941.

DAVISON, E. H.
Health visiting and case-work. *Nursing Times*, Oct. 26, 1956, p. 1087-8.

DERRYBERRY, MAYHEW, *editor*
A sampling of public health nurses' home visits. Washington, Govt. Printing Office, 1940.

DOYON, R.
The responsibilities of the public health nurse. *Canadian Nurse*, July 1959, p. 635-6.

DUNBAR, C., *and others*
Social workers look at public health nursing. *Nursing Outlook*, Feb. 1957, p. 70-2.

ELDER, A. T.
Why and wherefore of health visiting. *Nursing Times*, Dec. 19, 1953, p. 1286-7.

ELDRIDGE, R. W.
The health visitor in the social work field; care of the handicapped. *Royal Society for the Promotion of Health Journal*, Sept. 1956, p. 613-8.

EMORY, FLORENCE H. M.
Public health nursing in Canada: principles and practice. Toronto, Macmillan, 1945.
2nd edn., 1953.

EVE, ENID, *editor*
Manual for health visitors and infant welfare workers, by several writers. Bale, Sons & Danielssohn, 1921.

FERGUSON, MARION
Public health nursing service to patients. Washington, Govt. Printing Office, 1959.

FLETCHER, H. E.
Job satisfaction. *Canadian Nurse*, Sept. 1957, p. 812.

FREEMAN, RUTH B.
Public health nursing practice. Philadelphia, Saunders, 1950.
2nd edn., 1957.

FUJIKURA, Y. Y.
Public health nursing in Japan. *American Journal of Nursing*, Nov. 1956, p. 1416-9.

GARDNER, MARY SEWALL
Public health nursing. New York, Macmillan, 1916.
2nd edn., 1924.
3rd edn., 1937.

GILBERT, J.
Public health nurses for public health education. *Canadian Journal of Public Health*, Nov. 1956, p. 509-12.

GILBERT, RUTH
The public health nurse and her patient. Cambridge, Mass., Harvard U.P., for the Commonwealth Fund, 1940.
2nd edn., 1951.

GRANT, AMELIA HOWE
Nursing: a community health service. Philadelphia, Saunders, 1942.

HABEL, MARY LOUISE, *and* MILTON, H. D.
The graduate nurse in the home—meeting community needs. Philadelphia, Lippincott, 1939.

HALL, J. B.
The nurse in environmental sanitation. *Nursing Outlook*, Dec. 1957, p. 700-2.

HARTE, M. A.
Understanding within the public health nursing team—1. *Nursing Times*, Jan. 24, 1958, p. 96-7.

HILL, H. W.
Sanitation for public health nurses. New York, 1919.

HOLMES, THELMA M.
The changing role of public health nursing services in the rehabilitation of patients. *Nursing Outlook*, July 1960, p. 381-2.

HORMUTH, RUDOLPH P.
The public health nurse in community planning for the mentally retarded. Washington, Govt. Printing Office, 1957.

JONES, S. E., *and* PHILLIPS, M.
A pattern of co-operation. *Nursing Times*, Oct. 14, 1960, p. 1287-8.

JORDHEIM, A.
Public health nursing in Norway. *Nursing Outlook*, Nov. 1956, p. 628-30.

KERSHAW, J. D.
The public health nurse of the future. *Medical Officer*, July 22, 1955, p. 47; *Nursing Times*, July 29, 1955, p. 831-832; *Royal Society for the Promotion of Health Journal*, Dec. 1955, p. 825-33.

LAMONT, D. J., *and* MACQUEEN, I. A. G.
Health visiting: new tasks for old.
1. Promoting mental health.
2. Health education.
3. Social work.
Nursing Times, Oct. 23, 1959, p. 1027-8; Oct. 30, 1959, p. 1061-2 and Nov. 6, 1959, p. 1101-2.

LANGTON, B. M.
Some aspects of redeployment and the health visitor. *Nursing Times*, Dec. 7, 1956, p. 1254-6, and Dec. 14, 1956, p. 1282-6.

LEARMONT, D.
Health visiting: the challenge of 1960. *Royal Society of Health Journal*, July-Aug. 1960, p. 351-4.

LEASK, J.
The public health nursing assistant in the Toronto Department of Public Health. *Canadian Journal of Public Health*, May 1960, p. 194-9.

MACDONALD, V. MAY
Mental hygiene and the public health nurse: practical suggestions for the nurse of today. Philadelphia, Lippincott, 1923.

McEWAN, MARGARET
Health visiting: a textbook for health visitor students. Faber, 1951.
2nd edn., 1957.
3rd edn., 1959.

McEWAN, MARGARET
The training of the health visitor. Royal Sanitary Institute, 1935.

MACFIE, M.
The work of health visitors in connection with elderly people. *Medical Officer*, Mar. 13, 1959, p. 147.

McIver, Pearl
Public health nursing in a bi-county health department. Washington, Govt. Printing Office, 1935.

MacQueen, I. A. G.
The role of the health visitor in the prevention of mental and emotional disease. *Medical Officer*, Aug. 12, 1955, p. 83.

Ministry of Health *and others.*
Working Party on the Field of Work, Training and Recruitment of Health Visitors
An enquiry into health visiting: report of a Working Party on the Field of Work, Training and Recruitment of Health Visitors set up by the Ministry of Health, Department of Health for Scotland and Ministry of Education. H.M.S.O., 1956.
[Chairman: Sir Wilson Jameson.]

Monkhouse, Mary
The nurse as health visitor and sanitary inspector.
See
Nursing Times
The nurse and the nation: a survey of her position in the State today. *Nursing Times*, Nov. 5, 1910, p. 904-31.

Mullaney, Gertrude
The public health nurse and the exceptional child. *The Catholic Nurse*, June 1957, p. 48-52.

National League for Nursing.
Department of Public Health Nursing
Public health nurses for the nation. New York, The League, 1957.

National League for Nursing.
Department of Public Health Nursing
Public health nursing; achievements and goals. New York, The League, 1957.

National League for Nursing.
Department of Public Health Nursing
Public health nursing service manuals: a guide for their development. New York, The League, 1958.

National Organization for Public Health Nursing
How to enter the field of public health nursing. New York, The Organization, 1942.

National Organization for Public Health Nursing
Manual of public health nursing. New York, Macmillan, 1932.
2nd edn., 1937.
3rd edn., 1939.

National Organization for Public Health Nursing
Plan for study of public health nursing in a given community. New York, The Organization, [n.d.].

National Organization for Public Health Nursing
Principles and practices in public health nursing, including cost analysis. New York, Macmillan, 1932.

National Organization for Public Health Nursing
Recommended qualifications for public health nursing personnel (1940-1945). New York, The Organization, 1942.

National Organization for Public Health Nursing
Survey of public health nursing: administration and practice. New York, Commonwealth Fund, 1934.

Newington, D. K.
The use of health visitor resources in meeting new demands in home care. *Royal Society for the Promotion of Health Journal*, Sept. 1957, p. 603-7.

New York State. Department of Health
The public health nurse and the work she does. Albany, New York, Department of Health, [n.d.].

Nursing Times. Health Visiting
I. The work to be done: the right woman to do it. *Nursing Times*, Oct. 7, 1916, p. 1160-1.
II. How the work is done: the ins and outs of it. *Nursing Times*, Oct. 14, 1916, p. 1186-7.
III. The best and the worst of it. *Nursing Times*, Oct. 21, 1916, p. 1222-3.
IV. Cross currents and how to steer among them. *Nursing Times*, Oct. 28, 1916, p. 1273-4.

Philpott, Noreen
The public health nurse and mental hygiene. *Canadian Nurse*, Mar. 1960, p. 223-6.

Potter, M.
Health education and the health visitor. *Royal Society for the Promotion of Health Journal*, Aug. 1955, p. 616; *Nursing Times*, June 24, 1955, p. 701-2.

Public health nursing for Montana Indians. *Public Health Reports*, April 1959, p. 325-7.

Public health nursing practice in a family health service. *Nursing Outlook*, Sept. 1959, p. 518-20.

Ramos, L. F.
A man nurse in public health nursing. *American Journal of Nursing*, Sept. 1958, p. 1254.

Rice, G. U., Jr.
The role of the public health nurse in the hospitalization of mental patients and their follow-up after discharge. *American Journal of Public Health and the Nation's Health*, Feb. 1957, p. 210-4.

Richie, J.
Teaching health education to public health nursing aides. *American Journal of Public Health and the Nation's Health*, Jan. 1959, p. 28-33.

Roberts, Llywelyn, *and others*
Textbook for health visitors, by Llywelyn Roberts, I. G. Davies, Beryl D. Corner. Bailliere, Tindall & Cox, 1951. 2nd edn., 1960.

Rue, Clara B.
The public health nurse in the community. Philadelphia, Saunders, 1944.

Sheen, E. M., *and* Duncan, E. H. L.
A survey of a health visitor's work among the chronic sick and aged in Bristol. *Medical Officer*, Sept. 16, 1960, p. 175.

Slack, M.
Health visitor and social worker. *Nursing Times*, May 20, 1960, p. 630-1.

Sutherland, Dorothy G.
Nursing's new look in the public health service. *Nursing Outlook*, Oct. 1960, p. 571-2.

Tibbitts, C.
Social change, ageing and public health nursing. *Nursing Outlook*, Mar. 1958, p. 144-7.

Wales, Marguerite
The public health nurse in action. New York, Macmillan, 1941.

Walker, F. H.
The use of health visitor resources in meeting new demands in home care. *Royal Society for the Promotion of Health Journal*, Sept. 1957, p. 608-12.

Waterman, Theda L.
Nursing for community health. Philadelphia, Davis, 1944. 2nd edn., 1947.

Wearn, E. M.
A comprehensive community nursing service. *Royal Society for the Promotion of Health Journal*, Aug. 1956, p. 509-15.

Wensley, Edith
The community and public health nursing. New York, Macmillan, 1950.

Wilkins, Evelyn
An introduction to social science for health visitors. Arnold, 1932.

Willie, C. V.
The social class of patients that public health nurses prefer to serve. *American Journal of Public Health and the Nation's Health*, Aug. 1960, p. 1126-36.

WINDMULLER, I.
The health visitor in the changing field of social work. *Royal Society for the Promotion of Health Journal*, Sept. 1956, p. 618-25.

WOFINDEN, R. C.
Public health nursing—past, present and future. *District Nursing*, Jan. 1960, p. 202-4 and 210.

WOMEN PUBLIC HEALTH OFFICERS' ASSOCIATION *and* ROYAL COLLEGE OF NURSING. PUBLIC HEALTH SECTION
The duties of the health visitor in the national health service. The Association, 1952.

WORLD HEALTH ORGANIZATION
Report of a Working Conference for Public Health Nurses, Noordwijk, the Netherlands, 2-13 October, 1950. Geneva, W.H.O., 1951.

WORLD HEALTH ORGANIZATION.
EXPERT COMMITTEE ON NURSING
Public health nursing: fourth report of the Expert Committee on Nursing. Geneva, W.H.O., 1959.

WORLD HEALTH ORGANIZATION.
REGIONAL OFFICE FOR EUROPE
Public health nursing: report of a European Conference in Helsinki, 6-19 August, 1958. Copenhagen, W.H.O., 1959.

YOUNG, RUTH
Handbook for health visitors in India. Indian Red Cross Society, Maternity and Child Welfare Bureau, 1933.

Administration

ABBOTT, R. D.
New sight and insight for supervisors. *Nursing Outlook*, Aug. 1959, p. 476-8.

BRAINARD, ANNIE M.
Organization of public health nursing. New York, Macmillan, 1919.

BRODY, WILLIAM
Personnel administration in public health nursing. Kimpton, 1951.

DAVIES, M. E.
Reorganization within health visiting. *Nursing Times*, Sept. 9, 1955, p. 996-7.

EDWARDS, MARY P.
Public health nursing in Saskatchewan. *Canadian Nurse*, May 1960, p. 413-7.

FERGUSON, MARION
The service load of a staff nurse in one official public health agency. New York, Teachers' College, Columbia University, 1945.

FOLLMANN, J. F., JR.
Prepayment for public health nursing service . *Nursing Outlook*, July 1960, p. 384-7.

FREEMAN, RUTH B.
Principles of administration in public health nursing. *Nursing Outlook*, Sept. 1959, p. 514-7.

FREEMAN, RUTH B.
The public health nurse: co-ordinator. *Military Medicine*, Nov. 1958, p. 371-6.

FREEMAN, RUTH B.
Techniques of supervision in public health nursing. Philadelphia, Saunders, 1944.
2nd edn., 1949.

FREEMAN, RUTH B., *and* MCLAUGHLIN, M.
Leadership components in public health nursing. *American Journal of Nursing*, April 1958, p. 552-5.

GERSTENBURGER, H. J.
The question of smaller nursing districts for all kinds of public health work versus larger districts for specialized work. Cleveland, Ohio, 1915.

HALL, M. N.
What is a realistic case load? *Nursing Outlook*, Feb. 1959, p. 75-7.

HODGSON, VIOLET H.
Supervision in public health nursing. New York, Commonwealth Fund, 1939.

HUNTER, T. G.
Program design and evaluation in public health nursing. *Canadian Journal of Public Health*, May 1959, p. 206-11.

KELLOGG, W.
What public health nurses like about their jobs. *Public Health Reports*, Feb. 1957, p. 121-5.

KOHN, R.
A counseling program for public health nursing supervisors. *Nursing Outlook*, April 1958, p. 231-3.

LISTON, M. F.
Communications and their value in health nursing. *Military Medicine*, Nov. 1958, p. 366-70.

MALACHOWSKI, L. T.
The public health nurse as co-ordinator in a geriatric clinic. *Public Health Reports*, July 1959, p. 601-5.

NATIONAL LEAGUE FOR NURSING.
DEPARTMENT OF PUBLIC HEALTH NURSING
Nursing activities of public health nursing agencies. New York, The League, 1955.

NATIONAL LEAGUE FOR NURSING.
DEPARTMENT OF PUBLIC HEALTH NURSING
Progress report on combination services in public health nursing, New York. New York, The League, 1955.

NATIONAL ORGANIZATION FOR PUBLIC HEALTH NURSING
Handbook on records and statistics in the field of public health nursing, prepared by a joint committee of the N.O.P.H.N. and the Advisory Committee on Social Statistics and Child Welfare and related fields of the U.S. Children's Bureau. Washington, U.S. Govt. Printing Office, 1932.

NATIONAL ORGANIZATION FOR PUBLIC HEALTH NURSING
Public health nursing for your community: a guide to establishing a public health nursing service. New York, The Organization, 1950.

NATIONAL ORGANIZATION FOR PUBLIC HEALTH NURSING
Regional placement service. New York, The Organization, 1942.

NEWTON, MILDRED G.
Developing leadership potential. *Nursing Outlook*, July 1957, p. 400-3.

PERCY, D. M.
Integration and conservation of effort in public health nursing. *Canadian Journal of Public Health*, Mar. 1959, p. 111-6.

PICKENS, M. E., *and* TAYBACK, M.
A job satisfaction survey. *Nursing Outlook*, Mar. 1957, p. 157-9.

RANDALL, MARION G.
Personnel policies in public health nursing. New York, Macmillan, 1937.

REZLER, A.
The development of the health visitor and suggested redeployment. *Journal of the Royal Institute of Public Health and Hygiene*, Oct. 1957, p. 338-50.

SCHWARTZ, D. R.
Communication between hospital staff and community agencies: a study of referrals to the public health nurse. *American Journal of Public Health and the Nation's Health*, Aug. 1960, p. 1122-5.

SHETLAND, M. L.
A dynamic approach to evaluation. *Nursing Outlook*, Dec. 1957, p. 711-3.

YANKAUER, A., BOEK, W. E., and CAMPBELL, M.
How much do parents need and use public health nursing services? *Nursing Outlook*, Sept. 1958, p. 508-11.

Education

AFLECK, J. W., and others
In-service mental-health training for health visitors. *Lancet*, Sept. 17, 1960, p. 641-3.

AKESTER, J. M.
Post-certificate courses for health visitors. *Medical Officer*, Feb. 22, 1957, p. 110.

BURKETT, JESSE E.
Improving the professional qualifications of public health nurses. *Nursing Outlook*, Nov. 1958, p. 635-7.

COLUMBIA UNIVERSITY. TEACHERS' COLLEGE.
DIVISION OF NURSING EDUCATION, and others
The field practice period in the university public health nursing program of study: a report of an experiment in field experience in the official and voluntary agencies undertaken by the Division of Nursing Education, Teachers' College, Columbia University, the Bureau of Public Health Nursing, New York City Department of Health, and the Visiting Nurse Service of New York. New York, Columbia University, 1949.

EASTER, E. M., and FIUMARA, N. J.
A specialized agency for field instruction in public health. *Public Health Reports*, Mar. 1957, p. 217-22.

GLASGOW CITY CORPORATION
Glasgow Corporation training scheme for student health visitors. *Nursing Times*, July 29, 1955, p. 835-7.

GRING, A. C., and MAHER, M. A.
Regional planning for public health nursing education in New England. *Nursing Outlook*, July 1958, p. 374-6.

HEELY, P. I.
Public health assistants. *Nursing Outlook*, July 1957, p. 408-10.

KRISTAL, HELEN F., and MILES, HAROLD
Is on-the-job teaching effective. *American Journal of Nursing*, July 1960, p. 975-7.

LAMONT, D. J.
Health visitors' in-service training in mental health: a Scottish experiment. *Nursing Times*, April 29, 1955, p. 452-4.

LEAHY, KATHLEEN M., and BELL, AILEEN TUTTLE
Teaching methods in public health nursing. Philadelphia, Saunders, 1952.

MINISTRY OF EDUCATION
Regulations for the training of health visitors. H.M.S.O., 1919.

MURPHY, M.
Education for nurses already employed in public health; a new approach and old issues. *Nursing Outlook*, July 1959, p. 415-20.

NATIONAL LEAGUE FOR NURSING.
DEPARTMENT OF PUBLIC HEALTH NURSING
Staff education: a guide for public health nursing services. New York, The League, 1955.

NATIONAL ORGANIZATION FOR PUBLIC HEALTH NURSING
Report of a conference on graduate nurse education for public health nurses. New York, The Organization, 1951.

NATIONAL ORGANIZATION FOR PUBLIC HEALTH NURSING and UNITED STATES PUBLIC HEALTH SERVICE, *Joint Committee*
Public health nursing curriculum guide. New York, The Organization, 1942.

NEW YORK CITY, DEPARTMENT OF HEALTH
Manual of instructions for nurses, prepared by the Bureau of Nursing. New York, The Department, 1931.

O'CONNELL, P. E.
The education and training of health visitors. Royal Sanitary Institute, 1954.

OWEN, M. C.
Oxfordshire trains its health visitors. *Nursing Mirror*, Jan. 9, 1959, p. vi.

STEVENSON, D. M.
The health visitor—and her changing training. *Nursing Mirror*, Oct. 3, 1958, p. 35-6.

TSCHUDIN, MARY S., and NOTTER, LUCILLE
Preparation of basic students for public health nursing. *Nursing Outlook*, Jan. 1960, p. 16-21.

WHITE, M. R.
The art of application and interview: some suggestions principally for would-be student health visitors. *Nursing Mirror*, Aug. 19, 1955, p. v.

WILD, EDITH
A handbook for the student health visitor. Lewis, 1944.

WINSLOW, CHARLES EDWARD AMORY
The new profession of public health nursing and its educational needs. Washington, U.S. Govt. Printing Office, 1917.
[Paper presented before the second Pan American Scientific Congress, Washington, Dec. 27, 1915-Jan. 8, 1916.]

Health Visiting and General Practice

CHALKE, H. D., and FISHER, M.
Health visitor and family doctor. An exercise in liaison. *Lancet*, Oct. 5, 1957, p. 685-7.

CROMBIE, D. L., and CROSS, K. W.
The contribution of the nurse in general practice. *British Journal of Preventive and Social Medicine*, Jan. 1957, p. 41-4.

FORMAN, J. A.
A nurse in group practice. *Practitioner*, Sept. 1956, p. 325 and 324.

NICHOLSON, N. G.
A day with a health visitor: a general practitioner's point of view. *British Medical Journal*, June 25, 1955, p. 299 (supp.); *Nursing Times*, July 29, 1955, p. 828-30.

TAYLOR, S.
The general practitioner and domiciliary nursing. *Nursing Times*, June 19, 1954, p. 650-3.

WADHAM, M. A.
The Winchester experiment. *Nursing Times*, Sept. 30, 1960, p. 1202-4.

SCHOOL NURSING

AMERICAN RED CROSS SOCIETY
Rural school nursing. Washington, The Society, 1925.

BROOKS, LUCY
The work of the school nurse and medical inspection. *British Journal of Nursing*, April 16, 1911, p. 346-8.

CATCHINGS, MILDRED W.
The school nurse and accident prevention. *Nursing Outlook*, Feb. 1958, p. 108-11.

CHAYER, MARY ELLA
School nursing: a contribution to health education. New York, Putnam, 1931.

CROMWELL, GERTRUDE E.
School nursing is pediatric nursing. *Nursing Outlook*, Feb. 1957, p. 73-5.

EDWARDS, A. D.
The school nurse: her work among the children and parents. *British Journal of Nursing*, Aug. 29, 1908, p. 164-6.

FALTHER, ANNE R.
Family life education in the school health program. *Journal of School Health*, June 1958, p. 179-82.

GARSIDE, ALMA H.
The school nurse as a family health advisor. *Journal of School Health*, May 1958, p. 153-7.

GRAHAM, A. A.
The school nurse and the future. *Public Health*, April 1959, p. 263-6.

GROSSMAN, JEROME
The school nurse's perception of problems and responsibilities—implications for professional education. *Nursing Research*, June 1956, p. 18-26.

KELLEY, H. W., *and* BRADSHAW, M. C.
Handbook for school nurses. New York, Macmillan, 1918.

LEIPOLDT, C. LOUIS
The school nurse: her duties and responsibilities. Scientific Press, 1912.

LIPELES, J. C.
The school nurse represents medical and legal authority. *Nursing Outlook*, Nov. 1957, p. 652-4.

LOS ANGELES. COUNTY SUPERINTENDENT OF SCHOOLS
A handbook for school nurses. Los Angeles, The Office [of the County Superintendent], 1950.

"A MEDICAL OFFICER"
The school nurse.
See
NURSING TIMES
The nurse and the nation: a survey of her position in the State today. *Nursing Times*, Nov. 5, 1910, p. 904-31.

MICHIGAN DEPARTMENT OF HEALTH
The nurse in the school community. Lansing, The Department, 1949.

NATIONAL LEAGUE FOR NURSING.
DEPARTMENT OF PUBLIC HEALTH NURSING
Report of national conference on school nursing services. New York, The League, 1956.

NATIONAL ORGANIZATION FOR PUBLIC HEALTH NURSING.
SCHOOL NURSING SECTION
Trends in school nursing. . . . New York, National League for Nursing, [1952].

OBERTEUFFER, DELBERT
School health education: a textbook for teachers, nurses and other professional personnel. New York, Harper, 1949.
2nd edn., 1954.

PEARSE, HELEN L.
The place of the school nurse. *British Journal of Nursing*, Aug. 17, 1907, p. 124-5.

PETTY, ROSE
School nursing. *Nursing Times*, June 3, 1905, p. 80-1.

RANDLE, B. B.
Program of school nursing for Cattarangus County Schools, 1927-1928. New York, Cattarangus County School Health Service, 1928.

RAPPAPORT, MARY B.
Co-operation of the nurse and teacher in the health program in small communities. *Journal of School Health*, Feb. 1957, p. 48-52.

ROGERS, LINA L.
School nursing in Toronto, Canada. *British Journal of Nursing*, Nov. 9, 1912, p. 371-3, and Nov. 16, 1912, p. 392-3.

STOBO, ELIZABETH
Today's preparation for the nurse in the school. *Teachers' College Record*, Dec. 1955, p. 196-9.

STRUTHERS, LINA ROGERS
The school nurse: a survey of the duties and responsibilities of the nurse in the maintenance of health and physical perfection and the prevention of disease among school children. New York, Putnam, 1917.

SWANSON, MARIE
School nursing in the community program. New York, Macmillan, 1953.

SWANSON, MARIE
The work of the school nurse teacher. Albany, University of the State of New York, 1932.
Revised 1949.

TERMAN, LEWIS M., *and* ALMACK, JOHN C.
The hygiene of the school child. Boston, Houghton Mifflin, 1929.

TIPPLE, DOROTHY C.
The changing role of the school nurse. *Teachers' College Record*, Jan. 1958, p. 191-5.

TIPPLE, DOROTHY C.
The future of school nursing. *Journal of the American Medical Association*, Sept. 5, 1959, p. 59-62.

WOODS, N. A.
Teacher-nurse communications in an elementary school. *Canadian Nurse*, Feb. 1958, p. 122-4.

RESPIRATORY SYSTEM

ASHER, P.
Some common diseases of the chest. *Hospital and Social Service Journal*, May 22, 1959, p. 523-4.

FENWICK, BEDFORD
The nursing of patients suffering from diseases of the chest. *Nursing Record*, 1901.

SCIENCE

LEAVELL, L. C., *and* THOMPSON, L.
Science in the nursing curriculum: content and methods. *Nursing Outlook*, Oct. 1957, p. 604-7.

THOMPSON, L., *and* LEAVELL, L. C.
Science in the nursing curriculum: philosophy and principles. *Nursing Outlook*, Sept. 1957, p. 537-9.

SOCIAL PROBLEMS AND NURSING

BROWN, M. L.
Helping the alcoholic patient. *American Journal of Nursing*, Mar. 1958, p. 387-8.

CORK, R. M.
Alcoholism and nursing. *Canadian Journal of Occupational Therapy*, Aug. 1957, p. 372-8.

COULTER, E. B.
Nursing care problems associated with ataraxic drugs. *Hawaii Medical Journal and Inter-Island Nurses' Bulletin*, Jan.-Feb. 1957, p. 303-4.

GOLDER, GRACE M.
The alcoholic, his family and his nurse. *Nursing Outlook*, Oct. 1955, p. 528-30.

GOLDER, GRACE M.
The nurse and the alcoholic patient. *American Journal of Nursing*, April 1956, p. 436-8.

LEWIS, JOHN A.
Alcoholism. *American Journal of Nursing*, April 1956, p. 433-5.

QUIROS, ALYCE
Adjusting nursing techniques to the treatment of alcoholic patients. *Nursing Outlook*, May 1957, p. 276-9.

SURGERY

GENERAL WORKS

ALEXANDER, EDYTHE LOUISE
Operating room technique. Kimpton, 1943.
2nd edn., 1949.
3rd edn., 1958, entitled "The care of the patient in surgery, including techniques."

BAILEY, HAMILTON
Demonstrations of operative surgery for nurses. Edinburgh, Livingstone, 1945.
2nd edn., 1954.

BAILEY, HAMILTON, and LOVE, R. J. MCNEILL
Surgery for nurses. Lewis, 1933.
2nd edn., 1936.
3rd edn., 1938.
4th edn., 1940.
5th edn., 1942.
6th edn., 1946.
7th edn., 1950.
8th edn., 1954.

BELCHER, J. R., and GRANT, I. W. B.
Thoracic surgical management. Bailliere, Tindall & Cox, 1953. 2nd edn., 1955.

BERRY, EDNA CORNELIA, and KOHN, MARY LOUISE
Introduction to operating-room technique. New York, McGraw-Hill, 1955.
2nd edn., 1960.

BICKFORD, E., and BUDD, E.
Pulmonary resection. 2. Nursing care. American Journal of Nursing, Jan. 1952, p. 40-3.

BRISTOL ROYAL INFIRMARY
Staphylococcal cross-infection in surgery. Two-year study of preventive measures at Bristol Royal Infirmary described by John W. Bradbeer. Nursing Mirror, Oct. 28, 1960, p. ii.

BULMAN, MICHAEL W.
Surgery and surgical nursing. Faber, 1934.
2nd edn., 1938.
3rd edn., 1941.
4th edn., 1943.
8th edn., 1952.

CAIRNEY, JOHN
Surgery for students of nursing. Christchurch, N.Z., Peryer, 1952.
2nd edn., 1955.
3rd edn., 1958.

COLLIS, J. LEIGH, and MABBIT, L. E.
Chest surgery for nurses. Bailliere, Tindall & Cox, 1944.
2nd edn., 1946.
3rd edn., 1951.
4th edn., 1956.

D'ABREU, A. L.
Thoracic surgery and the nurse. Nursing Times, Feb. 23, 1952, p. 178-9.

DANIELS, D. W.
An outline of surgery for nurses. Bristol, Wright, 1933.

DUNN, MARY ANN
Nursing care of patients undergoing open-heart surgery. Hospital Topics, 1958.

HARLOW, F. WILSON, editor
Modern surgery for nurses. Heinemann, 1948.
2nd edn., 1951.
3rd edn., 1954.
4th edn., 1959.

HARVEY, J. E.
The nurse in neurosurgery. Canadian Nurse, Jan. 1953, p. 11-18.

HILLMAN, O. STANLEY
Operative surgery described for nurses. Faber, 1927.
2nd edn., 1944.

HOUGHTON, MARJORIE
Aids to theatre technique. Bailliere, Tindall & Cox, 1944.
2nd edn., 1952.

HUDD, JEAN
An operating theatre sterilizing unit. Nursing Times, Sept. 27, 1957, p. 1088-92.

ILGENFRITZ, HUGH CALVIN
Synopsis of the preparation and after-care of surgical patients. St. Louis, Mosby, 1941.
2nd edn., 1948, called "Preoperative and postoperative care of surgical patients".

KEMBLE, JAMES
Surgery for nurses: a textbook for the surgical nurse. Bristol, Wright, 1949.

LOWBURY, E. J. L., and LILLY, H. A.
Disinfection of the hands of surgeons and nurses. British Medical Journal, May 14, 1960, p. 1445-50.

MCLAUGHLIN, C. R.
Plastic surgery: an introduction for nurses, with special sections by other members of the East Grinstead Queen Victoria Hospital staff. Faber, 1951.

MAHOOD, N. P.
Nursing of patients after free skin grafts. Nursing Mirror, July 6, 1956, p. iii.

MORONEY, JAMES
Surgery for nurses. Edinburgh, Livingstone, 1950.
2nd edn., 1952.
3rd edn., 1955.
4th edn., 1956.
5th edn., 1958.
6th edn., 1959.

NATIONAL LEAGUE FOR NURSING, DEPARTMENT OF HOSPITAL NURSING, and AMERICAN HOSPITAL ASSOCIATION
The operating room supervisor at work, by Edna L. Prickett. New York, The League, 1955.

ROWBOTHAM, G. F., and HAMMERSLEY, D. P.
Pictorial introduction to neurological surgery. Edinburgh, Livingstone, 1953.

ST. MARY'S HOSPITAL, ROCHESTER, MINNESOTA
The operating room: instructions for nurses and assistants. Philadelphia, Saunders, 1924.
2nd edn., 1928.
3rd edn., 1937.
4th edn., 1952, called "Operating room technic".
5th edn., 1957.

SOLOMON, GLADYS
Theatre technique for nurses and students. Cape Town, Maskew Miller, [19?].

STAFFORD, EDWARD S., and DILLER, DORIS
A textbook of surgery for nurses. Philadelphia, Saunders, 1947.
2nd edn., 1954.
3rd edn., 1958.

TAYLOR, SELWYN
A summary of surgery for nurses. Faber, 1948.

WELLS, CHARLES
A manual of surgery for nurses. Edinburgh, Livingstone, 1938.

WOOLF, M. S.
Principles of surgery for nurses. Philadelphia, Saunders, 1930.

YEAGER, MARY ELLEN
Operating room manual: a guide for O.R. personnel. New York, Putnam, 1958.

ACCIDENTS, BURNS, ETC.

ALEXANDER, J.
The nurse and accidental poisoning cases. American Association of Industrial Nurses' Journal, March 1959, p. 13-14.

BAKER, T. J.
Open techniques in the management of burns. *American Journal of Nursing*, Sept. 1959, p. 1262-5.

BLOCKER, TRUMAN G., *and others*
The care of patients with burns. *Nursing Outlook*, July 1958, p. 382-7.

BRANTL, V. M., BROWN, B. J., *and* MOORELAND, M.
The case of patients with burns; comprehensive nursing care. *Nursing Outlook*, July 1958, p. 383-5.

CHAMPION, R.
The treatment of burns. *Journal for Industrial Nurses*, Spring 1953, p. 271-94.

CLARKSON, P.
Modern treatment of burns.
1. Introduction.
2. Treatment of primary phase.
3. Healing phase.
4. Rehabilitation.
Nursing Mirror, June 26, 1953, p. x; July 3, 1953, p. vi; July 10, 1953, p. xii.

CREWS, E. R., *and* BROWN, S.
Nursing care of massive burns. *Nursing World*, July 1957, p. 9-11.

HENDERSON, L. M.
Nursing care of patients with facial injuries. *American Journal of Nursing*, April 1957, p. 453-6.

LUB, A.
Nursing patients with burns. *Nursing Times*, Feb. 19, 1960, p 215-7.

MAHER, M. H., *and* DAVIS, J. H.
The nursing care of burns. *Nursing World*, Aug. 1954, p. 33-6.

NORMAN, L. G.
The nurse's part in road safety. *Nursing Mirror*, Dec. 2, 1960, p. 817-8.

RHODES, V. A., *and* SHANNON, A. M.
Nursing care of the burn patient. *American Journal of Nursing*, Sept. 1959, p. 1265-8.

SCHWEISHEIMER, W.
Occupational burns in industry: remarkable healing effects by modern methods. *Nursing Mirror*, Nov. 13, 1953, p. vii.

WALLACE, A. B.
The treatment of burns. *Nursing Mirror*, Oct. 15, 1954, p. iii.

WINDSOR GROUP OF HOSPITALS
Accident sisters in an after-care service. *Nursing Mirror*, Nov. 4, 1960, p. 451.

ORTHOPAEDICS

CALDERWOOD, CARMELITA
Orthopaedic nursing: content and method of the teaching program in schools of nursing. New York, Joint Orthopaedic Nursing Advisory Service, 1942.

ELLIS, M.
Needs of long-term orthopaedic patients. *Nursing Times*, Mar. 20, 1954, p. 309-11.

FUNSTEN, ROBERT V., *and* CALDERWOOD, CARMELITA
Orthopedic nursing. Kimpton, 1943.
2nd edn., 1949, by C. Calderwood, revised by Carroll B. Larson and Marjorie Gould.
3rd edn., 1953.
4th edn., 1957.

HUGHES, J. M.
Nursing care after intramedullary nailing. *American Journal of Nursing*, Feb. 1959, p. 239-40.

JOINT ORTHOPAEDIC NURSING ADVISORY SERVICE
Orthopaedic conditions at birth, nursing responsibilities. New York, National Organization for Public Health Nursing, 1943.

KERR, AVICE
Orthopaedic nursing procedures. New York, Springer, 1959.

KNOCKE, FREDERICK J., *and* KNOCKE, LAZELLE S.
Orthopedic nursing. Philadelphia, Davis, 1954.

LEWIN, PHILIP
A textbook of orthopedic surgery for nurses. Philadelphia, Saunders, 1928.
2nd edn., 1934.
3rd edn., 1940, called "Orthopedic surgery for nurses including nursing care".
4th edn., 1947.

MCBRIDE, EARL D.
Crippled children: their treatment and orthopedic nursing. Kimpton, 1931.

NATIONAL LEAGUE OF NURSING EDUCATION
Suggestions for content and instruction in orthopedic nursing. New York, The League, 1950.

NAYLOR, ARTHUR
Fractures and orthopaedic surgery for nurses and masseuses. Edinburgh, Livingstone, 1945.
2nd edn., 1948.
3rd edn., 1952.
4th edn., 1960.

PEARCE, EVELYN CLARE
A textbook of orthopaedic nursing. Faber & Gwyer, 1927.
3rd edn., 1943.

POWELL, MARY
Orthopaedic nursing. Edinburgh, Livingstone, 1951.
2nd edn., 1956.
3rd edn., 1959.

WALLER, BERTHA
Aids to orthopaedics for nurses. Bailliere, Tindall & Cox, 1945.
2nd edn., 1948.
3rd edn., 1959, by Winifred Talog Davies.

WEST, JESSIE STEVENSON
Congenital malformations and birth injuries: a handbook on nursing. New York, Association for the Aid of Crippled Children, 1954.

SURGICAL NURSING

ANDREWS, M. S.
Nursing care in maxillo-facial surgery. *Military Medicine*, July 1959, p. 520-5.

ARMSTRONG, KATHERINE F.
Aids to surgical nursing. Bailliere, Tindall & Cox, 1938.
2nd edn., 1941.
3rd edn., 1942.
4th edn., 1949.
5th edn., 1954.
6th edn., 1957.

ATKINS, HEDLEY JOHN BARNARD
After treatment: a guide to general practitioners, house-officers, ward-sisters and dressers in the care of patients after operation. Oxford, Blackwell, 1942.
2nd edn., 1944.
4th edn., 1952.

ATKINSON, W. J.
Nursing care in the management of head injuries. *Nursing Mirror*, May 18, 1956, p. ii.

AYLETT, S.
Colostomy and its nursing care. *Nursing Mirror*, May 25, 1956, p. ii; June 1, 1956, p. xi.

BEARDSLEY, J. M., *and* CARVISIGLIA, F. F.
A special care ward for surgical patients. *Nursing World*, Mar. 1957, p. 11.

BELL, JOSEPH
Notes on surgery for nurses. Simpkin Marshall, 1888.
5th edn., 1899.

BIRD, BRIAN
Psychological aspects of preoperative and postoperative nursing care. *American Journal of Nursing*, June 1955, p. 685-7.

BONELL, P. R.
Understanding surgical patients. *American Journal of Nursing*, Aug. 1959, p. 1148-9.

BRAGDON, JANE SHERBURN, *and* SHOLTIS, LILLIAN A.
Teaching medical and surgical nursing. Philadelphia, Lippincott, 1955.

BROOKES, HENRY S.
A textbook of surgical nursing. St. Louis, Mosby, 1937.
2nd edn., 1940, by Henry S. Brookes and Pearl Castile.

CABOT, HUGH, *and* GILES, MARY DODD
Surgical nursing. Philadelphia, Saunders, 1931.
2nd edn., 1934.
3rd edn., 1937.
4th edn., 1940.

CANTLIN, VERNITA L.
O.R. nursing is a professional speciality. *Nursing Outlook*, July 1960, p. 376-8.

COLP, RALPH, *and* KELLER, MANELVA WYLIE
Surgical nursing. New York, Macmillan, 1921.
2nd edn., 1929, by Ralph Colp and Manelva Wylie Keller, called "Textbook of surgical nursing".
3rd edn., 1936, by Manelva Wylie Keller.
4th edn., 1946, by William F. McFee and Manelva Wylie Keller.
5th edn., 1950, by John Pettit West, Manelva Wylie Keller and Elizabeth H. Harman, called "Nursing care of the surgical patient".
6th edn., 1957.

DARLING, H. C. RUTHERFORD
Surgical nursing and after treatment: a handbook for nurses and others. Churchill, 1917.
2nd edn., 1923.
3rd edn., 1928.
4th edn., 1932.
5th edn., 1935.
6th edn., 1938.
7th edn., 1941.
8th edn., 1944.
9th edn., 1946.
10th edn., 1951, by H. C. R. Darling and Edward Wilson.
11th edn., 1960, by Edward Wilson.

DE GUTIERREZ-MAHONEY, C. G., *and* CARINI, ESTA
Neurological and neurosurgical nursing. St. Louis, Mosby, 1949.
2nd edn., 1956.
3rd edn., 1960.

DUSSEAULT, RITA
Basic teaching in surgical nursing. *Canadian Nurse*, Oct. 1959, p. 891-2.

ELIASON, ELDRIDGE L., FERGUSON, L. K., *and* LEWIS, ELIZABETH K.
Surgical nursing. Philadelphia, Lippincott, 1929.
2nd edn., 1930.
3rd edn., 1931.
4th edn., 1934.
5th edn., 1936.
6th edn., 1940, by E. L. Eliason, L. K. Ferguson and A. M. Farrand.
7th edn., 1945, by E. L. Eliason, L. K. Ferguson and A. M. Farrand.
8th edn., 1947, by E. L. Eliason, L. K. Ferguson and A. M. Farrand.
9th edn., 1950, by E. L. Eliason, L. K. Ferguson and Lillian A. Sholtis.
10th edn., 1955.

FALK, HENRY C.
Operating room procedure for nurses and internes. New York Putnam, 1925.

FELTER, ROBERT K., *and others*
Surgical nursing, by Robert K. Felter, Frances West, Lydia M. Zetzsche and associates. Philadelphia, Davis, 1937.
2nd edn., 1940.
3rd edn., 1942.
4th edn., 1946.
5th edn., 1948.
6th edn., 1952.
7th edn., 1958.

FISK, JEAN E.
Nursing care of the patient with surgery of the biliary tract. *American Journal of Nursing*, Jan. 1960, p. 53-5.

FLANAGAN, EILEEN C., *and* HERDAN, IRENE M.
A preliminary study and analysis of nursing requirements in neurological and neurosurgical nursing: the Montreal Neurological Institute. Reprinted from the *Canadian Nurse*, Nov. 1955.

GEISTER, JANET
The operating room nurse and nursing organization. *Hospital Topics*, 1959.

GILLIS, L.
The nursing care of amputations. *Nursing Mirror*, Feb. 8, 1957, p. vii; Feb. 15, 1957, p. v; Feb. 22, 1957, p. v.

GLASSMAN, JACOB A., *and* MCNEALY, RAYMOND W.
Care of the surgical patient. Baltimore, Williams & Wilkins, 1959.

GRAFFAM, SHIRLEY
Care of the surgical patient: a textbook for nurses. New York, McGraw-Hill, 1960.

GRIFFIN, AMY E.
Evaluation of experience in the operating room. *Canadian Nurse*, Aug. 1960, p. 705-9.

HALL, EDITH D., *compiler*
Surgical instrument guide for nurses. New York, Edward Weck, 1953.

HAMBY, WALLACE B.
The hospital care of neurosurgical patients. Springfield, Illinois, Thomas, 1940.
2nd edn., 1948.

HAYNES, WALTER G., *and* MCGUIRE, MARY
Textbook of neurosurgical nursing. Philadelphia, Saunders, 1952.

HENDERSON, L. M.
Nursing care of patients with facial injuries. *American Journal of Nursing*, April 1957, p. 453-6.

HINSON, J. A., OLEKSYN, E. E., *and* DAFOE, C. A.
Nursing care of the thoracic surgical patient. *Canadian Nurse*, Mar. 1959, p. 218-22.

HOWARD, RUSSELL
Surgical nursing and the principles of surgery for nurses. Arnold, 1905.
6th edn., 1930.

HOWELL, CORNADE
A series of lectures on surgical nursing and hospital technic . . . delivered to nurses at Grant Hospital, Protestant Hospital, Columbus State Hospital, with fifty-five half-tone engravings throughout the text and six plates, illustrating the ideal operating room and its accessory rooms. Columbus, Ohio, Stoneman Press, 1913

JACKSON, M. L.
Nursing care of skin grafts. *Nursing World*, Sept. 1958, p. 16-17.

JOLLY, JEAN D.
Operating room procedures for nurses. Faber, 1936.
2nd edn., 1941.
3rd edn., 1951.

KLEMME, ROLAND M.
Nursing care of neurosurgical patients. Springfield, Illinois, Thomas, 1949.

LEWIN, W.
Recent developments in the nursing of head injuries. *Nursing Mirror*, April 5, 1957, p. v.

LINDSAY, W. F.
Outlines of general, surgical nursing. Lona Linda, California, . . . 1912.

LOCKWOOD, CHARLES D., *and* NEWTON, MILDRED E.
The principles and practice of surgical nursing. New York, Macmillan, 1932.

MARIE, EDGAR, SISTER
O.R. experience program aids professional student nurses. *Hospital Progress*, Feb. 1959, part I, p. 65-7.

MINTER, SARAH
Theatre technique for nurses. *Nursing Mirror*, 1952.

NASH, D. F. ELLISON
The principles and practice of surgical nursing. Arnold, 1955.

NEEF, FREDERICK E.
A textbook of surgical nursing. Philadelphia, Lea & Febiger, 1933.

NORTHCROFT, G. B.
Neurosurgical nursing and the role of the nurse.
1. Neurosurgery in the 20th century.
2. Nursing unconscious patient in neurosurgical unit.
3. Nursing paraplegic patient in neurosurgical unit.
4. Care of head injuries in the neurosurgical unit.
5. Care of cerebral tumours.
Nursing Mirror, Aug. 12, 1960, p. iv; Aug. 19, 1960, p. v; Aug. 26, 1960, p. x; Sept. 2, 1960, p. xii; Sept. 9, 1960, p. x.

NORTON, DOREEN
Aids to thoracic surgical nursing. Bailliere, Tindall & Cox, 1955.

NORWEGIAN NURSES' ASSOCIATION
General surgical nursing; paper prepared on behalf of the Norwegian Nurses' Association at the request of the Nursing Service Committee of the International Council of Nurses. Supplement to *International Nursing Review*, April 1959.

OUIMET, JACQUELINE
Clinical teaching in surgical nursing. *Canadian Nurse*, Oct. 1959, p. 893-5.

PARENT, ADRIENNE
Preparation for nursing in cardiac surgery. *Canadian Nurse*, Oct. 1959, p. 902-3.

PARKER, E. M., *and* BRECKENRIDGE, S. D.
Surgical and gynaecological nursing. 3rd edn. Philadelphia, . . . 1925.

PEARCE, EVELYN CLARE
Instruments, appliances and theatre technique. Faber, 1941.
2nd edn., 1943.
3rd edn., 1955.

PERKINS, ERLINE WEBB
Aseptic technique for operating room personnel. Philadelphia, Saunders, 1959.

REGARDIE, V. H., *and* HELLYER, E. M.
Recovery room experience for students. *Nursing Outlook*, Sept. 1957, p. 542-3.

SACHS, ERNEST
The care of the neurosurgical patient before, during and after operation. Kimpton, 1945.

SCOTT, R. B.
Cardiac surgery: nursing care before and after. *Nursing World*, Aug. 1955, p. 21-4.

SKELLERN, E. M.
Caring for bilateral adrenalectomy patients. *Nursing Times*, May 18, 1956, p. 436-7.

SKELLERN, E. M.
A post-operative observation ward. *Nursing Times*, Mar. 30, 1956, p. 243-5.

SWEDISH NURSES' ASSOCIATION
Acceptable standards of neurosurgical nursing service. *Australian Nurses' Journal*, July 1956, p. 161; *Nursing Mirror*, Nov. 30, 1956, p. ii; Dec. 7, 1956, p. ii; Dec. 14, 1956, p. vii.

THOREK, PHILIP
Illustrated preoperative and postoperative care. Pitman, 1958.

WAKELEY, CECIL
Nursing care and treatment of hernia.
1. External hernia. *Nursing Mirror*, Sept. 6, 1957, p. iii.
2. The treatment of femoral hernia. *Nursing Mirror*, Sept. 13, 1957, p. iii.
3. Umbilical hernia; its treatment and nursing care. *Nursing Mirror*, Sept. 20, 1957, p. ii.
4. Hernia of the bladder. *Nursing Mirror*, Sept. 27, 1957, p. xi.
5. Rare herniae. *Nursing Mirror*, Oct. 4, 1957, p. vi.

WAKELEY, CECIL
Pre- and post-operative care of cisternal puncture. *Nursing Mirror*, Dec. 28, 1956, p. ii.

WAKELEY, CECIL
Pre- and post-operative care of cases of subdural haematoma. *Nursing Mirror*, Jan. 4, 1957, p. v.

WAKELEY, CECIL
Pre- and post-operative nursing care of extradural haemorrhage. *Nursing Mirror*, Jan. 11, 1957, p. vii.

WAKELEY, CECIL
Pre- and post-operative care of cases of basal fractures of the skull and their nursing care. *Nursing Mirror*, Jan. 18, 1957, p. x.

WAKELEY, CECIL
Pre- and post-operative care of depressed fractures of the skull. *Nursing Mirror*, Jan. 25, 1957, p. vi.

WAKELEY, CECIL
The surgery of the pituitary gland, including pre- and post-operative nursing care. *Nursing Mirror*, Feb. 1, 1957, p. x.

WAKELEY, JOHN C. N.
Pre- and post-operative nursing care of the partial gastrectomy case. *Nursing Mirror*, June 13, 1958, p. 801.

WULFSOHN, N. L.
Aids to pre- and post-operative nursing. Bailliere, Tindall & Cox, 1958.

YAPP, C. SEYMOUR
Practical surgical nursing for probationers. (Description of common operations). Poor-Law Publications Ltd., [19?].

THERAPEUTICS
GENERAL WORKS

PARKER, NINETTE A.
Materia medica and therapeutics—a textbook for nurses. Philadelphia, . . . 1915.

ANAESTHETICS

FINNIE, W. J.
Anaesthetics and anaesthesia for nurses. *Nursing Mirror*, 1951.

GEISTER, JANET M.
The anesthetist as a professional nurse. *Journal of the American Association of Nurse-Anesthetists*, 1959, p. 18-27.

GODWIN, ERIC
Anaesthesia for nurses. Bristol, Wright, 1957.

HEWER, C. LANGTON
Outline of anaesthesia from the nurse's viewpoint. *Hospital and Social Service Journal*, [1950?].

HOULE, E. L.
The nurse anesthetist. What she does. How she does it. *Hospital Management*, Sept. 1960, p. 61.

HUNT, ALICE M.
Anaesthesia: principles and practice; a presentation for the nursing profession. New York, Putnam, 1949.

LETOURNEAU, CHARLES U.
What is the present status of the nurse anaesthetist. Chicago, *Hospital Management*, 1957.

REGAN, W. A.
A nurse-anaesthetist and the law. *Hospital Progress*, Sept. 1958, p. 76-7; II. *Hospital Progress*, Nov. 1958, p. 72-3.

THATCHER, VIRGINIA S.
History of anesthesia, with emphasis on the nurse specialist. Philadelphia, Lippincott, 1953.

WATSON, J. K.
Anaesthesia and analgesia for nurses and midwives. Bristol, Wright, 1938.

DIETETICS AND NUTRITION

AMERICAN DIETETIC ASSOCIATION.
PROFESSIONAL EDUCATION COMMITTEE
A manual for teaching dietetics to student nurses. Philadelphia, Saunders, 1949.

BIEN, RUTH V.
Nutrition and meal preparation for the practical nurse. Albany, Delmar, 1956.

BROWN, M. L.
The dietitian in a diploma nursing program. *Journal of the American Dietetic Association*, May 1960, p. 474-5.

DEEGAN, D.
Teaching nutrition in the basic nursing curriculum. *Journal of the American Dietetic Association*, Feb. 1958, p. 169-71.

GREENE, JESSIE C.
Nutrition in a collegiate basic nursing curriculum. *Nursing Outlook*, June 1960, p. 314-5.

GREENE, J. M.
Nutrition in nursing: a bookshelf review. *Journal of the American Dietetic Association*, July 1960, p. 38-44.

HARRIS, CATHERINE F.
Handbook of dietetics for nurses. Bailliere, Tindall & Cox, 1953.

HASSENPLUG, LULU WOLF
The teaching dietitian's place in nursing education. *Journal of the American Dietetic Association*, May 1960, p. 467-71.

HOWE, PHYLLIS S.
Nutrition for practical nurses. Philadelphia, Saunders, 1955.
2nd edn., 1958.

KRAUSE, MARIE V.
Nutrition and diet therapy in relation to nursing. Philadelphia, Saunders, 1952.
2nd edn., 1957.

LOANE, M.
Practical instruction in district sick cookery. *British Journal of Nursing*, May 13, 1905, p. 372-4.

METROPOLITAN LIFE INSURANCE COMPANY
Suggestions concerning food for normal nutrition for the use of nurses. New York, The Company, 1943.

MOLLESON, A.
Teaching nutrition to student nurses. *Journal of the American Dietetic Association*, Feb. 1958, p. 164-9.

MORRIS, ENA
How does a nurse teach nutrition to patients? *American Journal of Nursing*, Jan. 1960, p. 67-70.

MOWRY, LILLIAN
Basic nutrition and diet therapy for nurses. St. Louis, Mosby, 1958.

NEW YORK STATE DEPARTMENT OF HEALTH.
NUTRITION BUREAU
Nutrition reference for nurses. Albany, The Department, 1952.

NEWTON, MARJORIE E.
What every nurse needs to know about nutrition. *Nursing Outlook*, June 1960, p. 316-7.

PAVEY, AGNES E.
Nutrition and diet therapy. Faber, 1948.
2nd edn., 1956.

PEYTON, ALICE B.
Practical nutrition. Philadelphia, Lippincott, 1957.

PROUDFIT, FAIRFAX T.
Dietetics for nurses. New York, Macmillan, 1918.
2nd edn., 1922.
3rd edn., 1924.
4th edn., 1927.
5th edn., 1930.
6th edn., 1934.
7th edn., 1938.
8th edn., 1942.
5th-8th edns. called "Nutrition and diet therapy".
9th edn., 1946.
10th edn., 1950.
11th edn., 1955.
9th-11th edns., by F. T. Proudfit and Corine H. Robinson, called "Nutrition and diet therapy".

RYNBERGEN, HENDERIKA J.
Teaching nutrition in nursing. Philadelphia, Lippincott, 1948.
2nd edn., 1950.
3rd edn., 1953.
4th edn., 1956.

SHACKLETON, ALBERTA DENT
Practical nurse nutrition education. Philadelphia, Saunders, 1960.

STEWART, I.
Dietetics for the nurse. Faber, 1928.
2nd edn., 1930.
3rd edn., 1932.
4th edn., 1934.
5th edn., 1937.
6th edn., 1939.
7th edn., 1943.
8th edn., 1949.

THIGPEN, L. W., and MITCHELL, I. A.
Integrating nutrition into nursing education. *Journal of the American Dietetic Association*, April 1957, p. 378-80.

WANSBROUGH, ROSAMOND
"Preliminary" textbook of dietetics and cookery for nurses. Faber, 1939.
2nd edn., 1942.
3rd edn., 1944.
4th edn., 1951.

PHARMACOLOGY

ADELSON, DANIEL
Are nurses needed in pharmacological research? *American Journal of Nursing*, Sept. 1960, p. 1278-81.

BIDDLE, HARRY C., and SITLER, DISA W.
The mathematics of drugs and solutions: a workbook designed to supplement textbooks on drugs and solutions for schools of nursing. Philadelphia, Davis, 1934.
2nd edn., 1941.
3rd edn., 1945.
4th edn., 1947.
5th edn., 1951.
6th edn., 1956.

BLUMENTHAL, ANN
Principles of solutions and drugs—a textbook for nurses.
New York, 1916.

CRAWFORD, A. MUIR
Materia medica for nurses. Lewis, 1927.
2nd edn., 1932.
3rd edn., 1934.
4th edn., 1937.
5th edn., 1942.
6th edn., 1947.

CUNNINGHAM, P. J., editor
Practical preparations in common use. Faber, 1953.
[Originally issued as N. W. Powell's "Practical preparations mainly medical", 1933, q.v.].

DOOLEY, MARION SYLVESTER, and RAPPAPORT, JOSEPHINE
Pharmacology and therapeutics in nursing. New York, McGraw-Hill, 1948.
2nd edn., 1953.

FADDIS, MARGENE O.
How rational drug therapy affects nursing duties. Modern Hospital, July 1959, p. 92-6.

FADDIS, MARGENE O.
Textbook of pharmacology for nurses, assisted by Joseph M. Hayman. Philadelphia, Lippincott, 1940.
2nd edn., 1943.
3rd edn., 1949.
4th edn., 1953.
5th edn., 1959.

FALCONER, MARY W., and NORMAN, MABELCLAIRE RALSTON
The drug, the nurse, the patient. Philadelphia, Saunders, 1958.

FERGUSON, IRA LUNAN, and FERGUSON, ELIZABETH S.
The mathematics of dosages and solutions for nurses. Philadelphia, Saunders, 1956.

FORTESCUE-BRICKDALE, J. M.
A textbook of pharmacology and medical treatment for nurses. O.U.P. and Hodder & Stoughton, 1920.

GARNSEY, CHARLES EUGENE
Dosage and solutions: a textbook for nurses. Philadelphia, Saunders, 1924.
2nd edn., 1932.
3rd edn., 1937, revised by Hulda L. Gunther.
4th edn., 1942.
5th edn., 1959.

GILBERT, ALBERT J., and MOODY, SELMA
Essentials of pharmacology and materia medica for nurses. St. Louis, Mosby, 1941.
2nd edn., 1944.
3rd edn., 1951, by A. J. Gilbert and Selma Moody Brawner.

GOOSTRAY, STELLA
Drugs and solutions for nurses. New York, Macmillan, 1924.
2nd edn., 1927.

HINDES, GWENDOLEN, and ARDLEY, D. G.
Materia medica and pharmacology for nurses. Faber, 1924.
2nd edn., 1929.
3rd edn., 1933.
4th edn., 1940.
5th edn., 1944.
6th edn., 1947.

HOPKINS, S. J.
Storage and control of drugs in wards. Nursing Mirror, June 17, 1955, p. 793-4.

JAMISON, SARA
Solutions and dosage. New York, McGraw-Hill, 1947.
2nd edn., 1951.
3rd edn., 1956.

KRUG, ELSIE E., and McGUIGAN, HUGH ALISTER
Pharmacology in nursing. St. Louis, Mosby, 1936.
2nd edn., 1940.
3rd edn., 1942.
4th edn., 1945.
5th edn., 1948.
6th edn., 1951.
7th edn., 1955.
8th edn., 1960.

McGUIGAN, HUGH ALISTER, and BRODIE, E. P.
An introduction to materia medica and pharmacology. St. Louis, Mosby, 1936.

MALECKA, A. BLANCHE
An analysis of the basic mathematical skills needed in the nursing functions of preparing medications and external solutions. Washington, Catholic University of America Press, 1950.

MALONEY, E. M., and JOHANNESEN, L.
How the tranquilizers affect nursing practice. American Journal of Nursing, Sept. 1957, p. 1144-6.

MODELL, WALTER, and PLACE, DORIS J.
The use of drugs: a textbook of pharmacology and therapeutics for nurses. New York, Springer, 1954.
2nd edn., 1955.

MORTON, A. L.
Principal drugs and their uses. Faber, 1934.
13th edn., 1950.

NAST, MINETTE
Simplified drugs and solutions for nurses; including arithmetic. St. Louis, Mosby, 1957.
2nd edn., 1960.

OAKES, LOIS, and BENNETT, ARNOLD
Materia medica for nurses. Edinburgh, Livingstone, 1934.
2nd edn., 1947.
3rd edn., 1949.

PEEL, J. S.
Materia medica and pharmacology for nurses. Christchurch, New Zealand, Peryer, 1955.
2nd edn., 1957.

POWELL, N. W.
Practical preparations, mainly medical. Faber, 1933.
[Later issued as "Practical preparations in common use", by P. J. Cunningham, ed. q.v.]

SEARS, W. GORDON
Materia medica for nurses: a textbook of drugs and therapeutics. Arnold, 1943.
2nd edn., 1947.
3rd edn., 1955.
4th edn., 1959.

SHESTACK, ROBERT
Handbook of pharmacology for nurses. Philadelphia, Saunders, 1952.

SKELLEY, ESTHER G.
Medications for the nurse. 2nd edn. New York, Delmar, 1960.

SQUIBBS, AMY E. A.
Aids to materia medica for nurses. Bailliere, Tindall & Cox, 1942.
2nd edn., 1944.
3rd edn., 1949.
4th edn., 1953.
5th edn., 1957.

SQUIRE, JESSIE E.
Basic pharmacology for nurses. St. Louis, Mosby, 1957.

TROUNCE, J. R.
Pharmacology for nurses; with a chapter on anaesthetic drugs, by J. M. Hall. Churchill, 1958.

WILLIAMS, F. J.
Nurses have much to do about poison control. Nursing Outlook, Feb. 1958, p. 93-5.

OXYGEN THERAPY

LIVINGSTONE, HUBERTA M.
Nursing care in oxygen therapy. *American Journal of Nursing*, Jan. 1957, p. 65-8.

PHYSICAL MEDICINE

BEAUMONT, WILLIAM
Fundamental principles of ray therapy: an elementary textbook for nurses, students and practitioners. Lewis, 1931.

CHANDLER, E. M.
Nursing care in radiation therapy. *Canadian Nurse*, Nov. 1958, p. 1023-8.

DEAKIN, B. M.
Radiotherapeutic nursing. A new Australian post-basic course. *International Nursing Review*, Jan. 1959, p. 33-4.

KOVACS, RICHARD
Physical therapy for nurses. Boston, Lea & Febiger, 1936. 2nd edn., 1940.

NELSON, KATHRYN L. JEWEN
Massage in nursing care. New York, Macmillan, 1941. 2nd edn., 1947.

POCHIN, E. E.
Conduct of radio-isotope treatment. *Nursing Times*, Nov. 2, 1956, p. 1115-7.

SCHNEIDER, C. M.
Isotope therapy and nursing care precautions. *Military Medicine*, Nov. 1956, p. 303-7.

SKAGGS, L. S., *and* HAUGHEY, R.
Radioactive isotope therapy. *Nursing Outlook*, April 1956, p. 214-6.

SLOGGINS, M. L. C.
Preparing patients for X-ray examinations. *American Journal of Nursing*, Jan. 1957, p. 76-9.

TUDWAY, R. C.
Nursing aspects of radiotherapy. *Nursing Mirror*, June 22, 1956, p. ii.

VENNES, CAROL HOCKING, *and* WATSON, JOHN C.
Patient care and special procedures in X-ray technology. St. Louis, Mosby, 1959.

REHABILITATION

ALLGIRE, MILDRED J., *and* DENNEY, RUTH R.
Nurses can give and teach rehabilitation: a manual. New York, Springer, 1960.

CRAWFORD, M. E.
Rehabilitation in a teaching program. *Canadian Nurse*, Mar. 1959, p. 205-10.

DRAKE, MELBA F.
Rehabilitation: an added dimension in nursing care. *American Journal of Nursing*, Aug. 1960, p. 1105-6.

DUNTON, WILLIAM RUSH
Occupational therapy: a manual for nurses. Philadelphia, Saunders, 1915.

ENGLEFIELD, A. M.
The district nurse—her role in the rehabilitation process. *Rehabilitation*, Spring 1957, p. 18.

HAWKINS, K. L.
The role of the nurse in rehabilitation. *Canadian Nurse*, Nov. 1957, p. 1005-8.

HAYDEN, M. L.
After surgery; rehabilitation for a full life. *Nursing Outlook*, Jan. 1959, p. 21-3.

JENSEN, DEBORAH MacLURG, *editor*
Principles and technics of rehabilitation nursing, by Florence Jones Terry, Gladys S. Benz, Dorothy Mereness, Frank R. Kleffner; St. Louis, Mosby, 1957.

LANE, H. C.
Rehabilitation nurse. *Nursing Outlook*, Mar. 1958, p. 157-9.

MACARTHUR, C.
The role of the public health nurse in a rehabilitation programme. *Canadian Journal of Public Health*, Feb. 1957, p. 61-3.

MACARTHUR, C.
We teach; do our patients learn? *Canadian Nurse*, Mar. 1959, p. 205-10.

MANNINO, S. F.
The role of the nurse in recreational therapy. *Nursing World*, Mar. 1957, p. 14-16.

MORRISSEY, ALICE B.
Preparation of the nurse for her role in rehabilitation: the nurse's scope in rehabilitation. *International Nursing Review*, Oct. 1956, p. 28-33.

MORRISSEY, ALICE B.
Rehabilitation nursing. New York, Putnam, 1951.

PETERSON, R. I.
Overview of rehabilitation nursing: is it new or is it old? *Military Medicine*, April 1959, p. 884-8.

PHILLIPS, ELIZABETH C.
Nursing aspects in rehabilitation and care of chronically ill. New York, National League for Nursing, 1956.

PHILLIPS, ELIZABETH C.
The role of the nurse in rehabilitation. *Canadian Nurse*, Nov. 1956, p. 810-18.

SHIELDS, C. D., *and* GROVER, E. P.
Co-operation between rehabilitation and nursing services in the care of patients. *Bulletin of the Georgetown University Medical Center*, Sept. 1957, p. 19-21.

SHONTZ, F. C., *and* FINK, S. L.
The significance of patient-staff rapport in the rehabilitation of individuals with chronic physical illness. *Journal of Consulting Psychology*, Aug. 1957, p. 327-34.

SKELLERN, E.
A therapeutic community: aims and treatment at the social rehabilitation unit, Belmont Hospital, Surrey. *Nursing Times*, April 22, 1955, p. 426-7; May 13, 1955, p. 533-5; May 27, 1955, p. 593-4; June 10, 1955, p. 642-3; June 24, 1955, p. 688-9.

SPRINGER, D. M. M.
The role of the hospital nurse in the rehabilitation process. *Rehabilitation*, Spring 1957, p. 7.

TRACY, SUSAN EDITH
Studies in invalid occupation: a manual for nurses and attendants. Boston, Whitcomb & Barrows, 1910.

TREACY, J. M.
Nurses in general hospitals can contribute to rehabilitation. *Military Medicine*, Mar. 1959, p. 224-7.

WANDELT, MABEL A.
Teaching is more than telling. *American Journal of Nursing*, May 1957, p. 625-6.

ZAUFAS, IRMA E., *and* SCHWARTZ, BARBARA
Rehabilitation nursing in a sheltered workshop. *American Journal of Nursing*, Oct. 1959, p. 1428-31.

TUBERCULOSIS NURSING

AMERICAN PUBLIC HEALTH ASSOCIATION
Guide for the medical and public health nursing supervision of tuberculosis cases and contacts. New York, The Association, 1953.

BUCHANAN, SHEENA H.
The health visitor and tuberculosis. *Nursing Times*, July 12, 1957, p. 770-2.

BUCHANAN, SHEENA H.
The health visitor and tuberculosis. National Association for the Prevention of Tuberculosis, 1955.

BUXTON, O. V., and MACKAY, P. M. MACULLOCH
The nursing of tuberculosis. Bristol, Wright, 1947.

CADY, LOUISE LINCOLN
Nursing in tuberculosis. Philadelphia, Saunders, 1948.

CARTER, G. M. M.
Secondment of nurses for tuberculosis nursing. *Nursing Mirror*, Feb. 12, 1954, p. ii.

CONNOLLY, ELEANOR C.
Tuberculosis among hospital personnel. New York, National Tuberculosis Association, 1950.

DEMING, DOROTHY
Home care of tuberculosis: pointers for the nurse. New York, National Tuberculosis Association, 1943.

DOWNEY, E.
Tuberculosis nursing in hospitals. *Nursing Outlook*, Nov. 1956, p. 635-7.

ERWIN, G. S.
Tuberculosis and chest diseases for nurses. Churchill, 1946.

EYRE, JESSIE G.
Tuberculosis nursing. Lewis, 1949.
2nd edn., 1957.

GROSVENOR, A. G.
Problems of tuberculosis nursing. *Nursing Mirror*, Dec. 19, 1952, p. 253-4.

HEINEMANN, EDITH, and others
The study of student anxiety in a tuberculosis nursing situation. *Nursing Research*, Summer 1959, p. 155-9.

HEINEMANN, EDITH, and PATRICK, MAXINE
Reducing tuberculosis nursing experience. *Nursing Outlook*, Aug. 1960, p. 448-9.

HETHERINGTON, H. W., and ESHLEMAN, FANNIE
Nursing in prevention and control of tuberculosis. New York, Putnam, 1941.
2nd rev. edn., 1945.
3rd rev. edn., 1950.
4th edn., 1958, called "Tuberculosis: prevention and control".

HODGSON, VIOLET H.
Handbook on tuberculosis for public health nurses. New York, National Tuberculosis Association, 1939.
2nd edn., 1942.

HOUGHTON, L. E., and SELLORS, T. HOLMES
Aids to tuberculosis nursing. Bailliere, Tindall & Cox, 1945.
2nd edn., 1946.
3rd edn., 1949.
4th edn., 1953.
5th edn., 1957.

JOHNSON, M. L.
The visiting nurse's part in the anti-tuberculosis work of America. *British Journal of Nursing*, Aug. 24, 1907, p. 143-5, and Aug. 31, 1907, p. 164-6.

LONGHURST, G. M.
Tuberculosis nursing. Philadelphia, Davis, 1941.
2nd edn., 1947.

MEACHEN, G. NORMAN
Tuberculosis: a manual for tuberculosis nurses, health visitors and other workers. Scientific Press, 1920.

MYERS, J. ARTHUR
The care of tuberculosis: a treatise for nurses, public health workers, and all those who are interested in the care of the tuberculous. Philadelphia, Saunders, 1924.

NATIONAL LEAGUE FOR NURSING.
TUBERCULOSIS NURSING ADVISORY SERVICE
Abilities, basic concepts. Content in tuberculosis for public health nurses. New York, The League, 1956.

RANDLE, J.
Some aspects of the secondment of nurses to a chest hospital. *Nursing Mirror*, Oct. 14, 1955, p. v.

RENTON, B. H.
Post-graduate training of nurses in the tuberculosis field. *Nursing Mirror*, Oct. 16, 1953, p. 173-4.

RICHIE, JEANNE
The tuberculosis patient who refuses care. *Nursing } Outlook*, Nov. 1960, p. 621-3.

SOUTH, JEAN
Tuberculosis handbook for public health nurses. New York, National Tuberculosis Association, 1950.

WINDSOR, A. E.
The nurse in the fight against tuberculosis.
See
NURSING TIMES
The nurse and the nation: a survey of her position in the State today. *Nursing Times*, Nov. 5, 1910, p. 904-31.

VENEREAL DISEASE NURSING

BATCHELOR, R. C. L., and MURRELL, MARJORIE
Venereal diseases described for nurses. Edinburgh, Livingstone, 1951.

BUCH, FRANCIS S.
Venereal disease control manual for nurses. Washington, U.S. Public Health Service, 1948.

CLARKE, E. A.
Challenge of communicable disease today: venereal disease control. *American Journal of Public Health and the Nation's Health*, July 1959, p. 865-8.

DOCK, LAVINIA L.
Hygiene and morality: a manual for nurses and others, giving an outline of the medical, social and legal aspects of the venereal diseases. New York, Putnam, 1910.

MORRIS, EVANGELINE HALL
Public health nursing in syphilis and gonorrhea. Philadelphia, Saunders, 1946.

MORRIS, EVANGELINE HALL
Venereal disease nursing in the basic curriculum. *Nursing Outlook*, April 1957, p. 233-4.

ONTARIO. DEPARTMENT OF HEALTH.
DIVISION OF VENEREAL DISEASE CONTROL
Venereal diseases and their control; a manual for nurses. Toronto, Department of Health for Ontario, 1949.

RYLE-HORWOOD, E. M.
Aids to the nursing of venereal diseases. Bailliere, Tindall & Cox, 1949.
2nd edn., 1956.

WARWICK, TURNER
A handbook on venereal diseases: for nurses and others engaged in the routine treatment of these diseases. 2nd edn. Faber, 1941.

HOSPITALS

GENERAL WORKS

GREAT BRITAIN. MINISTRY OF HEALTH
Hospital survey: the hospital services of the North Eastern area, by Hugh Lett and A. E. Quine. H.M.S.O., 1946.

GREAT BRITAIN. MINISTRY OF HEALTH
Hospital survey: the hospital services of the North Western area, by Ernest Rock Carling. H.M.S.O., 1945.

GREAT BRITAIN. MINISTRY OF HEALTH
Hospital survey: the hospital services of the Sheffield and East Midlands area, by L. G. Parsons. H.M.S.O., 1945.

GREAT BRITAIN. MINISTRY OF HEALTH
Hospital survey: the hospital services of the Eastern area, by William G. Savage. H.M.S.O., 1945.

GREAT BRITAIN. MINISTRY OF HEALTH
Hospital survey: the hospital services of the Yorkshire area, by Herbert Eason [and others]. H.M.S.O., 1945.

GREAT BRITAIN. MINISTRY OF HEALTH
Hospital survey: the hospital services of Berkshire, Buckinghamshire and Oxfordshire, by E. C. Befers [and others]. H.M.S.O., 1945.

GREAT BRITAIN. MINISTRY OF HEALTH
Hospital survey: the hospital services of the West Midlands area, by John B. Hunter [and others]. H.M.S.O., 1945.

GREAT BRITAIN. MINISTRY OF HEALTH
Hospital survey: the hospital services of London and the surrounding area, by A. M. H. Gray and A. Topping. H.M.S.O., 1945.

GREAT BRITAIN. MINISTRY OF HEALTH.
Hospital survey: the hospital services of the South Western area, by V. Z. Cope [and others]. H.M.S.O., 1945.

GREAT BRITAIN. MINISTRY OF HEALTH
Papers as to the administration of the London Lock Hospital and Home. H.M.S.O., 1929.

GREAT BRITAIN. MINISTRY OF HEALTH.
VOLUNTARY HOSPITALS COMMISSION
Report on voluntary hospital accommodation in England and Wales. H.M.S.O., 1925.

GREAT BRITAIN. MINISTRY OF HEALTH.
VOLUNTARY HOSPITALS COMMITTEE
Interim report. H.M.S.O., 1921.

SCOTLAND. DEPARTMENT OF HEALTH
Scottish hospitals survey, general introduction to the reports by R. S. Aitken [and others]. Edinburgh, H.M.S.O., 1945.

SCOTLAND. DEPARTMENT OF HEALTH
Scottish hospitals survey: report on the Eastern region. Edinburgh, H.M.S.O., 1946.

SCOTLAND. DEPARTMENT OF HEALTH
Scottish hospitals survey: report on the North-Eastern region. Edinburgh, H.M.S.O., 1946.

SCOTLAND. DEPARTMENT OF HEALTH
Scottish hospitals survey: report on the Northern region. Edinburgh, H.M.S.O., 1946.

SCOTLAND. DEPARTMENT OF HEALTH
Scottish hospitals survey: report on the South-Eastern region. Edinburgh, H.M.S.O., 1946.

SCOTLAND DEPARTMENT OF HEALTH
Scottish hospitals survey: report on the Western region. Edinburgh, H.M.S.O., 1946.

SELECT COMMITTEE OF THE HOUSE OF LORDS ON METROPOLITAN HOSPITALS, ETC.
Report . . . together with the proceedings of the Committee, minutes of evidence and appendix. Eyre & Spottiswoode, 1890.

SELECT COMMITTEE OF THE HOUSE OF LORDS ON METROPOLITAN HOSPITALS, ETC.
Analysis of evidence taken before the Select Committee. . . . Eyre & Spottiswoode, 1890.
[This volume is the index to, and analyses the evidence given in, the first report of the Select Committee. Cover title—Index. . . .]

SELECT COMMITTEE OF THE HOUSE OF LORDS ON METROPOLITAN HOSPITALS, ETC.
Analysis of evidence taken before the Select Committee. . . . Vol. II. H.M.S.O., 1891.
[This volume is the index to, and analyses the evidence given in, the second report of the Select Committee.]

SELECT COMMITTEE OF THE HOUSE OF LORDS ON METROPOLITAN HOSPITALS, ETC.
General index to the reports on the metropolitan hospitals. Eyre & Spottiswoode for H.M.S.O., 1892.
[This volume is the index to, and analyses the evidence given in, all three of the reports of the Select Committee.]

SELECT COMMITTEE OF THE HOUSE OF LORDS ON METROPOLITAN HOSPITALS, ETC.
Second report . . . together with the proceedings of the Committee, minutes of evidence, and appendix. H.M.S.O., 1891.

SELECT COMMITTEE OF THE HOUSE OF LORDS ON METROPOLITAN HOSPITALS, ETC.
Third report . . . together with the proceedings of the Committee, minutes of evidence, and appendix. H.M.S.O., 1892.

WALES. BOARD OF HEALTH
Hospitals survey: the hospital service of South Wales and Monmouthshire, by A. Trevor Jones [and others]. H.M.S.O., 1945.

ADMINISTRATION

AIKENS, C. A.
Hospital housekeeping. Sutton, 1906.

BURDETT, HENRY C.
Hospitals and the State, with an account of the nursing at London hospitals and the actual and comparative cost of management and maintenance, and of work done by the principal hospitals, convalescent institutions and dispensaries throughout Great Britain and Ireland. Churchill, 1882.

BURLING, TEMPLE, and others
The give and take in hospitals: a study of human organization in hospitals, by Temple Burling, Edith M. Lentz, Robert N. Wilson; a study conducted by the New York State School of Industrial and Labour Relations . . . with the support and co-operation of the American Hospital Association. New York, Putnam, 1956.

DE CAMP GENERAL HOSPITAL
Regulations for the government of the De Camp General Hospital, U.S. Army at David's Island, New York Harbour. De Camp General Hospital Press, 1864.
[Contains orders for nurses and also contains note that money received from hospital sludge and swill could be used to buy books for the library.]

DOCK, LAVINIA L.
Hospital organisation. *British Journal of Nursing*, Mar. 21, 1903, p. 228-9, and Mar. 28, 1903, p. 249-50.

FORTMAN, A. G.
Ward records relative to the patient: what should be kept and why. *Nursing Mirror*, May 29, 1959, p. 677-8 and 680.

A HOSPITAL SECRETARY
The nurse and hospital management.
  I. Her relation to the outside public. *Nursing Times*, July 28, 1917, p. 891-2.
  II. How nurses can help the Secretary. *Nursing Times*, Aug. 4, 1917, p. 916-9.
  III. Her relation to the Board. *Nursing Times*, Aug. 11, 1917, p. 950-1.

KANDEL, PHOEBE MILLER
Hospital economics for nurses. New York, Harper, 1930.

MACMANUS, EMILY ELVIRA PRIMROSE
Hospital administration for women. Faber, 1934.
2nd edn., 1949.

MUSGROVE, J.
Noise control in hospital. *Nursing Mirror*, Dec. 28, 1956, p. 896.

PAVEY, AGNES
The housekeeper's department as a sphere for specialisation. *British Journal of Nursing*, Sept. 21, 1918, p. 180-1.

PERRY, I.
Hospital housekeeping: its relationship to nursing service. *Hospital Management*, Jan. 1957, p. 42-3.

POWELL, M. B.
A matron's view of hospital administration. *Hospital*, Dec. 1958, p. 872-5.

REVANS, R. W.
The sister and the hospital system: proposed study of her work and opinions. *Nursing Mirror*, April 25, 1958, p. 261-2.

SNOKE, A. W.
The responsibility of hospitals for nursing service. *Hospitals*, Aug. 1st, 1958, p. 28-32.

STEWART, ISLA
Hospital administration. *Nursing Record*, Oct. 12, 1901, p. 297-30.

WATKIN, BRIAN V.
Delegation—how and why. *Nursing Times*, Nov. 20, 1959, p. 1156-8.

WATKIN, BRIAN V.
Truly tripartite—a nurse's point of view. *Hospital*, Feb. 1957, p. 109-13.

WEBB, J.
The nurse and the medical records office. *Nursing Mirror*, April 15, 1955, p. xiii-xiv, and April 30, 1955, p. v-vi.

WEIL, T. P., *and* PARRISH, H. N.
How did it happen? An analysis of the causes of 2,036 patient accidents at New York's Mount Sinai Hospital. *Hospitals*, Sept. 1, 1958, p. 43-8.

WOODWARD, JOSEPH JANVIER
The hospital steward's manual: for the instruction of hospital stewards, ward masters and attendants in their several duties. Prepared in strict accordance with existing regulations and customs of service in the armies of U.S.A. and rendered authoritative by order of the Surgeon-General. Philadelphia, Lippincott, 1862.
[Contains section on female nurses in the army. Mentions Dorothea Dix as having been authorized by the War Department to employ "female nurses" in the army.]

YOUNG, M. L.
Work study and nursing. *Nursing Times*, Jan. 2, 1959, p. 10-11.

STAFF

BIRMINGHAM REGIONAL HOSPITAL BOARD.
MENTAL HEALTH SERVICES COMMITTEE
Report of a working party appointed to advise on standards of staffing in mental hospitals. The Board, 1954.

BIRMINGHAM REGIONAL HOSPITAL BOARD.
MENTAL HEALTH SERVICES COMMITTEE
Report of a working party appointed to advise on standards of staffing in mental deficiency hospitals. The Board, [1956].

BOMFORD, M. K.
Use of night orderlies to relieve nursing staff. *Nursing Mirror*, Nov. 15, 1957, p. viii-ix.

HODGKINSON, S.
Economy in woman-power. *Hospital and Social Service Journal*, Feb. 25, 1955, p. 181-2.

KING EDWARD'S HOSPITAL FUND FOR LONDON
Nursing staff: considerations on standards of staffing. George Barber (for the Fund), 1945.

MANCHESTER REGIONAL HOSPITAL BOARD
Report of the working party on standards of nursing staff for hospitals. [Manchester, The Board, 1957.]

NEWTON, MILDRED E.
The administrative assistant. *Nursing Outlook*, Feb. 1957, p. 78-9.

NUFFIELD PROVINCIAL HOSPITALS' TRUST.
SCOTTISH ADVISORY MEDICAL COMMITTEE
Summary report of Committee's discussions on nursing staffing in hospitals, 1946. Edinburgh, The Committee, 1946.

SHYNE, I. J., *and* AMIERIRO, M.
The advisability of employing ward secretaries. *Hospital Progress*, April 1951, p. 108-10.

SIMPSON, M. A.
"Monday to Friday" wards. *Nursing Mirror*, Oct. 7, 1960, p. 55-56.

EQUIPMENT AND PLANNING

BEAMS, R.
Helping to plan a new hospital. *American Journal of Nursing*, Feb. 1956, p. 202-4.

BROWN, L. G.
Designing a new hospital at Vale of Leven, Dumbartonshire. *Nursing Mirror*, Oct. 7, 1955, p. ix-xi.

BURDETT, HENRY C.
Cottage hospitals, general, fever, and convalescent: their progress, management, and work in Great Britain and Ireland and the United States of America.... Scientific Press, 1877.
2nd edn., 1880.
3rd edn., 1896.

BURDETT, HENRY C.
Hospitals and asylums of the world: their origin, history, construction, administration, management and legislation; with plans of the chief medical institutions accurately drawn to a uniform scale, in addition to those of all the hospitals of London in the jubilee year of Queen Victoria's reign. 4 vols. Churchill. Vols. 1-2, 1891; vols. 3-4, 1893.

COPE, ZACHARY
John Shaw Billings, Florence Nightingale and the Johns Hopkins Hospital. *Medical History*, Oct. 1957, p. 367-8.
[Letters from J.S.B. to F.N. about the construction of the hospital.]

DAVIES, RICHARD LLEWELLYN
Hospitals for the future. *Nursing Times*, July 29, 1960, p. 933-8.

FLANAGAN, E. C.
Ward planning for patients' satisfaction and ease of nursing in the new McConnell Wing of the Montreal Neurological Institute. *Nursing Mirror*, Feb. 18, 1955, p. vii-ix.

GOLDFINCH, DONALD A.
Hospital architecture. 1. Design and planning; a nursing matter? *International Nursing Review*, June 1960, p. 21-4.
2. Do's and don'ts for nurses advising on hospital planning, by P. H. Knighton. *International Nursing Review*, Aug. 1960, p. 41-5.
3. Planning the nursing unit, by Anne M. White. *International Nursing Review*, Oct. 1960, p. 53-7.

GOLDFINCH, DONALD A.
Hospital design, function and finance.
(a) Hospital furnishings and equipment—experiments in Northern Ireland, by Anne M. W. White, *Nursing Times*, Mar. 22, 1957, p. 321.
(b) Research in hospital planning. *Nursing Times*, Mar. 29, 1957, p. 346.
(c) Plans and problems in Scotland, by A. A. Hughes. *Nursing Times*, April 19, 1957, p. 434.
(d) Central supply services, by M. Brooksbank. *Nursing Times*, April 19, 1957, p. 435.
(e) General hospital planning. *Nursing Times*, April 26, 1957, p. 468.
(f) Long-term planning, by S. G. M. Francis. *Nursing Times*, April 26, 1957, p. 470.

GOLDFINCH, DONALD A.
Planning mental and mental deficiency hospitals. *Nursing Times*, Aug. 30, 1957, p. 979-80.

MODERN HOSPITAL
Circular nursing division runs rings round rectangle. *Modern Hospital*, Nov. 1958, p. 71-3.

NIGHTINGALE, FLORENCE
Notes on hospitals: being two papers read before the National Association for the Promotion of Social Science, at Liverpool, in October 1858. With evidence given to the Royal Commissioners on the state of the Army in 1857. John W. Parker, 1859.
3rd edn., enlarged and for the most part rewritten, Longmans, 1863.

PARSONS, H. FRANKLIN
Isolation hospitals. O.U.P., 1914.
2nd edn., 1922, revised and partly rewritten by R. Bruce Low.

ST. THOMAS'S HOSPITAL, LONDON
An experiment in ward layout carried out in Christian Ward, St. Thomas's Hospital. *Nursing Mirror*, Mar. 29, 1957, p. vi-vii.

SHELBY, B.
Central work corridor simplifies nurses' work. *Modern Hospital*, Dec. 1959, p. 65-70.

HISTORY OF HOSPITALS

GENERAL WORKS

BREAY, MARGARET
Some Bristol hospitals [The Royal Infirmary, the General Hospital, the Children's Hospital, St. Peter's Hospital and the Stapleton Infirmary]. *British Journal of Nursing*, June 8, 1912, p. 455-8.

CLAY, ROTHA MARY
The mediaeval hospitals of England. Methuen, 1909.

EATON, LEONARD K.
New England hospitals, 1790-1833. Ann Arbor, Michigan, University of Michigan Press, 1957.

EVANS, A. DELBERT, *and* HOWARD, L. G. REDMOND
The romance of the British voluntary hospital movement. Hutchinson, [1930?].

HACKNEY GROUP HOSPITAL MANAGEMENT COMMITTEE
Hackney Group of Hospitals: National Health Service Act, 1946: the first ten years, with a short historical survey. The Committee, 1958.

HOBSON, JOHN MORRISON
Some early and later houses of pity. Routledge, 1926.

HOWARD, JOHN
An account of the principle lazarettos in Europe: with various papers relative to the plague; together with further observations on some foreign prisons and hospitals; and additional remarks on the present state of those in Great Britain and Ireland. Warrington, Eyres, Printers, 1789.

HOWARD, JOHN
An account of the present state of the prisons, houses of correction, and hospitals in London and Westminster; taken from a late publication of . . . by permission of the author. London, printed by order of the Society lately instituted for giving effect to His Majesty's proclamation against vice and immorality, [1789].

IVES, A. G. L.
British hospitals. Collins, 1948.

LONDON COUNTY COUNCIL
The L.C.C. hospitals: a retrospect. Staples Press, 1949.

MCLAREN, EVA SHAW, *editor*
A history of the Scottish women's hospitals. Hodder & Stoughton, 1919.

WINGENT, R. M.
Historical notes on the Borough and the Borough hospitals. Ash, 1913.

WOOD, CATHERINE J.
Hospitals in New Zealand and Fiji. *Nursing Times*, Aug. 1, 1908, p. 593-4, and Aug. 15, 1908, p. 634-5.

WYLIE, W. GILL
Hospitals, their history, organization and construction. New York, Appleton, 1877.

HISTORY OF INDIVIDUAL HOSPITALS

AUCKLAND PSYCHIATRIC HOSPITAL
Historical notes on the Auckland Psychiatric Hospital, by R. M. Hunter. *New Zealand Nursing Journal*, Feb. 1957, p. 15.

BELLEVUE HOSPITAL, NEW YORK
The Bellevue story, by Page Cooper. New York, Crowell, 1948.

BETHLEHEM HOSPITAL
The story of Bethlehem Hospital from its foundation in 1247, by Edward Geoffrey O'Donoghue. Fisher Unwin, 1914.

BIRMINGHAM AND MIDLAND EYE HOSPITAL
Description, with account of life and work of nurses. *Nursing Record*, Feb. 25, 1892, p. 165-7, and Mar. 31, 1892, p. 264-7.

BIRMINGHAM GENERAL HOSPITAL
The General Hospital, Birmingham. *British Journal of Nursing*, June 6, 1914, p. 501-3.

BIRMINGHAM GENERAL HOSPITAL
History and description. *Nursing Record*, May 5, 1892, p. 365-7; May 19, 1892, p. 406-7; June 9, 1892, p. 468-70.

BLOCKLEY HOSPITAL, PHILADELPHIA
A history of Blockley: a history of Philadelphia General Hospital from its inception, 1731-1928, compiled by John Welsh Crosby. Philadelphia, Davis, 1929.

BOSTON CHILDREN'S HOSPITAL
The Children's Hospital, 1869-1939. School of Nursing, 1889-1939. 1939.

BOSTON FLOATING HOSPITAL
Boston Floating Hospital [for children]. *Nursing Record*, June 15, 1901, p. 472-4.

BRISTOL EYE HOSPITAL
Bristol Eye Hospital, 1810-1960. *Nursing Mirror*, June 17, 1960, p. viii-ix.

BRISTOL ROYAL INFIRMARY
A history of the Bristol Royal Infirmary, by George Munro Smith. Bristol, Arrowsmith, 1917.

BROMPTON HOSPITAL
The Brompton Hospital: the story of a great adventure, by Maurice Davidson and F. G. Rouvray. Lloyd-Luke, 1954.

CHESTER ROYAL INFIRMARY
Chester Royal Infirmary, 1756-1956, by Enid M. Mumford. The Infirmary, [1956?].

CHESTER ROYAL INFIRMARY
Chester Royal Infirmary. Nursing Mirror, July 15, 1960, p. viii-ix.

CITY OF LONDON HOSPITAL FOR DISEASES OF THE HEART AND LUNGS
The story of a city hospital, 1848-1925, by Lady Butterworth. City of London Hospital for Diseases of the Heart and Lungs, [1925].

CLAYBURY HOSPITAL.
Claybury Hospital. The Hospital, 1958.

COLONIAL HOSPITAL, PORT-OF-SPAIN, TRINIDAD
The centenary of the Colonial Hospital, Port-of-Spain, Trinidad, 1858-1958. Caribbean Medical Journal, 1958, p. 3-35.

COLORED HOME AND HOSPITAL, NEW YORK CITY
Colored Home and Hospital, New York City. Nursing Record, July 14, 1900, p. 14-15.

CORNELL UNIVERSITY—NEW YORK HOSPITAL
Cornell University—New York Hospital, by Helene Jamieson Jordan. New York, The Society of New York Hospital, 1952.

DR. STEEVENS' HOSPITAL, DUBLIN
The history of Dr. Steevens' Hospital, Dublin, 1720-1920, by T. Percy C. Kirkpatrick. Dublin, University Press, 1924.

DUNDEE ROYAL INFIRMARY
Dundee Royal Infirmary, 1798-1948. The story of the old infirmary, with a short account of more recent years, by Henry J. Gibson. Dundee, 1948.

EDINBURGH ROYAL INFIRMARY
Story of a great hospital, the Royal Infirmary of Edinburgh, 1720-1929, by A. Logan Turner. Edinburgh, Oliver & Boyd, 1937.

EMORY UNIVERSITY HOSPITAL
Until now: a brief history of the Emory University Hospital and School of Nursing, by Mabelle Jones Dewery. Emory University, Georgia, Banner Press, 1947.

FOREST GATE HOSPITAL
The history of Forest Gate Hospital; by E. R. Gamester. Friends of Forest Gate Hospital, 1954.

GLASGOW ROYAL INFIRMARY
The Royal Infirmary, Glasgow, by Margaret Breay. British Journal of Nursing, Feb. 28, 1914, p. 188-9.

GLASGOW ROYAL INFIRMARY
A short history of Glasgow Royal Infirmary, by John Patrick. Glasgow Royal Infirmary, 1940.

GLOUCESTER INFIRMARY
The General Infirmary at Gloucester and the Gloucestershire Eye Institution—its past and present, by George Whitcombe. Gloucester, John Bellows, [1903].

GLOUCESTERSHIRE ROYAL HOSPITAL
Gloucestershire Royal Hospital. Nursing Mirror, Feb. 5, 1960, p. viii-ix.

GRAND FORKS DEACONESS HOSPITAL
History and progress of the Grand Forks Deaconess Hospital, 1892-1942. Grand Forks, N. Dakota, Holt Printing Co., 1943.

GREY'S HOSPITAL, PIETERMARITZBURG
A hospital century: Grey's Hospital, Pietermaritzburg, 1855-1955, by Alan F. Hattersley. Cape Town, Balkema, 1955.

GUY'S HOSPITAL
Mr. Guy's hospital, 1726-1948, by H. C. Cameron. Longmans Green, 1954.

HEREFORD GENERAL HOSPITAL
Hereford General Hospital. Nursing Mirror, May 27, 1960, p. viii-ix.

HOSPITAL FOR JOINT DISEASES, NEW YORK CITY, NEW YORK
The first fifty years: a brief history . . . by A. Rosenberg. Bulletin of the Hospital for Joint Diseases, Oct. 1956, p. 105-9.

HOSPITAL FOR SICK CHILDREN, GREAT ORMOND STREET
"Great Ormond Street", 1852-1952, by Thomas Twistington Higgins. Odhams, for the Hospital for Sick Children, [1952].

HOSPITAL FOR WOMEN, LEEDS
A short history of the Hospital for Women at Leeds, 1853-1953, by Andrew M. Claye. [Leeds, The Hospital, 1953.]

HOSPITAL OF ST. JOHN AND ST. ELIZABETH
Hospital of St. John and St. Elizabeth, 1856-1956: the story of the hospital, its foundation based on Florence Nightingale's work in the Crimea, its achievements and growth. The Hospital Centenary Fund, 1956.

L'HOTEL DIEU, PARIS
The history of a great hospital: L'Hotel Dieu. Medical Journal of Australia, Mar. 30, 1957, p. 424-5.
L'Hotel Dieu and its functions. Medical Journal of Australia, April 6, 1957, p. 470-1.
L'Hotel Dieu and its surgeons. Medical Journal of Australia, April 13, 1957, p. 516-7.

HULL ROYAL INFIRMARY
The Hull Royal Infirmary, 1782-1932, by K. J. Lowson. [Hull, The Infirmary, 1932.]

IOWA METHODIST HOSPITAL
Wings in waiting. A history of Iowa Methodist Hospital, 1901-1951, by Edith M. Bjornstad. Desmoines, Iowa, 1952.

IYI ENU HOSPITAL, NIGERIA
High Spring: the story of the Iyi Enu Hospital, by Margaret P. Roseveare. C.M.S., 1946.

JAMAICA HOSPITAL, NEW YORK
The Jamaica Hospital—a history of the institution—1892-1942, by Francis Gerald Riley. [Jamaica—New York], Medical Board, Jamaica Hospital, [1942].

KENT COUNTY MENTAL HOSPITAL
A retrospect, 1828-1927. Maidstone, The Hospital, 1927.

KING EDWARD VII'S HOSPITAL FOR OFFICERS.
Historical record, 1899-1955. by S.C.I. The Hospital, 1956.

KING'S COLLEGE HOSPITAL, LONDON
A short account of King's College Hospital, by B. W. Thomas. Physiotherapy, May 10, 1958, p. 129-32.

LAMBETH HOSPITAL
Lambeth Hospital: fifty years retrospect, by P. J. Watkin. The Hospital, [1954].

LEEDS GENERAL INFIRMARY
Leeds General Infirmary. Nursing Mirror, Aug. 12, 1960, p. viii-ix.

LEEDS GENERAL INFIRMARY
A historical sketch of the General Infirmary of Leeds, 1767-1916, by Richard Jackson. Leeds, Jackson, 1917.

LOVELL GENERAL HOSPITAL, PORTSMOUTH GROVE, RHODE ISLAND
The hospital at Portsmouth Grove, by S. J. Goldowsky. Rhode Island Medical Journal, Nov. 1959, p. 733-43.

MAIDA VALE HOSPITAL
A history of the Maida Vale Hospital for Nervous Diseases, by Anthony Feiling. Butterworth, 1959.

MAINE GENERAL HOSPITAL
Maine General Hospital: an historical sketch, by G. O. Cummings. *Journal of the Maine Medical Association*, Aug. 1960, p. 267-72.

MANCHESTER NORTHERN HOSPITAL
The centenary of the ... hospital, 1856-1956. *The Hospital*, 1956.

MANCHESTER ROYAL INFIRMARY
Portrait of a hospital, 1752-1948: to commemorate the bi-centenary of the Royal Infirmary, Manchester, by William Brockbank. Heinemann, 1952.

MARY FLETCHER HOSPITAL, BURLINGTON, VERMONT
Mary Fletcher comes back: a brief account of the history, progress and future of Vermont's first general hospital. Burlington, Vermont, published for the Board of Directors of the Mary Fletcher Hospital, 1941.

MASSACHUSETTS GENERAL HOSPITAL
A history of the Massachusetts General Hospital, by Nathanial Ingersoll Bowditch. Privately printed in 1851. 2nd edn. with continuation to 1872. Prepared by request in a vote of trustees, chiefly from records of the annual reports. Boston, printed by the Trustees for the Bowditch Fund, 1872.

MASSACHUSETTS GENERAL HOSPITAL
The Massachusetts General Hospital, 1935-1955, by Nathaniel W. Faxon. Cambridge, Mass., Harvard U.P., 1959.

MASSACHUSETTS GENERAL HOSPITAL
History of the Massachusetts Hospital; June 1852 to December 1900, by Grace W. Myers. Boston, The Hospital, 1929.

MIDDLESEX HOSPITAL
The Middlesex Hospital, 1745-1948, by Hilary St. George Saunders. Max Parrish, 1949.

MIDDLESEX HOSPITAL
The history of the Middlesex Hospital during the first century of its existence, compiled from the hospital records, by Erasmus Wilson. Churchill, 1845.

MILDMAY MISSION HOSPITAL
Mildmay: or the story of the first deaconess institution, by Harriette J. Cooke. Stock, 1893.

MILLER HOSPITAL AND ROYAL KENT DISPENSARY
Records of the Miller Hospital and Royal Kent Dispensary, by John Poland. Richardson, 1893.

MONTEFIORE HOSPITAL, NEW YORK
Montefiore Hospital, 1884-1934; a brief history, by Milton Bracker. New York, Privately Printed, 1934.

MOORHAVEN HOSPITAL
Moorhaven Hospital, Ivybridge, South Devon: historical review, 1891-1958, by Francis Pilkington. The Hospital, 1958.

MOUNT SINAI HOSPITAL
The story of the first fifty years of the Mount Sinai Hospital, New York, 1852-1902, compiled by Jane Benedict. New York, The Mount Sinai Hospital, 1944.

MOUNT SINAI HOSPITAL
The first hundred years of the Mount Sinai Hospital of New York, 1852-1952, by Joseph Hirsh and Beks Doherty. New York, Random House, 1952.

MOUNT VERNON HOSPITAL, NORTHWOOD
The golden jubilee of Mount Vernon Hospital at Northwood, 1904-1954. Northwood, The Committee, [1954].

NATIONAL HEART HOSPITAL, LONDON
The National Heart Hospital, 1857-1957, by M. Campbell. *British Heart Journal*, Jan. 1958, p. 137-9.

NATIONAL HOSPITAL FOR NERVOUS DISEASES, LONDON
The National Hospital, Queen Square, 1860-1948, by Gordon Holmes. Edinburgh, Livingstone, 1954.

NATIONAL HOSPITAL FOR NERVOUS DISEASES, LONDON
National Hospital, Queen Square, 1860-1960. *Nursing Times*, July 1, 1960, p. 820-1.

NATIONAL HOSPITAL FOR NERVOUS DISEASES, LONDON
The beginnings of the National Hospital, Queen Square, (1859-1860), by M. Critchley. *British Medical Journal*, June 18, 1960, p. 1829-37.

NEW YORK CITY CHILDREN'S HOSPITAL, RANDALL'S ISLAND, NEW YORK
The story of Randall's Island and the New York Children's Hospital, by C. G. McGaffin. New York Department of Hospitals, 1929.

NEW YORK HOSPITAL
The New York Hospital: a history of the psychiatric service, 1771-1936, by William Logie Russell. Columbia University Press, 1945.

NEWCASTLE-UPON-TYNE INFIRMARY
The Infirmary, Newcastle-upon-Tyne, 1751-1951: a brief sketch, by W. E. Hume. Newcastle-upon-Tyne, The Infirmary, [1951].

NORFOLK AND NORWICH HOSPITAL
A history of the Norfolk and Norwich Hospital from 1900 to the end of 1946, by Arthur J. Cleveland. Norwich, Jarrold, 1948.

NORTH CAROLINA BAPTIST HOSPITAL
North Carolina Baptist Hospital. *Medical Times*, Feb. 1960, p. 256-9.

NORWALK HOSPITAL
Norwalk Hospital. *Medical Times*, May 1960, p. 645-9.

NOTTINGHAM GENERAL HOSPITAL
A history of the General Hospital, near Nottingham, open to the sick and lame poor of any county, by Frank H. Jacob. Bristol, Wright, 1951.

OUR LADY'S HOSPICE, DUBLIN
A city set on a hill: Our Lady's Mount, Harold's Cross, Dublin; to commemorate the centenary of its foundation by Mother Mary Augustine Aikenhead, 14th Sept., 1845. Dublin, [The Hospice], 1945.

PENNSYLVANIA HOSPITAL
The history of the Pennsylvania Hospital, 1751-1895, by Thomas G. Morton. Philadelphia, Times Printing House, 1897.

PHILADELPHIA EPISCOPAL HOSPITAL
A century of care—a history of Episcopal Hospital, 1852-1952. Philadelphia, The Hospital, 1953.

PORTLAND HOSPITAL
A civilian war hospital: being an account of the work of the Portland Hospital and of experience of wounds and sickness in South Africa, with a description of the equipment, cost, and management of a civilian base hospital in time of war, by Anthony A. Bowlby and others. Murray, 1901.

PRESBYTERIAN HOSPITAL, NEW YORK
Early days of the Presbyterian Hospital in the city of New York, by David Bryson Delavan. East Orange, New Jersey, Pub. Priv., 1926.

QUEEN CHARLOTTE'S LYING-IN HOSPITAL
The history of Queen Charlotte's Lying-In Hospital, from its foundation in 1752 to the present time; with an account of its objects and present state, by Thomas Ryan. [The Hospital], 1885.

RADCLIFFE INFIRMARY, OXFORD
The Radcliffe Infirmary, by Alexander George Gibson. O.U.P., 1926.

THE RETREAT, YORK
A retired habitation: a history of The Retreat, York, by Harold Capper Hunt. Lewis, 1932.

ROCHESTER GENERAL HOSPITAL, NEW YORK
A century of service: Rochester General Hospital, 1847-1947, by Virginia Jeffrey Smith. Rochester, New York, 1947.

ROTUNDA HOSPITAL, DUBLIN
The Rotunda Hospital, 1745-1945, by O'Donel T. D. Browne. Edinburgh, Livingstone, 1947.

ROYAL BERKSHIRE HOSPITAL
The story of the Royal Berkshire Hospital, 1837-1937, edited by Ernest W. Dormer. Poynder Press, 1937.

ROYAL EDINBURGH HOSPITAL FOR SICK CHILDREN
The Royal Edinburgh Hospital for Sick Children, 1860-1960 . . . by Douglas Guthrie, with various contributors. Edinburgh, Livingstone, 1960.

ROYAL EYE HOSPITAL, LONDON
The Royal Eye Hospital, 1857-1957, by Arnold Sorsby. Royal Eye Hospital, 1957.

ROYAL EYE HOSPITAL, LONDON
Centenary of the Royal Eye Hospital, by M.M.W. *Nursing Times*, Nov. 29, 1957, p. 1357.

ROYAL GWENT HOSPITAL
History of the Royal Gwent Hospital, by Thomas Baker Jones and William John Townsend Collins. Newport, Mon., [The Hospital], 1948.

ROYAL HOSPITAL, HASLAR
The Royal Hospital, Haslar, 1753-1953, by S. E. Barrington. [Haslar, The Hospital, 1953.]

ROYAL MELBOURNE HOSPITAL
Hospital and community: a history of the Royal Melbourne Hospital, by K. S. Inglis. Melbourne, University Press, 1958.

ROYAL NATIONAL HOSPITAL FOR RHEUMATIC DISEASES, BATH
The Royal National Hospital for Rheumatic Diseases, Bath (Royal Mineral Water Hospital): 1742 to the present day, by J. M. T. Kelsall. [Bath, The Hospital], 1948.

ROYAL NORTHERN HOSPITAL
The Royal Northern Hospital, 1856-1956: the story of a hundred years' work in North London, by Eric C. O. Jewesbury. Lewis, 1956.

ROYAL NORTHERN INFIRMARY, INVERNESS
The Royal Northern Infirmary, Inverness. The further history of a Scottish voluntary hospital . . . 1930-1948, by T. Mackenzie. [Inverness, The Infirmary?], 1950.

ROYAL UNITED HOSPITAL, BATH
Royal United Hospital, Bath. *Nursing Mirror*, April 8, 1960, p. viii-ix.

ROYAL VICTORIA HOSPITAL, BELFAST
Fifty years on the Grosvenor Road: an account of the rise and progress of the Royal Victoria Hospital, Belfast, during the years 1903-1953, by Robert Marshall. [Belfast, The Hospital, 1953?]

ROYAL WEST SUSSEX HOSPITAL
The Royal West Sussex Hospital: the first hundred years, 1784-1884, by Francis Steer. Chichester, City Council, 1960.

RUBERY HILL AND HOLLYMOOR HOSPITALS
The story of mental nursing and of Rubery Hill and Hollymoor Hospitals; compiled by H. A. Crick, edited by A. H. Buffham. Published under the authority of David Rhydderch. . . . [Birmingham], The Hospitals, [1956].

ST. ALFEGE'S HOSPITAL, GREENWICH
St. Alfege's Hospital, Greenwich, by G. K. Hewitt. *Physiotherapy*, July 10, 1958, p. 199-203.

ST. BARTHOLOMEW'S HOSPITAL, LONDON
An account of a book published in 1552 called "The Ordre of the hospital of S. Bartholemewes in West Smythfielde in London". *Nursing Record*, Jan. 27, 1894, p. 66-7.

ST. BARTHOLOMEW'S HOSPITAL, LONDON
The history of Saint Bartholomew's Hospital, by Norman Moore. 2 vols. Pearson, 1918.

ST. BARTHOLOMEW'S HOSPITAL, LONDON
The Royal Hospital of Saint Bartholomew, by Gweneth Whitteridge. The Hospital, 1952.

ST. GEORGE'S HOSPITAL, LONDON
St. George's, 1733-1933, by J. Blomfield. Published for St. George's Hospital by the Medici Society, 1933.

ST. JOSEPH'S HOSPITAL, BALTIMORE, MARYLAND
History of St. Joseph's Hospital, by Sister Pierre. *Maryland State Medical Journal*, July 1957, p. 363-6.

ST. LUKE'S HOSPITAL, WOODSIDE
The story of St. Luke's Hospital, by C. N. French. Heinemann, 1951.

ST. MARY'S HOSPITAL, LONDON
St. Mary's Hospital (Paddington), by Zachary Cope. *Physiotherapy*, July 1957, p. 193-5.

ST. MARY'S HOSPITAL, ROCHESTER, MINNESOTA
A history of St. Mary's Hospital, Rochester, Minnesota, by M. C. Holman. *Hospital Progress*, Mar. 1957, p. 88-93.

ST. PAUL'S HOSPITAL, LONDON
The history of St. Paul's Hospital, London, by A. R. Higham. *Proceedings of the Royal Society of Medicine*, Mar. 1957, p. 164-6.

ST. PETER'S HOSPITAL FOR STONE, LONDON
The history of St. Peter's Hospital for Stone, London, by C. E. Dukes. *Proceedings of the Royal Society of Medicine*, Mar. 1957, p. 161-4.

ST. PETER'S HOSPITAL FOR STONE, LONDON
St. Peter's Hospital for Stone, 1860-1960, edited by Clifford Morson. Edinburgh, Livingstone, 1960.

ST. THOMAS'S HOSPITAL, LONDON
The history of St. Thomas's Hospital, by F. G. Parsons. Methuen.
Vol. 1. From the earliest times until A.D. 1600. 1932.
Vol. 2. From 1600 to 1800. 1934.
Vol. 3. From 1800 to 1900. 1936.

ST. VINCENT'S HOSPITAL, DUBLIN
A century of service: the record of 100 years; published for the centenary of St. Vincent's Hospital, 23rd Jan., 1934. Dublin, Browne & Nolan, 1934.

SAMARITAN FREE HOSPITAL
The history of the Samaritan Free Hospital, by Arnold Whitaker Oxford. Cambridge U.P., 1931.

SELLY OAK INFIRMARY
The Infirmary, Selly Oak, by Margaret Breay. *British Journal of Nursing*, May 5, 1914, p. 486-7.

THE TAUNTON AND SOMERSET HOSPITAL
The Taunton and Somerset Hospital. 150th anniversary, by L. Dopson. *Hospital*, Nov. 1959, p. 907-12.

TORONTO WESTERN HOSPITAL
Toronto Western Hospital. *Canadian Hospital*, May 1960, p. 50-1.

ULSTER HOSPITAL, BELFAST
The story of the Ulster Hospital, by R. Marshall. *Ulster Medicine*, Nov. 1, 1959, p. 118-47.

UNIVERSITY OF PENNSYLVANIA HOSPITAL
University of Pennsylvania Hospital. *Medical Times*, Jan. 1959, p. 125-9.

WARLEY HOSPITAL, BRENTWOOD
Warley Hospital, Brentwood: the first hundred years, 1853-1953, by G. S. Nightingale. Brentwood, Warley Hospital, 1953.

WELLINGTON HOSPITAL, NEW ZEALAND
A hundred years of healing: Wellington Hospital, 1847-1947, by D. Macdonald Wilson. Wellington, New Zealand, Reed, 1948.